FRCS: COMPANION CASES FOR THE INTERCOLLEGIATE EXAM IN GENERAL SURGERY

D1581788

FRCS: COMPANION CASES FOR THE INTERCOLLEGIATE EXAM IN GENERAL SURGERY

Bhaskar Kumar MD FRCS
Alexander Phillips MA MRCSEd FHEA

FRCS: COMPANION CASES FOR THE INTERCOLLEGIATE EXAM IN GENERAL SURGERY

Edited by: Mr Bhaskar Kumar MD FRCS
and Mr Alexander Phillips MA MRCSEd FHEA

Published by:-
Anshan Ltd
6 Newlands Road
Tunbridge Wells
Kent. TN4 9AT

Tel: +44 (0) 1892 557767
Fax: +44 (0) 1892 530358
e-mail: info@anshan.co.uk
web site: www.anshan.co.uk

© 2016 Anshan Ltd   Reprinted 2019

ISBN: 978 1 848290 853

While every effort has been made to ensure the accuracy of the information contained within this publication, the publisher can give no guarantee for information about drug dosage and application thereof contained in this book. In every individual case the respective user must check current indications and accuracy by consulting other pharmaceutical literature and following the guidelines laid down by the manufacturers of specific products and the relevant authorities in the country in which they are practicing.

Every effort has been made to trace all copyright holders, but if any have been inadvertently overlooked the publishers will be pleased to make the necessary arrangements at the first opportunity. All images reproduced in this book have been provided by the contributors, with variable print quality. Their image content is important and relevant, despite imperfect clarity in some instances.

British Library Cataloguing in Publication Data
A catalogue record for this book is available from the British Library.

Copy Editor: Andrew White
Cover Design: Emma Randall
Cover Image: Shutterstock
Typeset by: Kerry Press Ltd

Acknowledgements

The completion of this book was inspired by the enthusiasm and belief of my co-author Alex Phillips who provided the driving force for making ideas into reality. I wish to thank all the contributors for their energetic input amidst very busy working schedules. I also wish to thank Andrew White for all of his patience throughout the preparation of this book, from Down Under to the UK.

This book is dedicated to my wife Loveena and my daughters Liviya and baby Laykha for their unwavering support which inspires me everyday. My heartfelt thanks to my family and friends, especially my younger sister Sandhya from whom I draw strength and courage to face and conquer the unexpected.

Bhaskar Kumar

Writing a textbook has proven no easy task. I must thank those that have contributed to this book, many of whom have inspired me through my training, and particularly Bhaskar, who is able to work in a relentless fashion.

This book is dedicated to my fantastic wife, Nicola, who is always patient and always loving despite having to cope with twins and a husband recovering from a serious illness, and to my parents who will always be an inspiration.

Alexander Phillips

CONTENTS

Foreword

Postgraduate surgical training in the United Kingdom and Ireland has evolved to a new and more structured endpoint defined by the FRCS exit examination. This examination has evolved a great deal in recent years. It specifically addresses surgical principles and practice and it is to the trainee approaching these exams that this book is aimed.

The authors, Mr Bhaskar Kumar and Mr Alexander Phillips, are to be congratulated for putting together a text that vividly brings to light clinical problems using a case history format. The book is well structured and easy to read. I have no doubt that those approaching the intercollegiate exit exam will find it of great benefit.

I also think this text will be of value to trainers. As it is based upon case histories, it is very easy for a trainer to take any of the examples given as a focus for discussion.

The opening chapter of the book gives some interesting insights into examination techniques and I think the trainees will find the comments expressed here of great value.

The mark of an expert is the ability to make one's own subject interesting and easily understood by everyone. This volume is a unique collection of surgical case histories written by experts for non-experts. The authors have done a magnificent job and I congratulate them on their achievement. I sincerely hope that the book will become popular. The format is such that it would be easily modified to adapt to the ever-changing face of surgical practice.

John MacFie MD, FRCS (Eng), FRCSEd (ad hom), FRCP (Edin)
Professor of Surgery / Consultant Surgeon
President, Federation Surgical Speciality Associations, UK and Ireland

Preface

Surgical textbooks are usually organized around disease processes and organ systems. They include a lot of facts, with the level of detail usually tailored to the seniority of the target readership. Whilst facts and breadth of coverage are important, textbooks have a reputation for being dry, and they can be very effective treatments for insomnia if read late at night! Journal articles can have a similar effect.

Our human minds are hard-wired to respond to stories. We find stories interesting, but not facts. We generally consider facts to be "dry". Great public speakers engage their audiences with anecdotes; i.e. stories, they don't just tell us facts and detail. Compelling stories engage readers, maintain interest, and the reader is left wanting more.

In this book, the authors, Mr Bhaskar Kumar and Mr Alexander Phillips, have taken a very different approach to writing a surgical textbook. They have reorganised the information base for General Surgery around case based discussions. In doing this, they have placed the facts within compelling case based stories and conversations. This approach succeeds and engages the reader to keep reading. This is a book that will be read by trainees when they have a break between cases in the operating theatre, when they have some down time whilst on call, and for some trainees it might even become bedtime reading!

Even though specifically targeted to trainees sitting the FRCS General Surgery exit examination in the UK, General Surgery trainees working in similar training systems in other parts of the world will also find great value within its pages. There is no doubt that trainees in Australia and New Zealand will find this book very useful for their examination preparation. The selected cases comprehensively address clinical scenarios which are frequently encountered in clinical practice, and also frequently explored in viva examinations. Through these case based discussions, the authors have succeeded in delivering the clinical perspective and context that is often hard to glean from conventional textbooks.

However, this is not just a book for trainees. Trainers will benefit from the case based discussions, and for established surgeons looking for a way to refresh their own knowledge base, the case discussions are equally engaging and compelling. They offer an opportunity to brush up on areas that are encountered less frequently, as well as a practical approach to case management.

I congratulate the authors on their achievement in writing this book. I wish it had been available when I was studying for the General Surgery exit examination in Australia.

Professor David I Watson MBBS, MD, FRACS, FAHMS
Flinders University Department of Surgery
Adelaide, South Australia.

Authors' Preface

This book is aimed at candidates who wish to succeed at the Intercollegiate Speciality Examination in general surgery or the Joint Surgical Colleges Fellowship Examination. The preparation for this book started during the authors' revision for the exit examination in general surgery through a belief that there should be a greater availability of textbooks specific to the exam. Although there are several established and renowned textbooks for surgery there has been a shortage of books geared towards achieving success in the exit FRCS. Furthermore other sub-specialities such as orthopaedics seemed to have bridged this gap.

This is by no means a comprehensive textbook of general surgery, but it serves the purpose of focusing the candidate's mind on the types of questions asked in the viva and clinical parts of the exam, as well as on exam technique. We have also tried to provide insightful comments and experience from candidates who have been successful in the exam.

We hope that readers of the book come to understand that by far the majority of questions can be answered through their clinical experience. The format of the text is case based discussion, akin to the format of section 2 of the exam. Emphasis is placed on decision making as well as clarity of thought. Trying to keep up with the pace of modern day surgery and its ever growing evidence base is very difficult, but we have tried our very best to provide as up to date information as possible. In addition we have tried wherever possible to structure the questions and answers so that questions aimed at sub-speciality candidates are distinct from the general candidate. It must be emphasised that this book is no substitute for face-to-face viva practice, but is your key companion through the preparation for the event.

Finally this book is about helping you the reader and others in the future to succeed at the final hurdle before attaining CCT. We welcome any constructive comments and criticisms aimed at contributing to the process of continuous improvement of the material provided.

We are indebted to all of our contributors for finding the time amidst very busy clinical schedules and family commitments to onerously provide their insight into their various sub-specialities. We wish to thank especially Andrew White for all of his patience, encouragement and guidance through the preparation of this book.

Bhaskar Kumar
Alexander Phillips

Contributors

Mohamed I. Ahmed MBBS FRCSEd
Registrar in Paediatric Surgery
Our Lady's Children's Hospital,
Crumlin, Dublin 12, Ireland

Brice A. Antao MBBS MRCSEd FRCSEd (Paed.Surg)
Consultant Paediatric Surgeon
Our Lady's Children's Hospital,
Crumlin, Dublin 12, Ireland

Mr Waleed Al-Singary MBChB Dip (Urol) MPhil (Urol) FEBU FRCS (Urol)
Consultant Urological Surgeon
Benenden Hospital Trust
Kent, UK

Mr. Sunil Amonkar FRCS
Consultant Oncoplastic Breast and General Surgeon
Northumbria Healthcare NHS Foundation Trust, UK

Jonathan Barnes MBBS (Hons), MRES
Senior House Officer
Department of Hepatobiliary Surgery
Freeman Hospital
Newcastle upon Tyne Hospitals NHS Foundation Trust, UK

Mr Edward Cheong MD FRCS
Consultant Oesophagogastric Surgeon
Norfolk & Norwich University Hospitals NHS Foundation Trust
Norwich, UK

Mr Adam Critchley FRCS
Consultant Breast and Oncoplastic Surgeon
Royal Victoria Infirmary
Newcastle upon Tyne Hospitals NHS Foundation Trust, UK

Titus Cvasciuc MD
Fellow in Endocrine Surgery
Churchill Cancer Centre
Oxford, UK

Michael Delbridge MD FRCS
Consultant Vascular / Endovascular surgeon
Norfolk & Norwich University Hospitals NHS Foundation Trust
Norwich, UK

Mr M Tariq Dosani MRCSEd, FICS
Department of Hepatobiliary Surgery
Freeman Hospital
Newcastle upon Tyne Hospitals NHS Foundation Trust, UK

Mr Shridhar Dronamraju FRCSEd (Gen.Surg)
Senior Clinical Fellow, Department of Hepatobiliary Surgery
Freeman Hospital
Newcastle upon Tyne Hospitals NHS Foundation Trust, UK

Mr Rodrigo Figuerido MRCS
Research Fellow, Institute of Transplantation,
Freeman Hospital
Newcastle upon Tyne Hospitals NHS Foundation Trust, UK

Dr Jonathon Francis FRCA
Consultant Anaesthetist
Norfolk & Norwich University Hospitals NHS Foundation Trust
Norwich, UK

Mr Jeremy J French BSc MD FRCS (Gen Surg)
Consultant in Transplantation, Hepatobiliary and Retroperitoneal Sarcoma
Surgery
Department of Hepatobiliary Surgery
Freeman Hospital
Newcastle upon Tyne Hospitals NHS Foundation Trust, UK

Professor Alan F Horgan MD FRCS
Consultant Laparoscopic and Colorectal Surgeon
Freeman Hospital
Newcastle upon Tyne Hospitals NHS Foundation Trust, UK

Mr Alun E Jones FRCS (Gen Surg) ChM
Specialty Registrar
Wessex Deanery
Winchester, UK

Mr Jakub Kadlec FRCS
Senior Registrar in Cardiothoracic Surgery
Department of Thoracic Surgery
Norfolk and Norwich University Hospitals NHS Foundation Trust
Norwich, UK

Mr. Bhaskar Kumar MD FRCS
Consultant Oesophagogastric Surgeon
Norfolk & Norwich University Hospitals NHS Foundation Trust
Norwich, UK

Mr Michael Lewis MS FRCS
Consultant Upper Gastrointestinal Surgeon
Norfolk & Norwich University Hospitals NHS Foundation Trust
Norwich, UK

Mr. Mike Lim MD FRCS
Consultant Colorectal Surgeon
Raigmore Hospital,
Inverness, Scotland

Ms Sonia Lockwood MBChB MA FRCS (Gen Surg)
Consultant Colorectal Surgeon
Bradford Teaching Hospitals NHS Trust
Bradford, UK

Mr Liam Masterson BM MRCS DOHNS
ENT Specialty Registrar
Norfolk & Norwich University Hospitals NHS Foundation Trust
Norwich, UK

Mr. Sudhakar Mangam
Consultant Surgeon, QEQM Hospital
East Kent University Hospital Trust
Margate, Kent UK

Dr Ben Messer MRCP FRCA DICM(UK)
Consultant in Intensive Care Medicine and Anaesthesia
Royal Victoria Infirmary
Newcastle upon Tyne Hospitals NHS Foundation Trust, UK

Mr Radu Mihai MD PhD FRCS (Gen Surg)
Consultant Endocrine Surgeon
Churchill Cancer Centre
Oxford, UK

Dr Saeed Mirsadraee MD FRCR
Consultant Radiologist
Edinburgh Royal Infirmary
Edinburgh, Scotland

Mr Reza Mohammed Motallebzadeh
Specialist Registrar in Hepatobiliary & Transplantation Surgery
East of England Deanery
Cambridge, UK

Mr Ramez George Nassif MRCS, FRCS (ORL-HNS)
ENT/Head & Neck Surgery Consultant
Norfolk & Norwich University Hospitals NHS Foundation Trust
Norwich, UK

Brendan R. O'Connor BSc (Hons) MB BCh BAO (Hons) DOHNS DCH MRCSI
Specialty Trainee in Paediatric Surgery
Our Lady's Children's Hospital,
Crumlin, Dublin 12, Ireland.

Mr Alexander W Phillips MA, FRCSEd (Gen Surg), FHEA, MFSTEd
Northern Oesophagogastric Unit
Royal Victoria Infirmary,
Newcastle upon Tyne Hospitals NHS Foundation Trust, UK

Dr Nicola L Phillips LLM MRCPsych
Consultant in Forensic Learning Disability Psychiatry
Northgate Hospital
Morpeth, UK

Mr Dimitri Pournaras PhD FRCS
Specialist Registrar in Surgery
Norfolk & Norwich University Hospitals NHS Foundation Trust,
Norwich, UK

Dr Ali Robb MBBS, MRCP(UK), FRCPath, DipClinEd
Consultant Microbiologist
Royal Victoria Infirmary
Newcastle upon Tyne Hospitals NHS Foundation Trust, UK

Mr Stuart Robinson PhD, MRCS
Specialty Registrar, Department of Hepatobiliary Surgery
Freeman Hospital
Newcastle upon Tyne Hospitals NHS Foundation Trust, UK

Mr Rehan Saif MS, FRCSEd (Gen.Surg)
Specialty Registrar, Department of Hepatobiliary Surgery
Freeman Hospital
Newcastle upon Tyne Hospitals NHS Foundation Trust, UK

Mr Avinash Sewpaul BMedSci, MBBS, FRCS
Specialty Registrar, Institute of Transplantation,
Freeman Hospital
Newcastle upon Tyne Hospitals NHS Foundation Trust, UK

Mr Irshad A A K Shaikh, MS, MD, FRCS, EBSQ
Consultant Colorectal Surgeon
Norfolk & Norwich University Hospitals NHS Foundation Trust
Norwich, UK

Ms Loveena Sreedharan MBBS MRCS
Specialist Registrar in General Surgery
East of England Deanery
Cambridge, UK

Dr Eunice Tan MB BCh MRCP
Consultant Dermatologist
Norfolk & Norwich University Hospitals NHS Foundation Trust
Norwich, UK

Ms Alice Townend BMedSci, FRCS (Gen.Surg)
Specialty Registrar in Breast/General Surgery
Northern Deanery
Newcastle, UK

Mr Filip Van Tornout MD (Leuven), FRCSEd(C/th), FCS (SA), MMED (Pret.)
Consultant Thoracic Surgeon
Norfolk & Norwich University Hospitals NHS Foundation Trust
Norwich, UK

Dr Daniel Weiand MBChB FRCPath
Specialty Registrar in Medical Microbiology
Royal Victoria Infirmary
Newcastle upon Tyne Hospitals NHS Foundation Trust, UK

Mr. Simon Wemyss-Holden DM FRCS
Consultant Hepatobiliary Surgeon
Norfolk & Norwich University Hospitals NHS Foundation Trust
Norwich, UK

Mr Colin Wilson FRCS, PhD
Consultant Hepatobiliary and Transplant Surgeon, Institute of Transplantation
Freeman Hospital
Newcastle upon Tyne Hospitals NHS Foundation Trust, UK

Mr Robert Winterton FRCS (Plast)
Consultant Plastic and Reconstructive Surgeon
University Hospital of South Manchester
Manchester, UK

Mr Peng Wong MBChB MD FRCSEd (Gen Surg)
Consultant Vascular Surgeon
James Cook University Hospital NHS Foundation Trust
Middlesbrough, UK

Abbreviations

A&E	Accident & Emergency
AAA	Abdominal Aortic Aneurysm
AAC	Acute Acalculous Cholecystitis
AAST	American Association Surgical Trauma
ABG	Arterial Blood Gas
ABPI	Ankle Brachial Pressure Index
ACAS	Asymptomatic Carotid Artery Stenosis
ACE	Angiotensin Converting Enzyme
ACPGBI	Association of Coloproctology for Great Britain & Ireland
ACS	Abdominal Compartment Syndrome
ACS	Acute Chest Syndrome
ACST	Asymptomatic Carotid Surgery Trial
ACTH	Adrenocorticotrophic Hormone
ACTx	Adjuvant Chemotherapy
ADH	Antidiuretic Hormone
ADH	Atypical Ductal Hyperplasia
ADQI	Acute Dialysis Quality Initiative
AF	Atrial Fibrillation
AI	Aromatase Inhibitor
AII	Angiotensin II
AIN	Anal Intraepithelial Neoplasia
AKIN	Acute Kidney Injury Network
ALI	Acute Lung Injury
ALP	Alkaline Phosphatase
ALT	Alanine Transaminase
AMR	Antibody Mediated Rejection
ANH	Acute Normovolaemic Haemodilution
AO	Adjuvant Online
APC	Argon Plasma Coagulation
APER	Abdomino-perineal Resection
ARDS	Acute Respiratory Distress Syndrome
ARF	Acute Renal Failure
ARR	Absolute Risk Reduction
ART	Axillary Radiotherapy
ASCO	American Society of Clinical Oncology
ATA	American Thyroid Association
ATG	AntiThymocyte Globulin
ATN	Acute Tubular Necrosis
ATP	Adenosine Triphosphate
AV	Atrioventricular Node
AVF	Arteriovenous Fistula

AVG	Arteriovenous Grafts
AVM	Arteriovenous Malformations
Axr	Abdominal x-ray
BAL	Bronchoalveolar Lavage
BBV	Blood Borne Viruses
BCS	Breast Conserving Surgery
BE	Barrett's Oesophagus
βHCG	Beta-Human Chorionic Gonadotrophin
BIPAP	Biphasic Positive Airway Pressure
BMI	Body Mass Index
BP	Blood Pressure
BPD/DS	Biliary Pancreatic Diversion / Duodenal Switch
BPH	Benign Prostatic Hypertrophy
Bpm	Beats per minute
BSG	British Society of Gastroenterology
CABG	Coronary Artery Bypass Graft
CALI	Chemotherapy Assisted Liver Injury
cAMP	Cyclic Adenosine Monophosphate
CAS	Carotid Artery Stenting
CBD	Common Bile Duct
CCF	Congestive Cardiac Failure
CCLND	Central Compartment Lymph Node Dissection
CDI	Clostridium Difficile Infection
CEA	Carotid Endartrectomy
CEA	Carcinoembryonic Antigen
CETC	Carotid Endarterectomy Trialists Collaboration
CFA	Common Femoral Artery
CgA	Chromogranin A
CHD	Common Hepatic Duct
CK	Creatine Kinase
CLI	Critical Limb Ischaemia
CMV	Cytomegalovirus
CO	Cardiac Output
CONSORT	Consolidated Standards for Reporting Trials
COPD	Chronic Obstructive Airways Disease
CP	Chronic Pancreatitis
CPAP	Continuous Positive Airway Pressure
CPP	Cerebral Perfusion Pressure
CPR	Cardiopulmonary Resuscitation
CPX	Cardiopulmonary Exercise Test
CRM	Circumferential Resection Margin
CRRT	Continuous Renal Replacement Therapy
CRT	Capillary Refill Time

CSF	Cerebrospinal Fluid
CT	Computed Tomography
CTA	Computed Tomography Angiogram
CVA	Cerebrovascular Accident
CVI	Chronic Venous Insufficiency
CVP	Central Venous Pressure
CVVH	Continuous Venovenous Haemofiltration
CXR	Chest X-ray
DBD	Donation after Brain Stem Death
DCD	Donation after Cardiac Death
DCIS	Ductal Carcinoma in Situ
DCL	Damage Control Laparotomy
DEXA	Dual Energy X-ray Absorption
DGH	District General Hospital
DIC	Disseminated Intravascular Coagulation
DJ Flexure	Duodenal Jejunal Flexure
DM	Diabetes Mellitus
DO2	Oxygen Delivery
(2,3) DPG	Diphosphoglycerate
DRIL	Distal Revascularization and Interval Ligation
DSA	Digital Subtraction Angiography
DU	Duodenal Ulcer
DVLA	Driver and Vehicle Licensing Agency
DVT	Deep Vein Thrombosis
EBV	Epstein Barr Virus
ECF	Extracellular Fluid
ECG	Electrocardiogram
ECMO	Extra Corporeal Membrane Oxygenation
ECST	European Carotid Surgery Trials
EMR	Endoscopic Mucosal Resection
ENT	Ear Nose and Throat
ER	Estrogen Receptor
ERAS	Enhanced Recovery After Surgery
ERCP	Endoscopic Retrograde Cholangiopancreatography
ESD	Endoscopic Submucosal Dissection
ESRD	End Stage Renal Disease
ETT	Endotracheal Tube
EUA	Examination Under Anaesthesia
EUS	Endoscopic Ultrasound
EVAR	Endovascular abdominal aortic aneurysm repair
FAP	Familial Adenomatous Polyposis
FAST	Focused Assessment of Sonography in Trauma

FBC	Full Blood Count
FEA	Flat Epithelial Atypia
FFP	Fresh Frozen Plasma
FLR	Future Liver Remnant
FNAB	Fine Needle Aspiration Biopsy
FNAC	Fine Needle Aspiration Cytology
FRC	Functional Residual Capacity
FRV	Functional Residual Volume
GA	General Anaesthesia
GB	Gallbladder Remnant
G-CSF	Granulocyte Colony Stimulating Factor
GCS	Glasgow Coma Scale
GDT	Goal Directed Therapy
GFR	Glomerular Filtration Rate
GI	Gastrointestinal
GOJ	Gastrooesophageal Junction
GORD	Gastrooesophageal Reflux Disease
GP	General Practitioner
GSV	Great Saphenous Vein
GTN	Glyceryl Trinitrate
Gy	Gray
HAI	Hospital Acquired Infection
HAP	Healthcare Associated Pneumonia
HAT	Hepatic Arterial Thrombosis
Hb	Haemoglobin
HCC	Hepatocellular Carcinoma
HCV	Hepatitis C Virus
HDU	High Dependency Unit
HER2	Herceptin
HGD	High Grade Dysplasia
HIAA	Hydroxyindoleacetic Acid
HIT	Heparin Induced Thrombocytopenia
HPS	Hyperplastic Pyloric Stenosis
HPV	Human Papilloma Virus
HTA	Human Tissue Authority
HU	Hounsfield Units
IAH	Intra Abdominal Hypertension
IAP	Intra Abdominal Pressure
IBD	Inflammatory Bowel Disease
ICD	Implantable Cardioverter Defibrillator
ICF	Intracellular Fluid
ICP	Intracerebral Pressure

ICP	Intracranial Pressure
ICS	Intraoperative Cell Salvage
ICU	Intensive Care Unit
IH	Intermittent Haemodialysis
IHD	Ischaemic Heart Disease
IJV	Internal Jugular Vein
INR	International Normalised Ratio
IPF	Initial Poor Function
IPMN	Intraductal papillary mucinous neoplasm
IPPV	Intermittent Positive Pressure Ventilation
ISCP	Intercollegiate Surgical Curriculum Programme
ISE	Intercollegiate Speciality Examination
ITC	Isolated tumour cells
ITP	Idiopathic Thrombocytopenic Purpura
IV	Intravenous
IVC	Inferior Vena Cava
JSCFE	Joint Surgical Colleges Fellowship Examination
kHz	Kilohertz
LBO	Large Bowel Obstruction
LC	Laparoscopic Cholecystectomy
LC-CRT	Long Course Chemoradiotherapy
LCIS	Lobular Carcinoma In Situ
LDH	Lactate Dehydrogenase
LFT	Liver Function Test
LGD	Low Grade Dysplasia
LGIB	Lower Gastrointestinal Bleed
LH	Lutenising Hormone
LHM	Laparoscopic Heller's Myotomy
LIF	Left Iliac Fossa
LMWH	Low Molecular Weight Heparin
LOS	Lower Oesophageal Sphincter
LRINEC	Laboratory Risk Indicator for Necrotising Fasciitis
LSV	Long Saphenous Vein
LVEDP	Left Ventricular End Diastolic Pressure
LVI	Lymphovascular invasion
MA	Microwave Ablation
MAP	Mean Arterial Pressure
MALT	Mucosa Associated Lymphoid Tissue
MBL	Massive Blood Loss
MDM	Multidisciplinary Team Meeting

MDRD	Modification of Diet in Renal Disease
MELD	Model for End-Stage Liver Disease
MEN	Multiple Endocrine Neoplasia
mHz	Megahertz
MI	Myocardial Infarction
MIBG	Meta-iodobenzylguanidine
MMF	Mycofenolate Mofetil
MODS	Multi Organ Dysfunction Syndrome
MOOSE	Meta-analysis Of Observational Studies in Epidemiology
MRA	Magnetic Resonance Angiogram
MRC	Medical Research Council
MRCP	Magnetic Resonance Cholangiopancreatography
MRE	Magnetic Resonance Enterogram
MRI	Magnetic Resonance Imaging
MRSA	Methicillin Resistant Staphylococcus Aureus
MSSA	Methicillin Sensitive Staphylococcus Aureus
MTC	Medullary Thyroid Carcinoma
NAC	Nipple Areolar Complex
NAI	Non Accidental Injury
NASCET	North American Symptomatic Carotid Endarterectomy Trial
NCTx	Neoadjuvant Chemotherapy
NET	Neuroendocrine Tumour
NEX	Neoadjuvant Endocrine Treatment
NFATc	Nuclear Factor of Activated T cells
NG	Nasogastric
NGT	Nasogastric tube
NHS	National Health Service
NICE	National Institute for Clinical Excellence
NIV	Non invasive Ventilation
NJ	Nasojejunal
NNT	Number Needed to Treat
NOGCA	National Oesophagogastric Cancer Audit
OCP	Oral Contraceptive Pill
OGD	Oesophagogastroduodenoscopy
OPSI	Overwhelming Post Splenectomy Infection
PA	Pulmonary Artery
PAD	Pre-deposit Autologous Blood Donation
PAWP	Pulmonary Artery Wedge Pressure
PCA	Patient Controlled Analgesia
PCC	Prothrombin Complex Concentrate
PCR	Pathological Complete Response
PCT	Percutaneous Tracheostomy

PD	Peritoneal Dialysis
PD	Pneumatic Dilatation
PDS	Polydiaxonone
PE	Pulmonary Embolism
PEC	Percutaneous Endoscopic Colostomy
PEEP	Positive End Expiratory Pressure
PEP	Post Exposure Proplylaxis
PET	Positron Emission Tomography
PFA	Profunda Femoris Artery
PFC	Peripancreatic Fluid Collection
PH	Primary Hyperhidrosis
PHPT	Primary Hyperparathyroidism
PICC	Peripheral Indwelling Central Catheter
PNF	Primary Non Function
POCT	Point of Care Testing
POEM	Per Oral Endoscopic Myotomy
PPH	Procedure for Prolapsed Haemorrhoids
PPI	Proton Pump Inhibitor
PPV	Patent Processus Vaginalis
Pr	Per rectum
PRISMA	Preferred Reporting Items for Systematic Reviews and Meta-Analyses
PTC	Percutaneous Transhepatic Cholangiography
PTFE	Polytetrafluoroethylene
PTH	Parathyroid Hormone
PTLD	Post Transplant Lymphoproliferative Disorder
PTT	Prothrombin Time
PTU	Propylthyouracil
PVE	Portal Vein Embolization
QALY	Quality Adjusted Life Year
QOL	Quality Of Life
RAAS	Renin Angiotensin Aldosterone System
RAI	RadioIodine Ablation
RCC	Renal Cell Carcinoma
RCT	Randomised Controlled Trial
RFA	Radiofrequency Ablation
RIF	Right Iliac Fossa
RIG	Radiologically Inserted Gastrostomy
RLN	Recurrent Laryngeal Nerve
RR	Respiratory Rate
RRR	Relative Risk Reduction
RRT	Renal Replacement Therapy
RUDI	Revision Using Distal Inflow

SCA	Sickle Cell Anaemia
SCC	Squamous Cell Carcinoma
SCIWORA	Spinal Cord Injury Without Radiological Abnormality
SCM	Sternocleidomastoid
SCPRT	Short Course Preoperative Radiotherapy
SFA	Superficial Femoral Artery
SIADH	Syndrome of Inappropriate Antidiuretic Hormone
SIRS	Systemic Inflammatory Response Syndrome
SIRT	Selective Internal Radiotherapy
SLE	Systemic Lupus Erythematosus
SMA	Superior Mesenteric Artery
SMG	Submandibular Gland
SLNB	Sentinel Lymph Node Biopsy
SRH	Stigmata of Recent Haemorrhage
SSI	Surgical Site Infection
SSV	Short Saphenous Vein
STROBE	STrengthening the Reporting of OBservational studies in Epidemiology
SVC	Superior Vena Cava
SVR	Systemic Vascular Resistance
TAMIS	Transanal Minimally Invasive Surgery
TACE	Transarterial Chemotherapy
TB	Tuberculosis
TBSA	Total Body Surface Area
TEDs	Thromboembolism Deterrant Stockings
TEG	Thromboelastogram
TEMS	Transanal Endoscopic Microsurgery
TEP	Totally Extraperitoneal
TIA	Transient Ischaemic Attack
TME	Total Mesorectal Excision
TNF	Tumour Necrosis Factor
TOS	Thoracic Outlet Syndrome
TPMT	Transpurine Methyl Transferase
TPN	Total Parenteral Nutrition
TRALI	Transfusion Related Acute Lung Injury
TSH	Thyroid Stimulating Hormone
TTS	Through The Scope
U&Es	Urea and Electrolytes
UC	Ulcerative Colitis
UDT	Congenital Undescended Testicle
UGFS	Ultrasound guided Foam Sclerotherapy
USS	Ultrasound Scan
UTI	Urinary Tract Infection

VAC	Vacuum Assisted Closure
VACB	Vacuum Assisted Core Biopsy
VAP	Ventilator Associated Pneumonia
VARD	Video Assisted Retroperitoneal Dissection
VOC	Vaso-Occlusive Crisis
VRE	Vancomycin Resistant Enterococci
VTE	Venous Thromboembolism
WBI	Whole Breast Irradiation
WOPN	Walled Off Pancreatic Necrosis
ZES	Zollinger Ellison Syndrome

Introduction

The Intercollegiate Specialty Examination in General Surgery

The Intercollegiate Speciality Examination (ISE) in General Surgery consists of two sections. This book is focused on how to prepare and pass Section 2 of the exam. Section 1 is a written test consisting of two papers. Paper 1 is composed of single best answer Multiple Choice Questions (MCQs) and lasts 2 hours. Paper 2 is composed of Extended Matching Item questions (EMIs) and lasts 2.5 hours. Although preparation for this part of the exam is beyond the scope of this book we have included a short section on how to prepare for it, as well as useful links.

The format for section two has changed recently. Candidates are required to choose their special interest from one of upper GI (includes both oesophagogastric and HPB), colorectal, breast, transplant or endocrine (or vascular – applicable only to trainees following the 2010 curriculum or those appointed before 1 January 2013 following the 2013 curriculum or to Republic of Ireland trainees). "General surgery" will no longer be accepted as a special interest, in keeping with the 2013 curriculum.

Section 2 comprises of clinical and oral exams. There are two clinical exams of 40 minutes each. One covers general surgery (including emergencies) and the other the candidate's special interest. Each has a 20 minute case along with 2 cases of 10 minutes each.

The oral examination consists of 4 viva sections each of 30 minutes, comprising 6 questions, each of 5 minutes (to replace the previous 3 vivas):

1. **Emergency Surgery / Trauma / Critical care**	**30 minutes**
2. **General Surgery Principles and Clinical Practice**	**30 minutes**
3. **Special Interest Surgery – Clinical Practice**	**30 minutes**
4. **Special Interest Surgery – Basic Principles**	**30 minutes**
(applied anatomy / physiology / pathology)	**(15 minutes each)**
and Academic Paper	

Knowledge of the seminal papers providing evidence for practice in Emergency Surgery and in the applicant's special interest is expected as is the ability to assess relevant radiographic images to the level expected of a consultant general surgeon. Applied Basic Science knowledge will also be expected throughout, as indicated in the curriculum.

The Joint Surgical Colleges Fellowship Examination

For the first time the four surgical royal colleges have introduced a new fellowship exam for the international surgical community. General surgery is the first speciality to do this and the exam is aimed at overseas candidates who are about to or have recently completed their training. The Joint Surgical Colleges Fellowship Examination (JSCFE) will be assessed to the same standard as the intercollegiate speciality examination (ISE). The syllabus for this exam is outlined on the JSCFE website – go to www.jscfe.co.uk/syllabus.

Section 1 is the same for both the JSCFE and ISE examinations. Section 2 of the JSCFE will be as follows:

Clinical Examination – two 40 minute short case sessions

Oral Examination – there will be 3 vivas:

1) **Emergency Surgery with critical care**   **30 minutes**

2) **General Surgery**   **30 minutes**

3) **Academic**   **20 minutes**

Unlike the ISE having only recently been introduced there are no immediate plans to change the JSCFE examination.

How is section 2 of the ISE marked?

The viva/oral examination begins with the academic viva. Topics to be examined are usually decided at the Examiners' meeting prior to the exam itself. Examiners are told to start off with an easier question to allow the candidate to settle in. As the viva progresses the questions will become more challenging – this also allows any outstanding candidates to shine. Expect each examiner to cover three or four topics.

The range of marks given are as follows:

8 (outstanding)

7 (good)

6 (pass)

5 (fail)

4 (poor)

For each topic each examiner will give a mark independently. There is no discussion between examiners until the marks have been awarded. The final mark awarded is the mean of all the individual marks in each of the sections. It is possible to compensate for a poor performance in one section with a good performance in another and still pass i.e. it is an aggregate score.

The allocation of marks for each station is as follows:

Section	Pass Mark	Highest mark (% weighting)
General Surgery - Clinical	120	160 (23%)
Special Interest- Clinical	120	160 (23%)
Special Interest Surgery – Clinical Practice Oral	72	96 (14%)
Special Interest Surgery- Basic Principles and Academic	60	80 (12%)
Emergency Surgery/Trauma/ Critical Care Oral	72	96 (14%)
General Surgery / Principles and Clinical Practice Oral	72	96 (14%)
TOTAL	516	688

Clinical Exams:

Both the General Surgery Clinical and the Special Interest Clinical comprise one long case lasting 20 minutes and two short cases lasting 10 minutes each. The long case is scored on four components: history taking and examination, investigations and clinical knowledge, treatment options and complications, and finally professionalism/communication/consent. Thus a candidate will score out of 32 for the long case from each examiner. The short cases are marked against three components: history taking and examination, investigations/differentials and management, and finally complications/ professionalism/ communication/ consent. Therefore candidates will score out of 24 for each short case from each examiner.

Oral exams:

The Special Interest- Basic Principles and Academic Oral exam is split into two sections. The basic principles component examines on applied anatomy, physiology and pathology, and candidates are asked three questions, thus a total of 8 marks for each question from each examiner makes this out of 48. The second half of this exam is based on discussion of a pre-read published journal article and scores out of 32.

The other three oral examinations each comprise six questions (5 minutes per question) and candidates are scored out of 8 by each examiner for each question. Thus each oral exam is out of 96.

When should I take the ISE exam?

There is never a perfect time to take the exam. More than likely you are ready to take the exam from ST6 onwards even if you don't feel ready to do so! Procrastination will only delay the inevitable. A commitment to send the application off in a 'come what may manner' followed by a structured approach to preparation will start you off on the right pathway.

The exam is certainly not a test of knowing absolutely everything in the textbook and ability to recite the very latest journal articles. Instead it is very much geared around assessing your thought process and decision making as a safe independent practitioner of surgery. Clarity of thought, recognition of limitations, prioritisation are all of utmost importance to convey to the examiner, rather than dry textbook knowledge. The candidates will be expected to discuss a case as if he or she has been referred the case by a consultant colleague.

Preparation for Section 2

Preparation is key

The examination is not an examination on operative skills. Therefore having a great log book and the confidence that you can operate well will not by itself get you through this hurdle. Thorough preparation is absolutely vital and the correct approach to your preparation even more important given the time constraints imposed by a demanding working schedule.

What is the best way to prepare for the exam?

The exam is not about in depth reading and knowing the fine details and rarities, but it will test your clinical decision making skills, judgement as well as knowledge. The most important approach to success in this exam is technique and presentation of your answers. Much of your examination preparation will not be adding new knowledge, but perfecting your presentation to convey clarity of thought.

Here are some of the ways we recommend you prepare:

- **Group revision** – there is much to be said for putting yourself on the line in front of colleagues/friends who are also preparing. Try to form a small revision group or even work in a pair. Not only will you be able to help each other through the process but it will give an opportunity to share knowledge, motivate each other and above all practice under pressure.

- **Viva practice** – although consultants who are *college examiners* are *not allowed* to provide you with this practice, there is a lot to gain by viva practice with a consultant. This can be done one to one but you may find consultants are more willing to help if a small group /pair of you approach them. This will also mean that you will cover more topics in that time.

- **Practice under pressure** - Even the most eloquent candidate in practice can be broken by pressure if he/she hasn't practiced under realistic conditions. Though organising a viva session with two consultants together is simply not always practical, going one to one for a set period of 30 minutes in an identical manner to the exam will be much more effective than a relaxed one hour of informal discussion. Choose your sparring partners wisely. There is little to be gained by approaching the nicest consultant who is not going to push you in the right direction. Equally do not take harsh criticism to heart, just take it objectively not personally.

- **Use the syllabus** – make sure you have covered each and every topic. You may be unpleasantly surprised as one candidate found out on the day:

"In my general surgery viva the examiner said that I was in a 'very general surgical clinic'. My first case was a patient with an undescended testicle, followed by a varicocele, then a hydrocele, then a neck lump. I was not expecting so much urology in a general surgical exam. Luckily I had covered these topics with a urology consultant a week before the exam. If I hadn't been guided by the syllabus I may not have covered these topics" **Candidate GK**

So try not to leave any blanks – even if you are not able to go into a huge amount of detail you need to be able to hold your own whatever they throw at you. The exam is based on the 2013 Intercollegiate Surgical Curriculum Programme (ISCP). It would be highly advisable to refer to it, in order to be familiar with this. We have tried to follow in this book the list of topics given in the curriculum. Please note that there may be few topics which have not been covered in this edition of the book.

- **Attend MDTs** – this is most relevant to the sub-speciality viva. For example the candidates who are primarily oesophagogastric surgery trainees are also expected to have some working hepatobiliary surgical knowledge. Contact the relevant consultant well ahead of time to seek permission to attend.

- **Look after your health** – it is an incredibly stressful time for you and your family during exam preparation. You will feel the clock ticking constantly through the process, but a bit of "down time" to look after your health and well being will not only be good for you but will enhance your performance. Do not underestimate the benefit of getting some fresh air and exercise. You will find yourself sharper, more alert and able to handle stress much better. We cannot emphasise enough to you the importance of down time. Don't cut off the rest of the world totally, but make sure you participate in all the things you enjoy in your normal down time whether this be cycling, cooking or just going to the cinema.

- **Know what works for you** – after all, you have been through medical school exams, membership exams and maybe a higher degree as well. So you already have a pedigree of success in tough exams and would have worked out some individual quirks that have historically worked in your favour.

- **Courses** – but don't expect to be spoonfed. The aim of the course should be to consolidate on the revision you have already done. Most courses will have a mock exam component. Even though the mock exams are not done by current examiners they are usually able to recreate a very realistic replication. Taking part in these mock exams may be the most beneficial aspect of a course as it will be very revealing what your strengths and weaknesses are before the real thing. It also gives an invaluable opportunity to watch and learn from others' performance as well as obtain feedback from the practice examiners.

Viva technique

What we are about to tell you in this paragraph is the singular most important and decisive step you can take towards passing the exam. The absolute key in passing this exam will be your viva technique and not necessarily the depth of your knowledge. Being able to deliver an answer with clarity and structure will take a lot of practice. It is absolutely essential for success to spend time developing your delivery skills so that you can talk in an organised, clear and structured manner. Confidence will develop with practice. As an example just try to read a topic in a book, then close the book and recite what you have just studied – you may be surprised how difficult this exercise can be. It is important that you integrate viva practice into your revision and focus on weak areas rather than be tempted to go over areas where you are strong. Surgery is a craft profession and is practical in its very nature therefore so should your preparation be. Substituting viva practice for reading text books cover to cover is a recipe for failure.

Sell your knowledge – broadly speaking there are two methods of delivery of answers by candidates. For example consider the popular question answered by two such candidates:

Examiner: How do you define shock?

Candidate 1: *Shock is defined as a condition of insufficient delivery of oxygen to meet the metabolic demands of a tissue.*

Examiner: Can you give me some examples?

Candidate 1: *Examples include hypovolaemic, septic, cardiogenic, neurogenic shock.*

Examiner: What are the causes of hypovolaemic shock?

Candidate 1: *Blood loss.*

Examiner: What examples can you state?

Candidate 1: *Bleeding from for example a ruptured abdominal aortic aneurysm.*

In sharp contrast candidate 2 performs as follows:

Examiner: How do you define shock?

Candidate 2: *Shock is defined as a condition of insufficient delivery of oxygen to meet the metabolic demands of a tissue. Examples include hypovolaemic, septic, cardiogenic, neurogenic shock. Hypovolaemic shock is the most commonly seen by a general surgeon and may be caused by profound loss of blood or plasma. This may be seen for example in a ruptured abdominal aortic aneurysm. Septic shock is also commonly seen particularly in the context of a ruptured intra-abdominal viscus. Though cardiogenic and neurogenic shock are less commonly seen it is important to understand the physiological response to each as this may explain any differences in clinical presentation between each.*

Though in reality it is almost impossible to speak as fluently and eloquently as candidate 2 the majority of candidates will be somewhere between these two styles. It is crucially important that the examiner is not having to drag the answer out of the candidate as seen in candidate 1.The approach given by candidate 2 also allows better use of the time in the viva to score as many points as possible. **To answer in a similar manner can only be achieved through repetitive practice verbalising to each other over and over again.** Remember in expanding your answer do not stray away to answer something totally remote from the question as this will only irritate the astute examiner who will be able to tell you are trying to lead him away from the question.

Expect to be nervous – everyone will be. It will take some time to settle in and you may find your first viva/encounter particularly hard. Do your very best to ignore any other candidates and accept that your destiny is in the hands of you yourself and the examiners, not other candidates. It can be very off putting to hear other candidates reeling off beautiful answers, but you have no idea how other parts of the exam have gone for them. The examiners are expecting you to be nervous just like any other ordinary human being. What they will look for is your ability under pressure to handle the nerves and not buckle.

Systematic answer – Always try to organise your answer and present it in a manner that demonstrates a clear, systematic thought process. This is the key to producing succinct answers. It is useful to consider what the examiner is asking you before indulging in the details. The opening phrase is crucial in this regard. Start your answers with phrases such as:

'My overwhelming priority in this situation is the safety of the patient....'

'My main concern in this situation would be establishing control of haemorrhage...'

Try to compartmentalise and categorise your answer as much as possible. This is particularly important when the content of an answer is packed with information. The examiners are always impressed with a candidate who demonstrates a system to their answer because this shows that you conduct your surgical practice in a systematic and safe manner.

Speak from experience – it is often advised to speak in the exam as if you are the consultant and not a trainee. Calling for help and asking for senior advice constantly is not only irritating for the examiner but perfectly demonstrates a lack of experience and confidence. There will be very few scenarios in the exam which are beyond your scope of practice and hard earned experience. There is nothing wrong to speak from your experience particularly when there is no absolute right or wrong answer to a question. For example:

'How would you perform the anastomosis following a small bowel resection?'

It is perfectly reasonable to state that you would perform one of either a hand sewn or stapled anastomosis. In reality the examiners may have their own preferences of technique (in fact they may disagree with each other!) but remember you are answering as a consultant colleague not a trainee.

'From my experience I am most comfortable in this scenario to perform a two layer hand sewn anastomosis using 3.0 PDS in a continuous seromuscular extramucosal manner'

The wrong answer in this scenario would be

'Yes I am happy to perform a small bowel anastomosis but would check what my consultant would like me to do'

Do not read into the examiner's body language – imagine sitting all day examining the same questions over and over again. Even the most enthusiastic examiner will eventually be worn down by the monotony of the process. The majority of examiners will derive much pleasure from your good performance and will be looking wherever possible to pass you. Those that fail have usually done so even before facing the examiners.

A whole variety of examiner expressions and mannerisms can be seen through the course of the exam.

'In my critical care viva the examiner asked me about management of high output stoma. I felt I was answering well but he gave me absolutely no eye contact and even started staring at the ceiling. Momentarily this threw me off track but I tried to convince myself that he was putting this on. I passed this station without any problems but could see how some may get put off'

On the whole the examiner will be poker faced and will certainly not give you much in the way of positive acknowledgement and encouragement. This is in sharp contrast to your practice sessions with most consultants who may try and give you much feedback – usually positive.

Ignore the other one – one examiner will be marking the performance whilst the other asks questions. Never go looking at the marking examiner's point scoring sheet in the hope of a sneak preview. This will distract you from the main exam and can be irritating for the examiner asking questions.

Never argue with the examiner – this will almost certainly end in tears. You are not in a position to argue, no matter how convinced you remain. Be diplomatic and simply state what you believe in from your own experience and accept that there may be other approaches to the same problem.

The vivas are structured – the days when the examiner could make up a question or bring in their favourite question are over. With the structured format of the exam an examiner will not be able to question you in unfair detail on one area in which he may be an expert. Don't forget that the examiner may be asking you a question on something which is remote from their own practice to which you may have substantially more experience! You should draw confidence from this but equally do not underestimate the examiner's experience and be respectful at all times.

How to get the most out of this book - The book is not designed to be a comprehensive textbook of surgery or its sub specialities. Instead it is a revision companion and guide. We encourage you to get the most out of our book by working with a partner or forming a small group with emphasis on revision through interaction. We hope you are able to use it as a revision companion to maximise your revision sessions. We suggest you take it in turns to fire questions at each other but to really concentrate on reflecting on your answers to see how they can be made clearer and more concise. Although the book is primarily aimed at the viva section, much of the clinical examination consists of similar questions. We have done our best to cover as many topics as possible but there may be some we have not covered which may be evident in the ISCP syllabus. Finally we welcome any feedback and suggestions on how the text can be improved or modified for the benefit of future generations of candidates.

Candidate quotes / comments

"The first thing I would say is that this is not really a knowledge exam. People said that to me beforehand, and I didn't really believe it. But it is true. It is about a structured approach to fairly straightforward patients that you would expect on an average take or clinic. It mainly revolves around clinical/management. You are expected to give an answer for how you would assess and manage patients, and come up with a definitive management plan which you can justify. I don't think they want a list of possible alternative plans, just what you would do. Trying to be clever is definitely a bad idea- eg don't say you'll do a lap washout or primary anastomosis for someone with perf diverticulitis... As far as knowledge is concerned, the companion series (general surgery + your subspecialty) is more than enough".

"I would strongly recommend a viva course- specifically one in which you do practice vivas. There are some courses that try to teach the entire syllabus in a week, mainly in a lecture format. I think that you are better off going with a course where they concentrate on viva skills. I did a 2 day course in RCS Edinburgh, which was excellent. People had attended the Manchester course (Alpine course in winter) and said that was fantastic. Apart from anything else, I think they re-assure you that the knowledge base required is not especially high and it is the technique that is vastly important".

"Spending a lot of time looking at relevant research/ trials is probably unnecessary as far as the exam goes (although may be a useful time to learn these things at some point anyway, so the exam is a good excuse). Certainly for me, I don't think I really was able to mention anything about research trials, and I got a good pass on each station".

"I got really put off by one of the stations where I thought I had performed really badly (critical care). I hardly slept the night before the clinicals day due to this, and felt really down about it. In fact I did fine. So, if you think you've done badly in one station, put it behind you and you can quite easily make up the marks in other sections anyway".

"Think carefully about hotels to stay in - the viva part is usually in a conference type hotel. I stayed in a room immediately above the dining hall where the examiners had their pre-exam shindig. I could hear all the laughing and cheering and it was quite unsettling, and I felt like a prisoner in the room. I had to get room service. Would strongly recommend staying elsewhere if possible".

"The marking system for the vivas seems to suggest that the lesser the candidate is prompted, the better the mark achieved. I did not find the latter statement to be entirely accurate. I found that the examiners would often prompt you, no matter how knowledgeable you are, in an attempt to steer the conversation in the direction they want."

"The general surgical viva dealt with bread and butter topics in general surgery and in a broad manner whereas the speciality viva was quite detailed and in depth."

"For the Upper GI clinical, be prepared to interpret endoscopic, radiological images (CT and EUS scans), as well as pH and Manometry studies. I was quizzed on all."

"I found that the critical care viva was the hardest of the vivas. I recommend that you invest in a basic intensive care revision book. The scenarios quizzed on in the viva dealt with co-morbid disease that one would encounter in ICU patients such as diabetes, acute coronary syndrome, dialysis, electrolyte abnormalities, transfusions etc......."

"Although the breast viva is predominantly based around oncology, an increasing part of the clinical exam involves reconstructive cases and testing candidates' knowledge and understanding of this. This is an essential skill of a new breast consultant with reconstructive cases from both breast and plastic surgery being likely to dominate the specialist breast clinical."

"I had a few friends and colleagues sitting the exam at the same time. This really made revision less painful and less stressful. We had viva practice with each other and arranged practice with several consultants beforehand. The examiners pressurise and interrupt you more than I had anticipated and this can disrupt your thoughts- be prepared!"

"My first general surgery viva felt very rushed and pressured. There appeared to be little time to think, but it is important to gather your thoughts before speaking. The case was a patient with a neck lump. My second patient also had a neck lump to find. These are not normally cases I come across in my specialty on a day-to-day basis but they are part of the syllabus. Getting to some clinics where more of these patients are referred to would have been beneficial."

"The reading time for the academic vivas will fly past. It's crucial to practice reading papers in the same time frame in the weeks leading up to the exam. The discussion on the specialty paper was absolutely fine. The examiner for the general paper appeared to have more of an agenda. It was difficult to know exactly what he was asking for at times. Remember the examiners have had much longer to read the paper and will have picked up some of the finer details."

ACADEMIC VIVA

Alexander Phillips Bhaskar Kumar

Contents

Introduction

The format for this chapter is a little different from others in this book. Rather than provide question and answer scenarios we will make some suggestions on how to "read" the academic paper along with providing a few definitions. Many candidates get very anxious about this part of the exam, which should be straightforward. It will be made even more straightforward if you try and read journal articles regularly, and critically, particularly as part of a journal club.

The academic viva now comprises half of the "Specialty Interest Surgery - Basic Principles and Academic Foundation Oral". This involves 15 minutes of this 30 minute viva marked on the knowledge and interpretation of a paper given in advance. Candidates are given a single published paper to read over 30 minutes prior to the viva.

We would suggest spending 25 minutes reading the paper with the final five minutes given to practising what you want to say and to identify the salient points. We would recommend highlighting and annotating the paper so that you do not have to keep referring to separate notes. Also the examiners are able to see that you have noted salient points. It has also been suggested that highlighting should be done in different colours- one to indicate positive points and one to indicate the negative aspects.

Reading the paper

There are a number of different ways of approaching reading the paper. It is important to have a system, and the next part is a suggestion of how to approach things.

Initial Assessment

Have an initial scan through the paper - pay particular attention to the title, note that aims have been stipulated and correspond with the title, and have a good look at the abstract to see if everything ties together. Also identify what type of research has been performed - a randomised control trial, cohort study, something else?

After having an initial scan through the paper and abstract so that you know what you are dealing with, the paper can be broken down into sections.

What journal is the paper in? Is it a mainstream paper with a high impact factor or in a "smaller" journal? Caution should be taken with this as publication in a journal with a high impact factor does not necessarily equate to quality.

Which institution/study group has the paper come from? Do you know them, are they well regarded in their field? Is the study from a large teaching hospital or university or a small study from a district general? Are the references appropriate - the number and how recent are they?

The introduction:

Have the authors made their aims clear, and does the introduction place the study in context, making the case for its importance and reviewing the other literature that is available on the subject? It should be brief, succinct and relevant.

The methods:

This is probably the most important component of any paper. Irrespective of how important the subject matter is, or how convincing results may be, if the methodology is flawed then little can actually be drawn from the study.

The type of study should be very clear from the methods employed, and they will determine the level of evidence it provides.

Questions that need to be asked include -are the methods appropriate to the study question, have the primary and any secondary end points been clearly stated, are inclusion and exclusion criteria stated, have appropriate statistics been used, is there any obvious bias in the methods employed?

The results:

The demographics and baseline data should be provided, and in comparison groups it should be noted whether these were similar or not.

Results should be clearly displayed and tables and graphs should be looked at closely. Are they appropriate for the data being displayed? It is also worth looking at the units on graphical representations. For instance, authors may choose to represent survival using Kaplan-Meier graphs, which look on inspection to be similar, but on closer inspection one graph may use weeks as a unit, the other months. As a reminder it is often worth highlighting these units- particularly if there is a discrepancy. Graphs and tables should also have clear titles to allow easy interpretation. Also you should ensure that all the subjects are accounted for with an appropriate CONSORT diagram for randomised trials or PRISMA diagram for meta-analyses.

The discussion and conclusions:

Have the authors drawn appropriate conclusions from the data they obtained and have they compared this with other studies? Discussions should normally critically evaluate their own methodology and suggest improvements as well as how the study could be developed.

Miscellaneous:

The above points should give you a good grasp of the paper, but there are other components that should be observed that may give an insight into the motivation behind the paper and its quality.

Finally it may be worth having a set way of how you want to start talking about the paper to get you started. Have a few summary sentences prepared and annotate a few pros and cons in the margins so you have something to say when asked. Form an opinion on whether this is a good or bad paper and why? Ultimately, would it change your practice and why? And perhaps most importantly, if you think the paper is terrible and you are ready to take it apart, ensure the person examining you is not one of the authors, and if he is do it tactfully!

Statistical definitions

Null hypothesis (H0): This is the initial hypothesis which stipulates that there is no difference between the items being studied.

P value: The *P value* or calculated probability is the estimated probability of rejecting the null hypothesis of a study question when that hypothesis is true. A p value of 0.05 is usually taken as being statistically significant i.e only a 5% (or 1 in 20) likelihood that a result this extreme is obtained by chance.

Mean: It is the total of all values divided by the sample size. This should be used in normally distributed data.

Median: It is the middle value in a sample sorted into ascending order. This should be used in non-normally distributed data.

Mode: It is the most frequent value in a sample.

Power: Power measures the test's ability to reject the null hypothesis when it is actually false i.e. to make a correct decision. Power is the probability of not committing a type II error.

Error: This is the natural variation occurring in a sample.

Type I error: Rejecting the null hypothesis when there is no difference (i.e finding a difference when one does not exist).

Type II error: Accepting the null hypothesis when a difference exists (i.e failing to spot a difference when one exists). This is usually because the sample size is too small.

Sensitivity: Proportion of true positives correctly identified.

Specificity: Proportion of true negatives correctly identified.

Positive predictive value: Proportion of patients with a positive test result who are correctly diagnosed.

Negative predictive value: Proportion of patients with a negative test result who are correctly diagnosed.

Absolute risk: The chance of a person developing a specific disease over a specified time period.

Absolute risk reduction: This is the difference between the event rates in the two groups, where the adverse event rate is less in the treatment group. This suggests the intervention is beneficial.

Relative risk: The probability of an event in the treatment group divided by the probability of the event in the control group. 1=equal risk.

Odds ratio: The odds of an event in the treatment group divided by the odds of an event in the control group.

Both the odds ratio and relative risk compare the likelihood of an event between two groups.

Correlation: Correlation tests are used to assess whether there is a relationship between two or more variables.

Regression: Regression attempts to describe the dependence of a variable on one (or more) other variable.

Number needed to treat: It is the average number of people who need to be treated with a specific intervention for a given period of time to prevent one additional adverse outcome or achieve one additional beneficial outcome. It is one measure of treatment effectiveness.

Bias: Bias is a form of systematic error that can effect scientific investigations and distort the measurement process (see below).

Incidence: Incidence of a disease is the number of new cases per population in a given time period.

Prevalence: Proportion of a population found to have a condition at a point in time.

Variance: A summary value indicating the amount of variation within the data.

Standard deviation (SD): It is the square root of variance. It is used to summarise how much variability there is in a sample or population. 68% of data lies within one standard deviation of the mean, and 95% within two standard deviations when data is normally distributed.

Confidence interval (CI): The purpose of a confidence interval is to indicate the precision of the sample study estimates as population values.

Difference between SD and CI: Standard deviation is a measure of central tendency for the sample study. Confidence intervals relate the sample characteristics to the population as a whole.

Jadad score (Oxford quality scoring system): This is a score that allows the assessment of quality of clinical trials. There are three questions which should be answered yes or no – scoring a point if the answer is yes. These are:

1) Was this a randomised study?

2) Was the study double blind?

3) Was there a description of dropouts and withdrawals?

Further points could be scored for an appropriate method of randomisation and appropriate blinding.

This gives a maximum score of five. However, points are deducted if either randomisation described and or blinding described were inappropriate.

Zero equates to poor quality and five a good quality trial.

Impact factor: This is used as a proxy for the "importance" of a journal and is based on the number of citations from that journal in the preceding two years. For example:

Number of times citable articles produced in 2001 and 2002 were cited in indexed journals in 2003 = A. Number of citable articles produced in 2001 and 2002 =B. Impact factor of the journal for 2003 = A/B.

Thus this may vary from year to year. It is also subject to manipulation as editors may wish to publish papers that are likely to be referenced, and indeed some editors may encourage authors to reference heavily from their own journal.

Impact factor and implications-

Journal	Impact Factor (2012)	Journal	Impact Factor (2012)
NEJM	53.3	Archives of Surg	4.24
JAMA	30	Surg Endoscopy	4.01
Lancet	38.28	Dis Colon Rectum	3.13
BMJ	14.1	Colorectal Dis	2.93
Annals of Surg	7.49	J Gastrointest Surg	3.16
BJS	4.6	EJVES	2.99
Annals Surg Oncol	4.17	J Am Coll Surgeons	4.55

Power calculations

Power calculations are performed to ensure that if a difference exists between tested samples it will be actually observed. This is related to sample size. A predetermined level of difference that is deemed significant (usually what would be regarded as clinically significant) is used to perform the calculation as to how many subjects are required in each group in order to determine if that level of difference actually exists.

Generally the larger the sample size the easier to detect small differences. Carrying out a power calculation allows the deemed significant difference to be obtained more efficiently. In order to carry out the calculation an anticipated response needs to be used. This can be estimated from previous studies or by running a pilot study.

Bias

Bias can fundamentally affect the results and subsequent interpretation of a study. In essence it is any error that might occur in the design, carrying out, and interpretation of a study.

Amongst these are:

Selection bias: an error in methodology that leads to study groups not being representative of the general population.

Attrition bias: drop out of subjects in each cohort can lead to a skew in outcomes.

Recall bias: this is related to information that has been collected often with patients in the "disease" group being better at recalling exposure than the control group. This may particularly affect retrospective studies.

Non-respondent bias: Often people that agree to participate in a study differ from those that refuse and have an underlying motivation.

Publication bias: Journals are more likely to publish papers that produce positive results- i.e results that demonstrate a significant difference than those with "negative" results. Thus the published literature may not actually represent what actually occurs.

Levels of evidence

The level of evidence, as graded below, represents the actual strength of the evidence rather than the clinical importance. An increased level of evidence suggests that the finding can be regarded with greater confidence.

Level	Description
Ia	Evidence from a meta-analysis of randomised controlled trials
Ib	Evidence from a randomised controlled trial
IIa	Evidence from a well designed controlled study without randomisation
IIb	Evidence from at least one well designed quasi-experimental study
III	Evidence from well-designed non-experimental descriptive studies such as comparative studies, correlation studies or case studies
IV	Evidence from expert committee reports or opinions or clinical experiences of respected authorities

Types of studies

Randomised Control Trials

These are used to test treatments or interventions and can provide the strongest evidence of impact of the actual intervention. Randomisation of the study subjects aims to eliminate many of the biases present in other types of observational study. They are limited by non-compliance of subjects, loss to follow-up, and can be time consuming and costly to set up. Care needs to be ensured that sufficient subjects are recruited to identify if a difference exists between the cohorts. This requires a power calculation and involves extrapolation from existing literature to determine what a clinically significant difference is.

Case Control Study

These are retrospective studies that review those who have a disease compared with a control group that do not, in order to determine causative factors that the cases have been exposed to. This type of study is reliant on subject recall and is thus subject to recall bias. Often they are short observational studies and have the benefit over cohort studies in that they are less expensive and can be carried out over a shorter time period.

Cohort

Cohort studies are prospective studies that follow a "cohort" that has been exposed to a causative factor to determine how many in each group get a disease. This can be expensive and time consuming but provides better data than retrospective case control studies as it aims to eliminate recall bias. They can be used to study disease aetiology and prognosis between groups with different exposures.

Meta analysis

This is the pooling of several different studies (RCTs) to achieve a greater statistical power.

The main disadvantage is that it does not overcome the limitations of the studies included in the analysis.

Systematic review

Systematic reviews are similar to meta-analyses in that they aim to provide stronger evidence to answer a clinical question by pooling results from several studies. A strict inclusion and exclusion protocol and explicit search strategy needs to be set up to determine which studies should be included. Ideally a meta-analysis may form part of the results.

Guidelines have been produced to support researchers who perform meta analysis and systematic reviews. These not only act as an aid but also provide a degree of standardisation as well as consistency. These include the CONSORT statement

(Consolidated Standards of Reporting Trials) which are required for RCTs. Further, RCTs should be registered whilst in their planning stage. The CONSORT statement is a 25 point list and flow chart which identifies how the trial was designed, analysed and interpreted, and the flow chart demonstrates the outcomes of all the patients enrolled in the study.

The PRISMA consists of 27 points and a flow diagram. It aims to help researchers improve the reporting of such studies and to aid transparency.

Other guidelines have been created for observational studies along similar principles including the MOOSE (Meta-analysis Of Observational Studies in Epidemiology) and STROBE (STrengthening the Reporting of OBservational studies in Epidemiology), which journals are increasingly encouraging authors to use.

Difference between clinical and statistical significance

Statistical significance indicates that a difference has been found between the groups being studied which the statistical tool being employed has demonstrated is unlikely to be due to chance. Clinical significance relates whether this difference will have any actual bearing in a real life (clinical) setting.

Graphical representation of data

Forest plots

A forest plot is used to illustrate the relative strength of each study included in a meta-analysis. It allows visualisation of how much weight each included study has in the analysis. Confidence intervals are included and if these cross the vertical line which delineates no-effect it suggests the sample size is too small or the result is not statistically significant.

Kaplan Meier Graphs

These are usually outcome plots that demonstrate survival over a time period. They are an excellent way of representing relative outcomes of different cohorts as disparity in survival can be easily visualised.

Regression analysis

Regression analysis is a statistical test used for determining the relationship of different factors. It allows determination of how the dependent variable will change if an independent variable is altered.

Common statistical tests:

Statistical tests are grossly divided into parametric and non-parametric tests for use on data that is normally distributed or not-normally distributed respectively.

In general parametric tests are more powerful, and involve using the actual data rather than a ranking of the data to obtain a statistical result. However, caution needs to be taken that the data being studied is indeed normally distributed.

Some common tests and their usage are included in the table below.

	Categorical data	Parametric	Non-Parametric
Single Sample	Chi-squared test Fishers exact test	One sample t-test	Wilcoxon Signed Rank
Two paired groups	McNemars	t-test	Wilcoxon matched pair
Two unpaired groups	Chi-squared test	t-test	Mann-Whitney
More than two paired groups	Chi-Squared	One-way ANOVA	Friedman's
More than two unpaired groups	Chi-Squared	One-way ANOVA	Kruskal Wallis

In order to get you started with practising your academic revision we have provided two free to access references with an example of an academic viva. We would also recommend keeping abreast of the current literature in your field and try to hold a regular "journal club" with your peers so that appraising a paper becomes second nature.

These papers can be accessed for free through PubMed by entering the PMID number as given.

Academic Viva questions:

Paper 1

Srinivasa S, Taylor MH, Singh PP, Yu TC, Soop M, Hill AG. Randomized clinical trial of goal-directed fluid therapy within an enhanced recovery protocol for elective colectomy. Br J Surg. 2013 Jan;100(1):66-74. doi: 10.1002/bjs.8940. (FREE ARTICLE) PMID: 23132508

Can you briefly summarise this paper?

This paper is from the BJS in 2012 from a group based in New Zealand.

They have carried out a randomised controlled trial evaluating two types of perioperative fluid management in patients undergoing colonic surgery: a goal directed regime versus standard enhanced recovery protocols, which involve fluid restriction. It involved 84 patients randomised equally between the groups with a primary outcome based on patient reported recovery, and a number of secondary outcomes including grip strength, peak flow, length of stay, complications and haematological and biochemical markers.

Patients and surgeons were blinded to the cohort allocation and patients had their surgical recovery score measured at four defined post-operative points. The results demonstrated that demographically the cohorts were similar, and the authors found that the goal directed regime conferred no benefit and that these patients actually received more fluid than the standard regime- although this did not affect the other parameters measured.

The conclusions appear to be appropriate, although the authors have not really demonstrated findings that would change clinical practice.

The references are largely recent and relevant and overall the paper is well constructed and well written.

You've mentioned this is in the BJS - is this a good journal?

This is one of the premier general surgical journals as guided by impact factor which is relatively high for a general surgical journal. Only really the Annals of Surgery is higher, and has a good reputation and is widely read, being the main general surgical journal of the UK and Europe.

What is its impact factor? What do you understand by the term impact factor?

The BJS usually has an impact factor usually somewhere between 4 and 5. The impact factor is a method of trying to objectively "rank" peer review journals and is based upon the number of citations received for its publications over the preceding two years. Essentially the impact factor for 2014 would be based on the number of citations of articles published in 2012 and 2013 divided by the number of published articles in those years.

What do you think of the methodology?

This has been clearly recorded and would allow easy replication. As a randomised trial they have, appropriately, obtained ethical approval and registered the trial. Exclusion criteria are clearly documented and how the intervention was implemented is clearly set out.

They have done their best to maintain the blinded nature of the study with only the anaesthetist and research assistant unblinded- with fluid administration being strictly protocol driven.

What is CONSORT?

CONSORT stands for Consolidated Standards of Reporting Trials, and is a 25 point list that RCTs need to follow for the reporting of a randomised trial. The CONSORT statement was originally created by an international group of researchers, statisticians and journal editors in order to improve the quality of reports of these studies.

And the statistics employed? What about their use of parametric and non-parametric investigations?

The authors have employed appropriate statistical tests. They have recorded data that is likely to be normally distributed (e.g heart rate/cardiac index) as mean and quoted the standard deviation, and have similarly recorded length of stay which is less likely to be normally distributed as median and range. The tests employed are the appropriate parametric and non parametric tests; t-test for parametric analysis, Mann-Whitney and Fisher's exact for non parametric analysis.

What do you think about their power calculation?

The authors performed a power calculation based on previous data - powered to detect a 20% difference on the surgical recovery score with an appropriate alpha of 0.05 and beta of 0.2. This led to a sample size of 80 patients. This was increased to 85 due to exclusions. Power calculations are a standard tool used to reduce errors without needing to over-recruit and allow for a reasonable magnitude of effect.

What do alpha and beta signify?

The alpha level signifies the risk of a type one error (false positive) and the beta level the risk of a type 2 error (false negative). It is common in most power calculations to allow for a beta level four times that of an alpha level.

You said that it is common to allow a beta level four times an alpha level in studies - is this always the case and why in medicine particularly might you want to change this?

Within medical studies it is sometimes more desirable to change these parameters, particularly when looking at diagnostic tests. It may be more acceptable to allow a false positive- with the caveat that further investigations and tests are required – rather than to employ a test that allows a false negative and hence inappropriate reassurance.

Any particular weaknesses or concerns that you have?

The use of colloids within the protocol, and the findings that those in the goal directed group received significantly more colloid during surgery than those in the restricted group. It may have been better to conduct the study so that the goal directed fluid could have used more crystalloid rather than colloid, with blood being permitted as stipulated.

IV fluids were stopped on return to the ward postoperatively unless assessment was made by a clinician to indicate that they needed to be continued. The authors have not indicated what proportion of patients in each group required further fluid to be continued. Although figure 3 demonstrates the volumes, this graph is not clear – it does not show if these are excess volumes of IV fluid required in a 24 hour period, and these numbers could involve different numbers of patients. The fluid restriction group does appear to have received more colloid than the postoperative group, but no figures are actually given and the authors have just stated that there were no other statistically significant differences between groups.

They have also chosen to document sodium levels, but neglected to mention chloride (which would help indicate possible hyperchloraemic acidosis - that may have an impact on renal blood flow) and also potassium and magnesium levels which would influence the return of normal gut function as well as have a possible effect on cardiac function.

Further, in the methodology they have recorded grip strength and peak flow, but neither of these have been included in their results.

Would this paper change your practice?

This study has not shown any improvement on outcomes from those commonly employed within enhanced recovery protocols and, as they have concluded, do not indicate the need for a change.

Paper 2

Brenner H, Stock C, Hoffmeister M. Effect of screening sigmoidoscopy and screening colonoscopy on colorectal cancer incidence and mortality: systematic review and meta-analysis of randomised controlled trials and observational studies *BMJ* 2014; 348 doi: http://dx.doi.org/10.1136/bmj.g2467 (FREE ARTICLE). PMID: 24922745

Have the authors asked a focused question?

The authors have sought to address the question of whether endoscopic screening for lower GI malignancy impacts on the incidence and mortality associated with this disease. This is an important question due to the high prevalence of colorectal cancer, and the fact that if found early it is treatable with a better outcome. However, as with any screening tool, benefits must be balanced against potential costs and risk. To this end the authors have asked a focused question - looking specifically at the impact of lower GI endoscopy, rather than asking simply what factors reduce colorectal cancer incidence and mortality.

Were the inclusion criteria for this study appropriate and could important studies have been missed out?

The authors included all randomised controlled trials and observational studies up to a set deadline. They searched the major databases using appropriate key words to obtain a large pool of articles, which could then be reviewed for appropriateness. Eligibility was rightly assessed by two people, with a third to resolve any disagreements. They have, however, excluded non-English language articles, which may exclude important studies, and they have also excluded abstracts. The latter would seem reasonable given the limited information contained in published abstracts.

What are PRISMA and MOOSE?

PRISMA - is the Preferred Reporting Items for Systematic Reviews and Meta-Analyses. It is a checklist of 27 items used for reporting systematic reviews and meta-analyses. The aim of the statement is to improve reporting of these studies. There is a four phase flow diagram which takes researchers through; Identification of appropriate studies (both in databases and other sources), Screening of the studies found (and exclusion), Eligibility assessment of remaining studies (by review of full manuscripts) and finalisation of studies to be included.

MOOSE-stands for Meta-analysis Of Observational Studies in Epidemiology and comprises a checklist for reporting meta-analyses of observational studies in epidemiology. It is now expected by most journal editors when submitting such studies.

Have the authors appropriately assessed the validity of the included studies?

Two authors extracted information from the studies that were deemed eligible with information being extracted independently. It appears that each study has been carefully evaluated - although they have included a mixture of randomised controlled trials, as well as observational studies. They have excluded a number of studies based on small size, and intent of the study. However, they did not set any criteria regarding participation rates.

They have included a table which reviews important components for each of the RCTs reviewed, but it would also have been useful to state numbers picked up on initial screening and also how complete follow up was with each study.

Both RCTs and observational studies had relative risk extracted according to the site of the colorectal cancer. RCTs only had results included on an intention to screen and per protocol.

Was there homogeneity of the included studies?

The authors particularly comment that the designs of the observational studies are heterogenous, as is the reporting of results in both the observational trials and the controlled trials. This could impact on any results drawn from them, and suggests using caution in interpreting the results.

What is the importance of this?

The implication of a lack of homogeneity is that caution must be employed when interpreting the results. It is reasonable to expect that the actual incidence of colorectal cancer should be the same in the screened and non-screened population, and not unsurprising that flexible sigmoidoscopy should decrease mortality from distal cancers. Results were even stronger in the "per protocol" i.e. patients that adhered to the protocol subgroup analysis when compared with the intention to treat groups. However, it should be noted that the greater the heterogeneity of study design the less reliable the subsequent meta-analysis. Care needs to be taken with pooling data in this way to ensure the results are valid.

The authors state they have used a "random effects model" to calculate confidence intervals and pooled effects. What do you understand by the term "random effects model"?

Meta-analyses attempt to estimate the combined effect of the studies included. Because studies are likely to differ in precision it is desirable to assign a different weighting to each study included within the analysis. There are two models used in meta-analyses - the "fixed effect" model and the "random effects" model. These differ in the assumptions they make about the included studies and thus will lead to different weightings.

Under the fixed effect model it is assumed that there is one true effect size common to all the studies. The random effects model allows for a variation of effect from study to study (which might be influenced by age of subjects, where they live etc)

Within a fixed effect model the weighting of the studies included will be related to their size. To contrast this, in a random effects model it is assumed that the impact of the intervention being investigated may differ from population to population and this model allows this difference to be taken into account, so that weighting of studies is not related completely to size. Hence large studies are less likely to dominate. (Incidentally this leads to a widening of the confidence intervals).

Is this an appropriate model?

The drawback with this model is that the more heterogeneous the studies, the less impact size of the study has, to a point where an analysis with very high heterogeneity will place equal weighting on each study irrespective of the size. It could be argued that this is not an appropriate model for this analysis and may skew the results.

What are the limitations of this study?

The authors have clearly stated this study has several limitations, including the possibility of missing out some studies, and that there may be underreporting due to publication bias. Further, they have commented on the heterogeneity of the studies included and mentioned that many of the studies involved screening programmes with endoscopy that was carried out many years ago. Better technology may lead to better pick up rates, and thus the included studies may underestimate the benefit.

Do you think screening lower GI endoscopy is appropriate based on this study?

There is no comment regarding side effects or cost, but based purely on the data presented it could be said that the intervention reduces mortality from colonic malignancy.

CRITICAL CARE SURGERY

**Jonathon Francis Alun Jones Bhaskar Kumar
Ben Messer Ali Robb Daniel Weiand**

Contents

Abdominal Compartment Syndrome

You perform a complex laparotomy on a 35 year old female patient with small bowel obstruction several years following a subtotal colectomy for Crohn's disease. It is a very difficult operation due to dense adhesions, and the patient had grossly dilated small bowel for days. Abdominal entry is complicated by multiple enterotomies. After several hours of operating you decide to close the abdomen despite very distended bowel loops and tension in the abdominal wall. Postoperatively the critical care staff inform you that ventilation has been an issue and they are having to use particularly high ventilatory pressures, and the patient has been oliguric for four hours. They suggest she now has abdominal compartment syndrome (ACS).

What factors in this case have contributed to the development of ACS?

Failure to recognise patients at risk of developing ACS is one of the main factors for developing it. Closing the abdomen under tension after a long complex laparotomy is likely to provoke Intra-abdominal Hypertension (IAH) and subsequent ACS. The patient has had a complex long abdominal operation on swollen, distended and obstructed loops of bowel. Other disturbance to multiple physiological parameters (hypothermia/acidosis/coagulopathy) may also contribute. In addition the patient may have received large volumes of fluid perioperatively. Fluid volume administered is a strong predictor of the development of ACS.

Other conditions where early fascial closure may place the patient at risk of IAH/ ACS include peritonitis, intra-abdomonial trauma, and acute mesenteric ischaemia. Such patients are best managed with a damage control approach which involves abbreviated operating times and use of a laparostomy.

What is normal intra-abdominal pressure (IAP)? What is the definition of intra-abdominal hypertension?

IAP is approximately 5-7 mmHg in critically ill adult patients. Intra-abdominal hypertension (IAH) is defined by a sustained elevation in IAP > 12mmHg.

How is IAH graded?

- Grade I (12-15mmHg)
- Grade II (16-20mmHg)
- Grade III (21-25mmHg)
- Grade IV (>25mmHg)

How is IAH different to abdominal compartment syndrome (ACS)?

IAH is an intra-abdominal pressure >12mmHg but does not result in organ dysfunction. ACS is defined as a sustained IAP > 25mmHg that is associated with new organ dysfunction/failure.

What are the risk factors for IAH and ACS?

Increased intra-luminal contents

- Ileus / Gastric distention
- Colonic pseudo-obstruction
- Volvulus

Increased intra-abdominal contents

- Acute pancreatitis
- Haemoperitoneum / pneumoperitoneum
- Intra-peritoneal fluid collections e.g. gross ascites

Capillary leak / fluid resuscitation

- Overzealous fluid resuscitation
- Acidosis
- Massive blood transfusion
- Damage control laparotomy*

Miscellaneous

- Reduction/repair of massive incisional/abdominal wall herniae
- Peritonitis
- Obesity

What are the effects of abdominal compartment syndrome?

As IAP rises venous return is impaired and subsequently cardiac output is reduced progressive effects are seen on multiple organ systems, particularly renal, mesenteric and pulmonary circulations. Oliguria and raised ventilatory pressures are the commonest clinical features. Others include mesenteric ischaemia, raised intra-cranial pressure, diaphragmatic splinting. The increased IAP reduces the FRC (Functional Residual Capacity) and can result in hypoxaemia and an increasing oxygen requirement.

It must be remembered that leaving the abdomen open can still lead to ACS particularly when the abdomen is packed for bleeding and this continues.

How can intra-abdominal pressure be measured?

IAP is measured at end-expiration in the supine position. The transducer is zeroed at the level of the mid-axillary line and the standard for IAP measurements is via the bladder (transvesical method) with a maximal instillation volume of 25mls of sterile saline. There are usually dedicated kits available for this purpose. There are other means of measuring IAP, including transgastric pressure measurements, but transvesical measurements have gained the widest clinical application.

What treatment strategies to manage ACS do you know of?

In all cases aiming to prevent ACS should always be the aim, but measures to reduce IAH include:

Improve abdominal wall compliance

- Neuromuscular blockade
- Positioning: Keep head of bed at 30 degrees
- Optimisation of sedation and analgesia

Evacuate intra-luminal contents

- Nasogastric / colonic decompression
- Prokinetic agents

Evacuate abdominal fluid collections

- Percutaneous drainage of collections
- Paracentesis

Correct positive fluid balance

- Avoid excessive iv fluids

Organ support

- Optimise ventilation
- Haemodialysis

Decompressive laparotomy

Only for extremes of refractory ACS

You take the patient back to theatre to perform a decompressive laparotomy. Tell me your chosen method for performing a temporary abdominal closure.

My preference would be to use a negative pressure system such as vacuum-assisted closure (VAC®). The negative pressure allows removal of exudate thereby helping to prevent further ACS – patients are still at risk of ACS even after decompression. The system also allows easy access to the abdomen again should it be required.

For the next 3 weeks the patient remains on ICU and makes slow but steady progress. The abdomen has remained on a VAC® system for the duration of time. A decision is made to attempt abdominal closure. What are your potential options?

Loss of domain is one of the major factors which prevent tension free closure of the abdomen. A staged approach may be required and may also need involvement of teams that deal with this problem e.g. plastic surgeons.

Reference

Kirkpatrick AW, Roberts DJ, De Waele J, Jaeschke R et al. Intra-abdominal hypertension and the abdominal compartment syndrome: updated consensus definitions and clinical practice guidelines from the World Society of the Abdominal Compartment Syndrome. Intensive Care Medicine 2013 ;39(7):1190-206.

Acute Lung Injury / ARDS

A 53 year old man is admitted to ICU with acute gallstone pancreatitis. He is in respiratory distress with severe hypoxaemia (pO_2 6.5kPa) and hypotension (85/60mmHg). For the past day he has had abdominal bloating and vomiting. You obtain a chest x-ray.

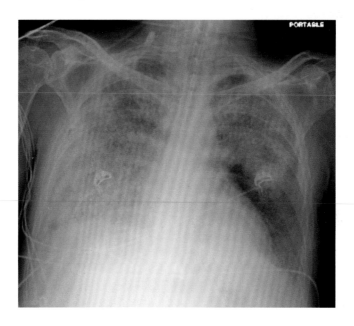

What are the findings on this portable chest x-ray?

There are diffuse bilateral infiltrates in both lung fields.

What is your differential diagnosis here?

Given the history of acute pancreatitis and the chest x-ray findings, one of the main differential diagnoses is that of Acute Lung Injury/Acute Respiratory Distress Syndrome (ARDS). Other possibilities include aspiration, particularly as the patient has been vomiting, though this tends to be a unilateral process. Other possibilities include pulmonary oedema or pulmonary embolus. Pneumonia tends to produce lobar infiltrates rather than a diffuse bilateral pattern.

What do you understand by the term acute lung injury (ALI)?

The term "Acute Lung Injury" is an umbrella term encompassing hypoxaemic respiratory failure, a severe version of which is "Acute Respiratory Distress Syndrome" (ARDS). ARDS is defined as:

- Bilateral pulmonary infiltrates on chest x-ray
- No clinical evidence of left atrial hypertension (previously a pulmonary wedge pressure <18mmHg was used)
- PaO_2/FiO_2 <300mmHg = ALI
- PaO_2/FiO_2 <200mmHg (26.6 kPa) = ARDS

What are the causes of ALI?

ALI is most commonly caused by pneumonia. Other causes include:

Direct Causes:-

- Aspiration
- Inhalation injury e.g. smoke / fumes
- Intrathoracic sepsis eg. Leak from oesophagectomy

Indirect Causes:

- Sepsis
- Acute pancreatitis
- Fat embolism
- Amniotic fluid embolism
- Major multisystem trauma
- Massive transfusion including use of FFP
- Burns

What do you understand by the term lung compliance and how is it affected in ALI?

Lung compliance is defined as the change in lung volume for a unit rise in pressure. Reduced lung compliance is seen in ALI leading to difficulty with ventilation, which leads to hypercarbia and also exposes the patient to the risks of trauma to the lung from overventilation (barotraumas/volutrauma).

How would you ventilate this patient?

The main proven ventilation strategy of ALI treatment is to keep the PaO_2 >60mmHg, without causing injury to the lungs with excessive O_2 or volutrauma i.e. low tidal volumes. In general tidal volumes should not exceed 6ml/kg. No intervention other than reducing tidal volumes has consistently been shown to improve outcome. Limiting tidal volumes will obviously result in hypercapnia, but as long as this does not cause significant myocardial depression due to acidosis then it is usually tolerated down to a pH of 7.20 (permissive hypercapnia).

What is ventilator induced lung injury?

Ventilator induced lung injury can result from higher distending pressures (barotraumas) or from higher distending volumes (volutrauma). If normal lungs are exposed to tidal volumes of >10-15ml/kg there is parenchymal inflammation, increased vascular permeability, accumulation of fluid in the lung and alveolar space and atelectasis – similar to that seen in ALI. Another source of lung injury is oxygen. High FiO_2 can cause lung injury through the formation of oxygen-free radicals which are cytotoxic. FiO_2 of greater than 50% may have a deleterious effect on the lung parenchyma. Alveolar overdistention may also result in macroscopic injuries such as pneumothorax, pneumomediastinum and pneumoperitoneum.

What are the major pathological changes of ALI?

There are two major pathological stages in ALI:-

- The acute phase is characterized by leakage of protein rich fluid into the interstitium through disruption of the alveolar-capillary interface. Damage occurs mainly to Type I pneumocytes, with Type II pneumocytes being more resistant to damage. Therefore fluid filled airspaces develop, there is loss of surfactant through damaged pneumocytes and microvascular thrombosis.

- A later reparative phase called the 'fibrotic phase' of ARDS is characterized by disorganized repair, fibroproliferation, and organization of lung tissue. However this phase does not always occur.

It should be understood that the pathological changes of ALI are diffuse and heterogenous such that not all lung units are affected equally. Therefore normal and diseased tissue may co-exist.

What are the physiological changes in the lung from ALI?

- Reduction of resting lung volumes (especially FRC which favours collapse of the airways during expiration and consequent hypoxaemia)

- Decreased compliance

- Increased ventilation-perfusion mismatch

- Shunt (due to atelectatic areas of lung still being perfused)

- Increased work of breathing

- Lymphatic drainage is compromised – contributing to the build up of extravascular fluid

Despite a low tidal volume based ventilation strategy the patient continues to have severe hypoxaemia. What alternative strategies are available?

The patient has refractory hypoxia and may benefit from adjunctive therapies. However, the role of adjunct therapies is limited as none have proven to be consistently effective - prone positioning, steroids and inhaled nitric oxide being the most commonly tried. Prone positioning may improve ventilation-perfusion matching but the exact mechanism is not known. Inhaled nitric oxide may act as a local vasodilator, around well-ventilated alveoli, thereby improving ventilation-perfusion matching. Due to the high cost of administering this agent, nebulized prostacyclin has been used as an alternative. Other strategies include steroids, high frequency oscillation and extracorporeal membrane oxygenation (ECMO). The first two have been shown to be ineffective in recent trials, but ECMO may have a role in refractory ARDS although it is limited to specialist centres currently.

There is limited data to support the use of steroids in chronic ARDS with high O_2 requirements days to weeks into the disease but not in the acute phase.

Why is it important to understand the pathology of ALI?

Through an understanding of this process it can be appreciated that some patients may fully recover but others have permanent sequelae. There is good follow up data to suggest reduced physiological reserve and health related QOL (Quality of Life) at 5 years following ALI/ARDS. Recent studies report that the in-hospital mortality rate is in the range of 40%.

Acute Renal Failure

Scenario 1

An 84 year old female undergoes a Hartmann's procedure for a sigmoid colon stercoral perforation with gross faecal peritonitis. On return to intensive care, the patient is intubated and ventilated, and on high doses of noradrenaline. Her urinary output is just 10ml in the first hour. She is given a litre of Hartmann's solution with a transient rise in CVP which is not sustained.

What is the pathophysiology leading to her oliguria?

Oliguria has been precipitated by profound sepsis from faecal soiling. This has led to marked vasodilatation, which leads to relative hypovolaemia and hypotension with reduced renal perfusion. Oliguria is also a consequence of the stress response to critical illness and surgery. Patients may be oliguric despite often having normal mean arterial pressures. The stress response leads to increases in anti diuretic hormone (ADH) and steroids which favour fluid retention as well as catecholamines which can vasoconstrict the renal vasculature.

What do you understand by the term auto-regulation and why is it important in the kidney?

Auto-regulation refers to the ability of an organ to regulate its own perfusion through a number of local mechanisms. It is a phenomenon seen in the brain as well as kidneys and allows a degree of self-regulation of perfusion.

Renal auto-regulation allows the production of urine in as efficient a manner as possible despite marked fluctuations in perfusion pressure, thereby allowing the body to excrete any waste materials. The kidneys work most effectively when there is a continuous flow of blood which allows the production of an ultra-filtrate.

Which part of the kidney is most vulnerable to ischaemia?

Renal tubular cells are oxygenated by blood in the vasa-recta - which supplies blood with a high haematocrit. The tubular cells in the renal medulla have a very high oxygen consumption and are relatively poorly perfused, thereby rendering them vulnerable to ischaemic damage. If medullary blood flow falls below 20% of normal, then ischaemic damage and necrosis will ensue. Thus below a certain mean arterial pressure, the kidney switches off a considerable amount of its filtration activities, and the patient becomes oliguric.

How is acute renal failure defined?

ARF is an acute-onset, often reversible, sustained loss of renal function resulting in a failure of the kidney to perform its normal functions / maintain homeostasis, including accumulation of urea and creatinine, acid-base imbalance and failure to regulate fluid and electrolyte balance.

There are two recent consensus group definitions that have attempted to create a more universal definition:

Acute kidney injury network (AKIN) definition:

- Rapid onset (less than 48 hours)

- Reduction in kidney function measured by either a rise in creatinine of > 50% of baseline or fall in urine output to < 0.5ml/kg for > 6 hours.

- Acute dialysis quality initiative (ADQI) definition: Uses the RIFLE acronym and describes using either the GFR or urine output (UO):

- **R** - risk - fall in GFR of up to 25% of normal; UO < 0.5ml/kg/hr for 6hrs

- **I** - injury - fall in GFR of up to 50% of normal; UO < 0.5ml/kg/hr for 12hrs

- **F** - failure - fall in GFR of up to 75% of normal; UO < 0.3ml/kg/hr for 24hrs

- **L** - loss of function for up to four weeks (requiring dialysis)

- **E** - end stage renal failure; complete loss of renal function for 3 months   (requiring dialysis)

How can we estimate a patient's expected GFR?

By using the universal Modification of Diet in Renal Disease (MDRD) formula, which estimates GFR based on age, race and sex.

What are the causes of acute renal failure?

- **Pre-renal** The most common type. Once post-renal / obstructive causes have been excluded, consider pre-renal causes, which commonly include sepsis or SIRS, often on the background of a kidney with pre-existing renovascular disease.

- **Post-renal** - usually easily identifiable by the bedside, e.g bladder outflow obstruction (blocked catheter, BPH, in combination with post-op urinary retention - common - is there a palpable bladder?); renal outflow obstruction (iatrogenic ureteral damage intra-op, renal stones).

- **Intra-renal** Once post-renal and pre-renal causes have been excluded, consider causes within the renal parenchyma. They can be further subclassified into causes affecting the renal tubule (glomerulonephritis), the vessels (vasculitis) and interstitium (interstitial nephritis). Specific causes include drugs / toxins and iodinated contrast media for CT and MRI scans.

- Both pre- and post- renal causes will eventually cause intra-renal failure if left untreated, and it can be regarded as a spectrum of initially reversible impairment, leading to irreversible failure without intervention.

What is acute tubular necrosis (ATN)?

Acute tubular necrosis (ATN) occurs when there is damage to the tubular cells from injury. The injurious insult may occur when the oxygen supply to the kidney is inadequate to meet its requirements or from nephrotoxic injury. Dead tubular cells may be represented as casts that may accumulate in the tubular space and obstruct urine flow, creating back-pressure which further reduces renal perfusion.

Scenario 2

A 75 year old man underwent repair of a ruptured supra-renal abdominal aortic aneurysm 6 hours ago and is intubated and ventilated on ICU. The operation was complex and over ten hours in duration. He has been transfused a total of 15 units of packed red cells. He has been oliguric since returning from theatre and increasingly difficult to ventilate. During the course of his admission he has become gradually oliguric and eventually becomes anuric despite fluid challenges.

What may be the cause of anuria and how is it managed?

As fluid challenges have been unsuccessful one needs to think about likely other causes. Post renal causes need to be urgently ruled out with imaging on the basis that they are often amenable to treatment.

The intraabdominal pressure was subsequently measured and recorded at 40mmHg. What is the diagnosis and what would you do?

This is consistent with abdominal compartment syndrome. I would take the patient back to theatre and fashion a laparostomy which should lead to recovery of urine output.

Scenario 3

A 92 year old female (50kg) undergoes an emergency aorto-bifemoral graft. It is a long complex operation and the patient transfers to ICU post-operatively. Her BP is 85/50mmHg and she is given a 1litre fluid challenge and the urine output increases transiently to 10ml/hr.

What further information do you need to correct her urine output?

Although pre-renal failure from hypovolaemia is by far the commonest cause of oliguria in the surgical patient, a careful approach is needed in an elderly patient as giving irrational fluid challenges will overload her.

It would be very useful to know:

1) What is her normal preoperative BP?

2) Was she on any antihypertensive medication?

3) What was her BP during the complex vascular operation?

In this case review of the notes revealed that her normal blood pressure at the preoperative screening clinic was 165/95mmHg (MAP = 115mmHg). Intra-operatively her pressure was on average 80/60mmHg (MAP 66mmHg) (she was given multiple boluses of phenylephrine), and her systolic pressure never rose above 90mmHg. Her MAP has been between 65 and 70mmHg. This patient developed acute renal failure and required dialysis.

What was the cause of her ARF?

The cause of the ARF here was renal hypoperfusion due to intraoperative hypotension relative to her normal blood pressure.

At what point would you consider renal replacement therapy?

Renal replacement therapy may be indicated in the acute or chronic settings.

Indications in the acute setting are:

- Fluid overload

- Biochemical abnormalities including K > 6.5, pH < 7.1, hypo- or hyper- natraemia, Ur > 40mmol/l or uraemia with uraemic pericarditis, encephalopathy.

- Drug overdose or toxin poisoning

In the setting of chronic renal failure, patients will require renal replacement therapy when their GFR reaches 15ml/min.

Atrial Fibrillation

A 66 year old man is on day five following an elective reversal of a Hartmann's procedure. He has been progressing well but has developed Atrial Fibrillation (AF) at 120bpm – confirmed on 12 lead ECG and a BP of 110/70mmHg. He has no chest pain and looks well. He has no symptoms of fever or abdominal pain and is opening his bowels to flatus. Preoperatively he was in sinus rhythm and has no significant past medical history.

How will you manage his AF?

As the patient is haemodynamically stable he is best managed by pharmacological treatment aiming to cardiovert him back to sinus rhythm. This can be achieved by class II (beta-blockers) or class III (amiodarone) anti-arrhythmic agents. In all cases the patient's electrolytes including K and Mg should be checked and corrected as necessary.

AF is a common postoperative arrhythmia but can represent a major source of morbidity and mortality in surgical patients. The aim of treating AF should be to:-

 1) Achieve control of the ventricular rate

 2) Prevent thromboembolic events

 3) Maintain sinus rhythm

When are patients particularly at risk of developing thromboembolic events?

When AF persists for more than 48 hours it is associated with an increased risk of thromboembolism e.g. stroke, or Transient Ischemic Attack (TIA). Therefore anticoagulation should be considered in these patients, but can be a difficult decision to make in a surgical patient due to the risk of bleeding.

How do you assess a patient's risk of developing thromboembolism?

I would liaise with the on call medical/cardiology team to discuss the case, but as a guide the CHADS2 scoring system can be used to assess this risk and help direct anticoagulation therapy.

Patients with total scores of 2 or higher should be considered for anticoagulation:

Risk Factor	Points
Congestive heart failure	1
Hypertension	1
Age > 75 years	1
Diabetes mellitus	1
Prior stroke or TIA	2

In high risk groups (i.e. score >2) long term anticoagulation has been shown to reduce stroke risk by 67%.

Remember anticoagulation is not required if the patient is in AF for less than 48 hours.

What pharmacological agents do you know of to convert AF to sinus rhythm?

There is no single pharmacological agent that has been deemed the drug of choice for converting AF to sinus rhythm.

Beta blockers (e.g.metoprolol) are effective and many consider it to be first line treatment in surgical patients. They can be given orally or intravenously with caution. They are particularly useful for patients who are on preoperative beta blockers that were withdrawn temporarily following surgery.

Amiodarone is usually commenced intravenously but generally can only be administered through a central venous line. In many centers it is only permissible to use this in an ICU/HDU setting and not on a general ward. It acts through reduction of AV nodal conductivity. This can lead to profound bradycardia and is best delivered with cardiac monitoring.

Digoxin even when given intravenously has a slow onset of action and is less effective in the hyperadrenergic post op state of surgical patients. It can be given orally or intravenously peripherally but has more of a role in chronic rate control.

In all these cases management is best done by close liaison and involvement of the critical care team as well as the surgical team. For patients with complex cardiac history advice should be sought from the on call cardiologist.

Scenario 2

A 71 year old man has undergone an emergency open cholecystectomy for a perforated gallbladder. He has a history of ischaemic heart disease. On day 2 post operatively he develops fast AF at a rate of 140 bpm with chest pain and clamminess. His systolic blood pressure is 60/40mmHg and not responding to a fluid challenge. He is semi-conscious and extremely clammy and sweaty.

How would you manage him?

This is a peri-arrest situation and requires urgent intervention. I would call for help immediately by putting out a cardiac arrest call. As he is haemodynamically unstable I anticipate he may require direct current cardioversion as the first line treatment with adjunctive pharmacotherapy. Adverse signs that pertain to impaired cardiac output include: chest pain, SBP<90mmHg, altered conscious level including confusion and pulmonary oedema.

As well as adherence to ALS based cardiac resuscitation a bolus dose of amiodarone can be given. Should he recover, review by the cardiology team is crucial, as he may well have sustained a peri-operative myocardial infarction. A transthoracic ECHO may be performed at the bedside, looking for motion abnormalities in keeping with an MI.

Brain Stem Death and Organ Donation

A 45 year old man has collapsed at home at the kitchen table. Ten minutes later the paramedic crew arrive and find the patient unconscious. The patient is intubated and ventilated on scene. Upon arrival at the resus room he has fixed dilated pupils. A head CT confirms a subarachnoid haemorrhage.

Which patients are identified as potential organ donors?

Organ donation should be considered as a usual part of 'end-of-life care' planning. Potential donors should be identified as early as possible using the following criteria:

- Patients who have had a catastrophic brain injury and absence of one or more cranial nerve reflexes, and a Glasgow Coma Scale (GCS) score of 4 or less that is not explained by sedation

- The intention to withdraw life-sustaining treatment in patients with a life-threatening or life-limiting condition that will, or is expected to, result in circulatory death

What is the meaning of "brain stem death"?

Brain stem death is the irreversible cessation of brain stem function (midbrain, pons, medulla) and therefore death of the person as a whole. It leads to an irreversible loss of capacity for consciousness and irreversible loss of capacity to breathe.

Brain stem death differs from a persistent vegetative state in that in the latter, although patients have irreversible unconsciousness, they have the capacity to breathe spontaneously.

The criteria in the UK used to establish brain stem death have been produced by a collaboration of UK medical colleges - the Academy of Medical Royal Colleges (2008): A code of practice for the diagnosis and confirmation of death.

What are the legal requirements for a clinician to be able to certify death prior to organ donation with in the UK?

The diagnosis of death by brain-stem testing should be made by at least two medical practitioners who have been registered for greater than five years and are competent in the conduct and interpretation of brain-stem testing. At least one of the doctors must be a consultant. Those carrying out the tests must not have, or be perceived to have, any clinical conflict of interest and neither doctor should be a member of the transplant team. Neither doctor must be potentially involved in the care of patients who might be in receipt of organs donated by the patient. Testing should be undertaken by the nominated doctors acting together and must always be performed on two occasions.

In children over the age of two months, the criteria used to establish death should be the same as those in adults. Between thirty-seven weeks of gestation and two months of age, it is rarely possible confidently to diagnose death as a result of cessation of brain-stem reflexes.

At what stage should the patient's family be approached to discuss organ donation?

Organ donation should be considered as part of 'end of life care planning'. If the patient meets specific referral criteria (see above) then the specialist nurse for organ donation may be contacted.

The family should only be approached after checking the NHS organ donor register and any advance statements of lasting power of attorney for health, as well as clarifying any safeguarding issues.

Where should this patient be managed for brain stem death testing?

The patient should be transferred under the care of the intensive care team and transferred to a critical care bed.

Describe the tests needed to establish a diagnosis of brain stem death.

The tests are of nerve reflexes that originate within the brain stem. Therefore:

- pupils fixed and dilated (no response to light)

- no corneal reflex: care should be taken to avoid damage to the cornea

- no gag reflex or cough reflex in response to bronchial stimulation by a suction catheter placed down the trachea to the carina, or gag response to stimulation of the posterior pharynx with a spatula

- no motor response to painful stimulation of cranial nerves (eg supraorbital pressure): within the cranial nerve distribution can be elicited by adequate stimulation of any somatic area or by supraorbital pressure

- no vestibular-ocular reflex: no eye movements are seen during or following the slow injection of at least 50mls of ice cold water over one minute into each external auditory meatus in turn. Clear access to the tympanic membrane must be established by direct inspection and the head should be at 30^0 to the horizontal plane, unless this positioning is contraindicated by the presence of an unstable spinal injury

- Apnoea test: no respiratory effort when pre-oxygenated and $PaCO_2 > 6.5$kPa. The apnoea test should only be considered once brain-stem areflexia has been confirmed. The apnoea test involves inducing a state of moderate hypercarbia and mild acidaemia [$PaCO_2$ is at least 6.0kPa and pH < 7.40 (in patients with COPD $PaCO_2$ of 6.5kPa and pH<

7.40)] by lowering the minute volume ventilation. The patient should then be disconnected from the ventilator and attached to an oxygen flow of 5L/min via an endotracheal catheter and observed for five minutes. If, after five minutes, there has been no spontaneous respiratory response, a presumption of no respiratory centre activity can be documented.

These tests should be clearly explained to the patient's relatives prior to being carried out.

What are the preconditions that need to be satisfied before these tests are undertaken?

A definitive diagnosis of the cause of brain stem death (may be evident from history, examination or from imaging).

Exclusion of "reversible" causes of coma including:

- hypothermia (core temperature must be >34°C)
- sedatives or depressant medications (eg alcohol, opiates, benzodiazepines, especially with concurrent renal or liver failure)
- neuromuscular blocking agents
- severe biochemical or electrolyte abnormalities (sodium, potassium, magnesium, phosphate excess of deficiency)
- endocrine abnormalities (hypoglycaemia)
- acid-base abnormalities

Assuming all the criteria are met, what is the legal time of death?

Following completion of the second set of tests, the legal time of death is the time at which the first set of tests was completed.

The patient is a potential organ donor, how would you proceed?

If the patient is a potential organ donor; they must remain connected to the ventilator with biological support. The transplant co-ordinator should be contacted. They will be able to establish whether the patient was on the Organ Donor Register and whether the organs are suitable for transplantation. The patient's relatives should then be approached and the process discussed with them. Currently, the assent of the relatives determines whether the patient is able to proceed to organ donation although assent is strictly not legally required. These discussions should be a normal part of the dying process.

How is death confirmed following cessation of cardio-respiratory function?

A suitably qualified medical practitioner must establish irreversible loss of cardiopulmonary function for at least five minutes (absence of central pulse or heart sounds or asystolic ECG tracing), with absence of neurological (pupillary) activity.

Reference

Organ donation for transplantation: improving donor identification and consent rates for deceased organ donation
www.nice.org.uk/guidance/CG 135

Burns

A 10-year-old girl was admitted for severe second and third-degree burns following her rescue from a burning house. It is believed that she was trapped in her bedroom and exposed to smoke inhalation. On arrival she was unconscious. She had second-degree burns over 5% of her body and third-degree burns over 15% of her body.

What are the principles of resuscitation of burns?

First aid at the scene includes extinguishing the flame, the removal of chemicals or switching off a power source etc. Cooling of the burn is then important as it reduces direct thermal injury, reduces release of inflammatory mediators and provides pain relief. 15°C water is ideal, but the ambient temperature should be kept warm so the patient does not become hypothermic.

In A & E the patient should be approached as any other multiply-injured patient (ABC). 100% oxygen should be administered and the airway checked – talk to the patient. A Yankauer sucker may be needed to remove debris from the mouth and a chin lift or jaw thrust manoeuvre needed. The airway may need to be protected with a Guedel airway, nasopharyngeal airway or endotracheal tube.

Breathing assessment should look carefully for signs of inhalational injury, which may necessitate invasive ventilatory support, such as soot in the airway, or carboxyhaemoglobin levels (though these can be falsely reassuring and a normal level does not exclude, neither does a high level confirm). A severely burned victim may require chest escharotomy. Circulatory collapse should be treated initially as for any other injury. The victim's whole body should be examined for burns. The patient may need a secondary survey/trauma series CT if mechanism supports the possibility of other injuries.

Other adjuncts that need to be considered include:

- NG tube for burns > 20% - gastric ileus is common
- Tetanus status
- Fluorescein eyes if facial burns are present
- Avoid hypothermia

How can the percentage total body surface area (%TBSA) be estimated?

Various charts are available in A & E to assess the TBSA involved in a burn. Only the burned skin should be included. Simple erythema should not be included. Lund and Browder charts are commonly used, and there are separate charts for children and adults, to account for the proportionally different sizes of body components. The Wallace "rule of nines" may also be useful. 9% TBSA is represented by each arm, front of back of each leg, and head, 18% by the front of the trunk, and back of the trunk, and 1% for the genitalia.

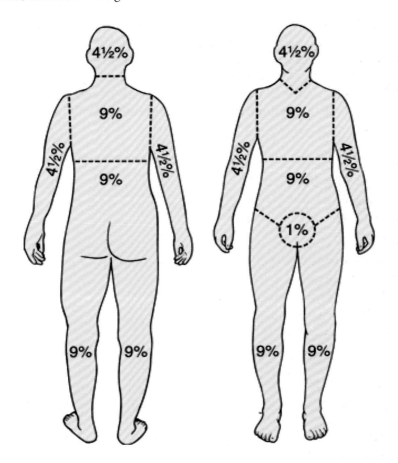

How do you calculate the fluid resuscitation needed for a 90kg man with a 40% TBSA burn?

Parkland's formula is used:

3-4ml x mass in kg x %TBSA burned

(4ml is used if there is inhalation injury, it is a child, delay in transfer, prior dehydration, loss of circulating volume from other injury etc)

Therefore:

3ml x 90kg x 40% = 10,800mls of fluid

Half of the fluid (5,400ml) is given in the first 8 hours (backdated to the time of the burn) and the remaining half over the subsequent 16 hours. Hartmann's solution is used in adults).

It is important to note that this may under- or overestimate the adequacy of resuscitation. Regular reassessment is required, looking at urine output (>0.5ml/kg/hour), warmth of peripheries/capillary, refill lactate and haemoglobin levels (high levels suggest haemoconcentration and under-resuscitation).

Scenario 2

A 34 year old 70kg man is admitted to A&E resus with 2nd and 3rd degree burns of both arms and entire anterior trunk. What are his initial IV fluid requirements?

The size of the burn is 9 + 9 + 18 = 36%

Using Parkland's formula: 3-4ml x mass in kg x %TBSA burned

Thus 4 x 70 x 36 = 10,080 ml

Half of the fluid in the first 8 hours = 5,040ml

Thus the rate required = 5040/8 = 630 ml/hr

In which circumstances does the Parkland formula tend to under-estimate fluid requirements?

Estimating fluid requirements is one of the most difficult aspects of burns management. The Parkland formula is an estimate and commonly underestimated fluid requirements occur in:

- Inhalation injury
- Delayed resuscitation
- Hyperglycaemia
- Alcohol intoxication
- Chronic diuretic therapy

Therefore the fluid rate may need to be adjusted depending on whether these circumstances are in existence or not. Under-resuscitation may convert a partial thickness burn to full thickness through hypoperfusion. Equally over-resuscitation may exacerbate tissue oedema.

What criteria necessitate transfer to a burns unit?

- Burns at the extremes of age
- Full thickness or partial thickness burn >10% in child
- Full thickness or partial thickness burn >15% in adult
- Inhalation injury
- Special areas (face, perineum, hands and feet)
- Electrical or chemical burns

- Burns requiring escharotomy
- Burns in children when NAI is considered

What are the indications for escharotomies?

Escharotomies may be required for circumferential third degree burns in situations associated with raised compartmental pressures in limbs as well as increased airway pressure associated with difficult ventilation.

Scenario 3

A 32 year old tree surgeon is admitted after contact with a 15,000V wire. He was unconscious for a minute but now has GCS of 15. He has paraesthesia of both hands. The palms of both hands have charred full thickness burns and are insensate. Insertion of a urinary catheter drained pink tinged urine.

What was the loss of consciousness in this patient due to?

Loss of consciousness was most likely from an arrhythmia and prompts the use of telemetry for this patient. Low voltage (< 1,000 volts) may cause death due to ventricular fibrillation at time of contact but results in little soft tissue damage and no permanent cardiac injury. High voltage (> 1,000 volts) may result in injury to the conduction system of the heart, and persistent arrhythmias. Significant soft tissue injury occurs, with 25% of patients requiring major amputation.

What is the significance of paraesthesia in both hands?

In the presence of full thickness hand burns a neurological exam may suggest significant nerve and soft-tissue damage. This may prompt fasciotomy of both forearms and release of the median and ulnar nerves at the wrist.

Why does the urine have a pink tinged appearance?

The patient with electrical burns is at high risk of developing rhabdomyolysis through muscle tissue necrosis. This is characterised by the appearance of pink tinged urine which is indicative of myoglobinuria.

How can rhabdomyolysis be prevented in such a patient?

Maintaining a urine output of >100ml/hr may help to clear myoglobin from the renal tubules where it may bind. Some units may use mannitol to force an osmotic diuresis. Crystallization of myoglobin in the renal tubule may be prevented by alkalinizing urine, or by administering sodium bicarbonate. Debridement of nonviable muscle may further decrease the severity of the rhabdomyolysis.

Cardiovascular Monitoring

What is Central Venous Pressure (CVP)?

The CVP is a measure of the hydrostatic pressure in the great vessels and is normally 0-8mmHg using the sternal angle as the reference point.

How useful is CVP as an assessment of left ventricular filling?

As there are several structures between the SVC and the left ventricle that could affect the CVP it does not truly reflect left ventricular volume and therefore fluid responsiveness.

What information does reading the CVP provide about left ventricular function?

The CVP should not be used to provide information on left ventricular function as the CVP is a right-sided pressure, and the desired measurement is really a left sided volume. This depends on several more factors including the mitral / tricuspid valves, right ventricle, pulmonary artery and the pulmonary circulation, not to mention whether the pressure in any of the chambers reflects the volume (this is defined by the compliance curve in these chambers). Therefore it is important to be aware of this limitation when extrapolating LV function from the CVP.

Why is the CVP indicative of a patient's volaemic status?

Neither the CVP value nor changes in CVP have been shown in studies to accurately predict fluid responsiveness in the critically ill. However as two thirds of the total blood volume is held within the great capacitance vessels i.e. vena cava, large veins of abdomen and proximal limbs, the CVP is therefore indirectly influenced by this volume.

A CVP line tip should be positioned at the junction of the superior vena cava (SVC) and entrance into the right atrium for accurate measurements.

What factors may increase the CVP?

- Raised intra-thoracic pressure e.g. coughing, Intermittent Positive Pressure Ventilation (IPPV), PEEP and CPAP
- Impaired right heart function e.g. cardiac failure, cardiac tamponade, large PE, SVC obstruction

What factors may decrease CVP?

- Hypovolaemia – leading to reduced venous return

What are the indications for inserting a CVP line?

These are classified into short and long-term access

Short term:

- Monitoring of CVP e.g. patients with acute renal failure to monitor fluid balance
- Intravenous access e.g. patients with very poor peripheral access
- Infusion of special medications e.g. inotropes, vasopressors, amiodarone, concentrated potassium
- Insertion of a pulmonary artery catheter
- Temporary transvenous cardiac pacing
- Access for haemofiltration

Long term:

- TPN
- Hickmann line e.g. for chemotherapeutic agents

What are the possible insertion sites for a CVP line? What are the potential problems with each site?

- Internal Jugular Vein (IJV): Though uncomfortable for the patient it is the most reliable and consistent site. There is a risk of carotid arterial puncture, but usually it can be stopped with direct pressure.
- Subclavian Vein: Most comfortable particularly for long term use but has a higher risk of pneumothorax. Should arterial trauma occur to the subclavian artery then it would not be possible to apply pressure to stop it. For both subclavian and IJV lines the patient needs to be in a head down (Trendelenburg) position.
- Femoral vein: Generally thought to be associated with a higher risk of infection. No risk of pneumo or haemothorax. Thromboembolism and femoral arterial puncture are risks.
- Cephalic, axillary and external jugular veins may also be used but rarely in day to day practice.

What are the complications of inserting a CVP line?

Immediate

- Malplacement – this comprises of the completely wrong position as well as the tip of the line being too far short of the correct position, or too far into the heart
- Bleeding / haematoma – with arterial puncture

- Arrhythmias – usually due to the guide wire irritating the myocardium or the line being too far in
- Pneumothorax
- Haemothorax
- Air embolism - Particularly in the hypovolaemic patient
- Chylothorax – due to damage to the thoracic duct
- Myocardial perforation which can lead to cardiac tamponade
- Catheter embolisation – parts of the catheter may shear off and embolise during insertion
- Guide wire embolism – parts of or the whole guide wire has been lost during insertion. Such a situation may require input from the interventional radiologist or cardiothoracic team for retrieval and removal

Late

- Occlusion
- Infection of cannulation site
- Systemic sepsis – line tip infection has even been associated with septic shock. Infective complications are reduced by aseptic technique, monitoring the number of days a line has been inserted and changing the line at an appropriate time
- Thrombosis of vein – commonest with femoral route

How does the CVP change with fluid resuscitation in the hypovolaemic, normovolaemic and overloaded patient?

- In the hypovolaemic patient a 500ml fluid bolus will lead to a rise of CVP which is not sustained and falls after 10 minutes
- In the normovolaemia patient there will be a rise of CVP above baseline, which then gradually returns to baseline levels
- In an overloaded patient the same fluid bolus will lead to a persistent rise of CVP

What is the correct technique for removing a CVP line?

Many units now have a policy of checking coagulation/clotting prior to line removal. When removing a CVP line the most important thing is to lie the patient down and apply pressure to the removal site (lying might increase bleeding from the site but will reduce the risk of air embolism).

What does a pulmonary artery (PA) catheter measure?

PA catheters provide both direct and indirect haemodynamic measurements.

- Direct: The most useful direct measurement is the pulmonary artery wedge pressure (PAWP) which is an indirect measure of the left ventricular end diastolic pressure i.e. preload. This is usually 8-12 mmHg

- PA catheters can also directly provide measurements of cardiac output, mixed venous saturation and temperature

Indirect:

- Cardiac index = Cardiac Output /Body Surface Area

- Systemic vascular resistance

- Pulmonary vascular resistance

- Oxygen delivery

What would happen to the PAWP in:

Septic Shock?

PAWP would fall and there would be an associated increase of cardiac index due to the hyperdynamic circulation of sepsis. PAWP falls due to a relative hypovolaemia through peripheral vasodilatation and leaky capillary membranes. Peripheral oxygen delivery is normal but oxygen extraction is impaired, hence mixed venous saturation may be high. In late sepsis there will be a rise in SVR and fall in oxygen delivery.

Pulmonary oedema?

Cardiac failure leading to pulmonary oedema is associated with a high PAWP due to LV dysfunction. Pulmonary oedema is likely with PAWP above 18-20mmHg.

Non cardiogenic pulmonary oedema?

Non cardiogenic pulmonary oedema as seen in ALI/ARDS may be associated with a normal PAWP.

Hypovolaemia?

With intravascular depletion there will be a fall in preload, hence a fall in left ventricular end diastolic pressure (LVEDP), and thus a fall in PAWP. This leads to a compensatory rise in SVR and reduced oxygen delivery.

What is cardiac output?

This is defined as the volume of blood pumped by the heart per minute.

- Cardiac output = stroke volume (litres) x heart rate (beats per minute)
- The stroke volume is the volume of blood ejected by the heart in a single beat
- Thus for a 70kg man the cardiac output = 0.07 litres x 70 bpm = 5 litres/ min

What is the cardiac index?

This is defined as the cardiac output per body surface area:

Cardiac index= cardiac output (l/min) / Body surface area (m^2)

Normal range = 2.2-3 L/min/min^2

What is Starling's law of the heart? Can you illustrate it?

Starling's law states that the force of myocardial contraction is proportional to stretch exerted on the myocardial fibre up to but not beyond a physiological limit.

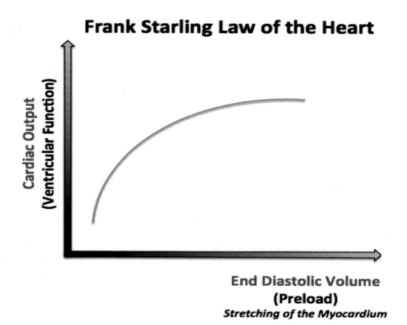

The y axis may be represented by CO, stroke volume and the x axis by left ventricular end diastolic volume (Preload).

Note this is *not* Starling's law of the capillaries – which relates to the movement of fluid across a capillary endothelium.

What factors may change the position of the curve?

- Heart failure moves the curve downwards and to the right

- Inotropic agents move the curve upwards

How do you measure cardiac output in an ICU setting?

- Thermodilution using a PA catheter used to be the most commonly used method in an ICU setting, but nowadays use of an Oesophageal Doppler Monitor (ODM)/LiDCO® / PICCO® is the most common

- 5-10mls of cold saline is injected as fast as possible through the peripheral port of a PA catheter

- The temperature will be expected to fall over time. A thermistor at the end of the catheter measures the drop in temperature

- A plot of temperature against time is produced and a computer uses an equation to measure cardiac output

- The procedure is repeated three times and the average of three measurements used

What is blood pressure?

- Blood pressure is defined as the product of cardiac output and systemic vascular resistance

- The pulsatile nature of the stroke volume produces an arterial waveform

What is the mean arterial blood pressure?

Mean arterial BP (MAP) = Diastolic BP + 1/3 (Pulse pressure)

How is BP measured?

- Direct: this is obtained through arterial cannulation and produces real time readings which are continuous. It also defines the shape of the waveform that has practical importance.

- Indirect: Using an automated measurement e.g. Dinamap or sphygmomanometer and detecting Korotkoff sounds. It is important that the correct cuff size is used, the width of which should be 20% greater than the arm's diameter.

What is the difference in the arterial tracing at the level of the radial artery compared to the aorta?

- Larger arteries such as the aorta are more distensible due to greater elasticity than the peripheral arteries. Therefore the peak pressure is less within them.

- Due to elastic recoil they are able to maintain diastolic flow better and so achieve a higher diastolic pressure than the peripheral vessel.

- Consequently the MAP achieved in the larger vessels is higher than the peripheral vessel.

Heparin Induced Thrombocytopenia

A 55 year old man has recovered from a major laparotomy for perforated diverticular disease. He has been on ICU for nearly 3 weeks and has been discharged to the ward. The junior doctor has alerted you that the platelet count is 50 x 10^9/L. There are no obvious causes for this (e.g. sepsis or medications etc.). He has been on CVVH for which the circuit was clotting off more frequently than expected.

What are you suspecting he may have?

It is possible he has Heparin Induced Thrombocytopenia (HIT) which typically manifests as a drop of >50% in the platelet count. Postoperatively HIT usually develops approximately 5 to 14 days post-heparin in those with no previous exposure to heparin. The tendency for the CVVH circuit to clot off more than expected may also consistent with HIT.

Patients with HIT classically present with a low platelet count (less than 100×10^9/L) or a relative decrease of 50% or more from a previous count. Platelet counts may remain within the normal range (between 150 to 400×10^9/L) even though there has been a drop of >50%. This is especially true in postoperative states and sepsis where thrombocytosis may be present.

What is Heparin Induced Thrombocytopenia (HIT)?

HIT is a rare but potentially life threatening complication of heparin treatment, of which there are two types.

HIT Type I: is clinically irrelevant as it is nothing more than a transient fall in platelet count. It is not due to an immune reaction.

HIT Type II: is due to an autoimmune reaction with antibodies formed against the platelet factor 4 and heparin complex.

Both forms are commoner with the use of unfractionated heparin than low molecular weight heparin, but can occur with both. Type II HIT is seen in approximately 0.1% of patients on LMWH and 2-3% of patients on unfractionated heparin.

Is the incidence of HIT higher with unfractionated heparin?

HIT can develop with any form of heparin. Although both low-molecular-weight heparin (LMWH) and unfractionated heparin (UFH) have been implicated, the incidence is ten times higher with UFH.

The incidence of HIT appears particularly high after orthopaedic surgery and is higher among surgical patients than medical patients.

How is a diagnosis of HIT made?

All patients with suspected HIT should be discussed with a senior member of the haematology team. A HIT screen using an antibody assay may be used.

Warkentin and colleagues have developed a '4T' scoring system to help assess the clinical probability of HIT:

Low scores (0-3) suggest that the probability of HIT is less than 5%.

High scores (6-8) suggest a probability of greater than 80%.

What are the complications of HIT type II?

The most dangerous complication is the development of thrombosis which can affect the arterial and/or venous system. It can occur even if the platelet count is within normal range. Also, the greater the reduction in platelet count, the more severe the thrombosis risk. Thrombosis can occur at any vascular bed but most frequently at sites of vascular injury such as central venous line sites. Arterial thrombosis can involve large arteries and cause acute arterial occlusion, with limb amputation required in up to 10% of patients with HIT. Heparin induced skin necrosis may rarely be seen and is associated with HIT-antibodies.

What complications of an extracorporeal circuit may occur in patients with HIT?

HIT induced occlusion of the extracorporeal circuit may manifest as:

- increased circuit pressure
- formation of clot in the drip chambers
- clotted dialyser fibres
- acute thrombocytopenia with more than 20% decrease in platelet count
- unexpected filter clotting during continuous venovenous haemofiltration

What are the principles of treating HIT?

- Stop ALL forms of heparin including small amounts for catheter flushing
- Send blood samples for HIT antibodies
- Early and urgent involvement of senior haematologist
- Start an alternative anticoagulant at treatment dose as HIT is a prothrombotic disorder
- Continue the alternative anticoagulant until the platelet count has stabilised
- Start warfarin while continuing alternative anticoagulant for at least five days

- Do not re-challenge with heparin at least in the next 100 days
- Prophylactic platelet transfusions are relatively contra-indicated as platelets may become activated and promote thrombosis

Possible alternative non-heparin anticoagulants used for the treatment of HIT are direct thrombin inhibitors (lepirudin and argatroban) or heparinoids (danaparoid). Two other agents, bivalirudin (another direct thrombin inhibitor) and fondaparinux, are lacking controlled studies for their use.

Reference

Warkentin TE, Heddle NM. Laboratory Diagnosis of Immune Heparin-Induced Thrombocytopenia. Current Hematology Reports. 2003; 2:148-157.

Inotropes and Circulatory Support

A 75 year old man on surgical HDU is being managed conservatively for a perforated gastric ulcer. He has become peritonitic in the past few hours and hypotensive (70/40mmHg), tachycardic (110bpm) and oliguric. You decide to proceed to an urgent laparotomy but need to fully resuscitate the patient.

How would you proceed?

Full resuscitation starts with assessment and management of this patient's airway, breathing and circulation. Specifically in terms of his circulation his intravascular volume must be optimised with an aim to produce a MAP of >65mmHg. Unless he has a sustained and stable response to fluids he should have a central venous line inserted to allow infusion of vasoactive medications.

Which vasopressors are the agents of choice for the management of septic shock?

Noradrenaline is the vasopressor of choice in septic shock as stated in the Surviving Sepsis Campaign. It is a potent alpha-1 agonist with minimal beta effect. It is used mainly as a vasopressor on the peripheral circulation rather than an inotrope to maintain mean BP >65mmHg. In this scenario a central venous line needs to be inserted prior to its use. Vasopressors should be given centrally due to the risks of skin necrosis with extravasation.

Which vasoactive agents can be used in addition to noradrenaline if a patient's BP is poorly responsive?

Vasopressin (ADH) can be added to norepinephrine to either raise mean arterial pressure to target or to decrease the norepinephrine dose (e.g. peripheral ischaemia) but should not be used as the initial vasopressor. This is particularly important in catecholamine resistant vasodilatory shock. Although dopamine has positive effects on the blood pressure, in this setting it is not recommended except in highly selected circumstances, as it is arrhythmogenic and causes more tachycardia.

Although the choice of vasopressor has been a matter of debate a meta-analysis of RCTs has recently shown that noradrenaline or noradrenaline plus low dose vasopressin use are associated with significantly reduced mortality compared with dopamine. The addition of an inotropic agent such as dobutamine or dopexamine did not reduce mortality.

What is the action of dopamine?

Dopamine is an endogenous precursor of noradrenaline and acts on dopaminergic receptors (D1 and D2). The effects of dopamine are dose dependent. Low dose dopamine stimulates mainly dopaminergic receptors leading to renal vasodilatation – the so-called renal dose dopamine. Between 5 and 10 μg/kg/min it causes a beta-1 mediated increase in CO and contractility. At higher doses it produces alpha-1 mediated vasoconstriction.

What is the definition of an inotrope?

An inotrope is defined as a drug which increases the force of myocardial contraction.

Through what mechanism do inotropes achieve this effect?

Most inotropes act to increase the availability of calcium within the cardiac myocyte. This is achieved through activation of adenylyl cyclase, which leads to an increase in the production of cAMP from ATP leading to the activation of protein kinase A. This leads to a rise in calcium influx and an increase in myocardial contractility. Almost all inotropes in common use have this cAMP dependent mechanism.

In general what are the problems in using inotropes?

All these agents will require central venous access for administration. They are all arrythmogenic, with some more so than others. They can also cause tachycardia which increases myocardial work and O_2 demand therefore causes cardiac ischaemia. Prolonged use of these agents can lead to a reduced therapeutic effect (down-regulation of receptors).

What is the action of dobutamine?

This synthetic catecholamine is predominantly a beta-1 adrenoreceptor agonist which increases myocardial contractility with minimal effect on heart rate.

What is the action of adrenaline?

This is an endogenous catecholamine which acts as an agonist on both alpha-1 and beta-1 adrenoreceptors. In low doses adrenaline acts as an inotrope through beta-1 adrenoreceptors and has a vasodilatory effect via beta-2 receptors. As the dose is increased alpha and beta effects are seen, but at higher doses alpha-1 vasoconstriction is the predominant pharmacological effect.

What is the action of dopexamine?

Dopexamine is a synthetic analogue of dopamine and is an inodilator. It acts on dopaminergic receptors to cause vasodilatation as well as increasing myocardial contractility, but is less likely to produce the beta-1 mediated tachycardia seen with dopamine. It has a protective effect on causing splanchnic vasodilatation making it a popular drug on some ICU settings.

What are milrinone and enoximone? In which clinical circumstances would you find them being used?

These are phosphodiesterase II inhibitors which through their action lead to an increase in cAMP. They are inodilators causing increase in myocardial contractility while causing peripheral vasodilation. These drugs are especially useful in the setting of right heart failure due to their inotropic action and their effect of pulmonary vasodilatation. They are often used in cardiothoracic intensive care units. Their use in general intensive care units is limited by their hypotensive effect mediated via systemic vasodilatation.

Reference

Oba Y, Lone NA. Mortality benefit of vasopressor and inotropic agents in septic shock: a Bayesian network meta-analysis of randomized controlled trials. J Crit Care. 2014 Oct;29(5):706-10.

Intravenous Fluids and Electrolytes

A 49 year old man with a long history of peptic ulcer disease has intractable non-healing distal gastric ulcers despite maximal medical management. He continues with symptoms of gastric outlet obstruction. A NG tube has drained 1.5 litres of gastric content. The serum potassium is 2.8 mmol/L, chloride 84 mmol/L and bicarbonate 45mmol/L.

What are the electrolyte and acid base changes that occur with gastric outlet obstruction?

Prolonged vomiting causes loss of potassium and hydrochloric acid and produces an increase of bicarbonate in the plasma to compensate for the lost chloride. This leads to a hypokalemic hypochloremic metabolic alkalosis.

With continued vomiting, the renal excretion of potassium increases in order to preserve sodium, and the adrenocortical response to hypovolemia intensifies the exchange of potassium for sodium at the distal tubule, with subsequent aggravation of hypokalemia.

What is the mechanism behind paradoxical aciduria?

Initially, the urine has a low chloride and high bicarbonate content, reflecting the primary metabolic abnormality. This bicarbonate is excreted along with sodium and so, with time, the patient becomes progressively hyponatraemic and more profoundly dehydrated. Because of the dehydration, a phase of sodium retention follows and potassium and hydrogen are excreted in preference. This results in the urine becoming paradoxically acidic.

How is fluid distributed between the normal body compartments in a 70kg patient?

- 42 litres of water in a 70kg patient
- Total body water is divided:
    - 2/3rd - Intracellular (ICF)   28 litres
    - 1/3rd - Extracellular (ECF)   14 litres
        - Intravascular: 3 litres
        - Interstitial: 10 litres
        - Transcellular (CSF, intraocular fluid)   1 litre

What are the daily basal requirements of water and electrolytes?

- Water 30-40 ml/kg/day

- Sodium 50-100 mmol/day

- Potassium 40-80 mmol/day

Additional requirements will depend on continuing losses and deficits.

Scenario 2

A 77 year old lady is admitted with small bowel obstruction from an incisional hernia. She has a sodium of 112 on admission. The on call team overnight have given her two one litre bags of normal saline. Her sodium remains at 112. How would you correct this lady's sodium level?

- First check her medication chart to see if she is on any medications that would promote sodium excretion such as diuretics, and stop them

- Secondly aim to correct her sodium levels but avoid over-rapid correction. Given she is most likely hypovolaemic Hartmann's can be used in a controlled manner

What are the clinical features of hyponatraemia?

Sodium is the main extracellular ion. A low sodium leads to water influx into cells.

This may manifest as cerebral oedema, presenting as confusion, headache, coma and even convulsions. Pulmonary oedema may also be a feature. Pre-menopausal women are particularly at risk of severe neurological effects of hyponatraemia.

What may occur if her sodium is corrected too rapidly?

Sodium correction should be slow as central pontine myelonosis and cardiac failure through fluid overload and pulmonary oedema may occur with rapid correction. A correction should be no more than by 0.5mmol/l/day. Neurological effects are more likely with rapid correction if the sodium has been chronically low.

What remains the commonest cause of hyponatraemia in surgical patients?

Dilution remains the commonest cause in surgical patients with the use of large volumes of glucose infusions such as 5% dextrose.

What is ADH and how does it act?

Anti-diuretic hormone (ADH) is released from the posterior pituitary in response to a rise in plasma osmolality sensed by osmoreceptors in the supraoptic nuclei of the hypothalamus. ADH then acts on the distal renal tubule to increase the conservation of water and to a lesser extent sodium.

What is SIADH?

The Syndrome of Inappropriate ADH (SIADH) secretion occurs by the autonomous and non-osmotic release of ADH leading to effects of hyponatraemia. It has several causes but the commonest are lung neoplasms as well as lung infections and intracranial malignancy.

What is a crystalloid? What is a colloid?

A crystalloid is a solution containing low molecular weight salts or sugars that dissolve completely in water and pass freely between the intravascular and interstitial compartments. A colloid contains larger molecular weight substances that do not dissolve completely and remain for a longer period in the vascular compartment than crystalloid solutions.

What can happen biochemically if large volumes of normal saline are infused?

A hyperchloraemic metabolic acidosis may occur from the large volume of chloride infused. Although large volumes of "normal saline" can result in hyperchloraemic acidosis the clinical importance of this is debated. It can definitely increase the uncertainty as to the cause of an acidosis and is therefore often avoided and balanced crystalloids such as Hartmann's are often used instead.

What other crystalloids do you know of?

Hartmann's solution is a balanced physiological solution with a composition similar to ECF. It does contain lactate, which is gluconeogenic and may contribute to hyperglycaemia in diabetics.

5% dextrose and 4%/0.18% dextrose-saline are considered free water and useful to resuscitate the ICF compartment. They have a limited clinical application and should be used with caution, as excessive amounts may cause dangerous hyponatraemia, especially in the elderly.

What does a bag of normal saline contain?

Na 154 mmol/l

Cl 154 mmol/l

What does a 1litre bag of Hartmann's contain?

Na 131 mmol/l

Cl 111 mmol/l

K 5 mmol/l

Ca 2 mmol/l

Lactate 29 mmol/l

What are the advantages and disadvantages of using crystalloids?

Advantages

- Crystalloids are cheaper than colloids and more readily available

Disadvantages

- They have a short duration in the circulation with only 50% being intravascular after 20 minutes from infusion
- No oxygen carrying capacity
- Interstitial oedema due to the free transfer between intravascular space and interstitial space
- All the commonly used crystalloids even Hartmann's are relatively hyperchloraemic

What is a colloid and what colloids do you know of?

- Colloids contain substances which are unable to pass through a semi-permeable membrane and are effectively a suspension of particles rather than a true solution (crystalloid)
- Generally all colloids contain large molecules >30 000kda which exert an oncotic pressure
- Gelatins (Gelofusine, Haemaccel) have a half life in the circulation of a few hours (approx 3 hours)
- Starches (hetastarch, hexastarch, pentastarch) remain in circulation much longer with a half life of 24 hours. Intractable pruritis has been described as a complication of its use
- Dextrans are rarely used in the UK but have a long half life as well (up to and beyond 3 hours) but may interfere with blood cross matching as well as renal problems
- Human Albumin Solution (HAS) is derived from pooled human plasma but is sterile. There are some concerns about the risk of prion transmission and its use is limited by expense

What are the potential advantages and disadvantages of using colloids in resuscitation?

- Colloids have a greater retention within the intravascular space than a crystalloid. Therefore less volume is required for resuscitation thereby minimising fluid overload. Approximately 2-3 times the volume of crystalloid is need to have the same effect as a colloid

- Colloids also have a risk of allergic reactions with rare instances of anaphylaxis described

- Colloids, particularly starches have been subject to several RCTs in critical care and have been shown to be at best associated with an equivalent outcome to crystalloids and at worst an increased mortality and an increased risk of renal failure and the need for RRT. Some starches have been withdrawn from the market on this basis

Scenario 3

A 65 year old man underwent an emergency small bowel resection for mesenteric ischaemia. From the DJ flexure approximately 3 metres of small bowel was left in situ and delivered as an end ileostomy. The patient made a quick recovery from HDU and has been transferred to the ward. On day 5 post op he has developed acute renal failure with a creatinine of 586.

What may be the aetiology of his acute renal failure?

Although a variety of causes are possible, pre-renal causes are by far the most common. In this case attention should be paid to his stoma output as it is possible, particularly at this stage following the operation (day 5), that he has a high output stoma with subsequent hypovolaemia leading to ARF.

The daily stoma output has been between 1.5 to 2 litres daily. He is receiving Hartmann's solution 1 litre every 8 hours. Why are ileostomies prone to high output? What biochemical abnormalities might you expect with a high output ileostomy?

An ileostomy would typically be expected to begin function between 1 and 3 days after surgery. Impaired fluid absorption across the mucosa occurs due to bowel wall oedema and this leads to a high volume output. A period of adaptation takes place over several days to weeks and this will lead to a decreased stoma output to somewhere between 400 to 800 ml/day. The typical electrolyte abnormalities seen are hypokalaemia, hypomagnasaemia and hypocalcaemia.

What are the essential steps in managing a high output ileostomy?

- Strict recording of daily stoma output. Ensure underlying infection is excluded by stool culture

- Daily bloods for serum electrolytes and renal function

- Maintaining adequate iv fluid replacement as guided by renal function and fluid balance

- Correction / replacement of electrolyte abnormalities

- Avoidance of drinking hypotonic fluids (e.g. water / fruit juice, soft drinks, tea and coffee), which can lead to sodium efflux into bowel lumen thereby exacerbating hyponatraemia. Use glucose-electrolyte balanced solutions e.g. commercially available sports drinks

- Fibre supplementation may help to slow intestinal transit – aiming for 20-30 gm of fibre per day

- Pharmacologic treatments include antidiarrheal agents, such as loperamide (2–4 mg tds to qds) as well as codeine phosphate. A PPI should be added for its antisecretory effect

- Involvement of a stoma nurse specialist

Massive Blood Loss

What is the definition of massive blood loss (MBL)?

Massive blood loss is defined as blood loss equivalent to the patient's total blood volume within 24 hours.

What is the blood volume in an adult and in children?

Adult = 70 ml/Kg

Children = 75 ml/Kg

What haematological parameters would you aim to achieve during treatment of MBL?

Aim to maintain Hb > 8g/dl

Aim for PT and APTT < 1.5x control

Aim for platelet count >75 x 10^9/L

Aim for fibrinogen > 1g/L

Aim for ionized calcium > 1.13 mmol/L

O Negative blood is always immediately available. Group specific blood is available within 25 minutes and cross-matched blood available in 45 minutes.

What strategies do you know of to reduce the use of stored blood?

Intraoperative Cell Salvage (ICS): autologous recovery of blood spilled during surgery using a cell saver can provide rapidly available blood. The cost effectiveness of using cell savers is a contentious issue.

Blood lost into the surgical field is filtered to remove particulate matter and aspirated into a collection reservoir where it is anticoagulated with heparin or citrate. Salvaged blood can be centrifuged and washed in a closed, automated system and red cells suspended in sterile saline solution are transfused to the patient within 4 hours of processing. (Most Jehovah's Witnesses would accept and consent to ICS). ICS should not be used when bowel contents contaminate the operation site, and blood should not be aspirated from bacterially infected surgical fields. Because of concerns about cancer cell reinfusion and spread, manufacturers do not recommend ICS in patients having surgery for malignant disease.

Pre-deposit autologous blood donation (PAD) – patients donate their own blood leading up to the time of surgery. The ideal patient for this strategy should have a window of two or more weeks before surgery to donate. Given the current remote risk of viral transfusion-transmitted infection by donor blood in developed countries, the rationale and cost-effectiveness of routine PAD has been questioned. Therefore it is rarely practiced in the UK.

Acute Normovolaemic Haemodilution (ANH)- this involves the removal of 1 to 4 units of the patient's own blood just before or immediately after induction of anaesthesia. The blood removed is replaced by crystalloid or colloid, and this results in a reduction of haematocrit to between 20% to 30%. The blood is stored in the operating theatre at room temperature and reinfused at the end of surgery or if significant bleeding occurs. ANH can be considered for patients with normal initial hemoglobin (Hb) and is safest when used in healthy young adults. (It is a good option for Jehovah's Witnesses who will consent to ANH if the blood is maintained in a closed circuit continuous flow system.) ANH is most often used in cardiac bypass surgery where the immediate postoperative transfusion of 'fresh whole blood' containing platelets and clotting factors is seen as an advantage.

What do you know of the role of tranexamic acid in major haemorrhage?

The CRASH-2 trial published in 2010 clearly showed that early administration of the antifibrinolytic drug tranexamic acid improves the survival of patients with major traumatic haemorrhage or those at risk of significant bleeding after trauma. Maximum benefit is obtained if tranexamic acid is given as soon as possible after the injury in a dose of 1 g over 10 minutes followed by a maintenance infusion of 1g over 8 hours. Tranexamic acid should not be given more than 3 hours after injury. Given its good safety profile, ease of administration and low cost, tranexamic acid should be considered as a component of most major haemorrhage protocols.

What ratio of blood products (packed cells, FFP and platelets) should be given to those with massive blood loss?

Conventional teaching suggested transfusing one FFP for every six units of packed cells. Studies in military trauma (and latterly in civilian populations) have indicated that transfusion in a 1:1:1 ratio is associated with improved outcomes. This is because massive blood loss is associated with dilution, consumption of clotting factors, hypothermia and acidosis, which leads to coagulopathy. Timely early transfusion of all blood products helps to minimize this problem. However it is hard to generalise the results from military studies to the everyday population who are much older and have more co-morbidities.

What is FFP?

- This is produced from plasma from a single donation

- Each 150 ml bag contains all clotting factors, albumin and gamma-globulin. It is usually able to replace fibrinogen without having to use cryoprecipitate

- FFP must be used immediately after thawing due to the labile factors V and VIII

- If it is stored it must be used within 24 hours at 4°C

- It must be ABO compatible

- Plasma is frozen to -30°C and can be stored for up to a year
- The dose of FFP is weight dependent and the usual starting dose is 10-15 ml/kg (equivalent to four packs of FFP for a 70kg person)
- Immediate reversal of warfarin effect, in the presence of life-threatening bleeding
- FFP only has a partial effect and is not the optimal treatment; prothrombin complex concentrates are recommended as a first line when major bleeding is from anticoagulant therapy
- Risk of transmission with FFP is very small but present

What are the indications for using FFP?
- Single clotting factor deficiency e.g. factor V deficiency
- Corrects coagulopathy
- Reverses warfarin
- DIC
- Massive blood transfusion

Does FFP need cross-matching?
The first choice would be the same ABO group as the patient. If this is not available then FFP of a different ABO group is acceptable so as long as it has been shown not to possess anti-A or anti-B activity in high titres. Group O FFP should only be given to O recipients as it has caused haemolysis in non O patients. FFP does not need to be Rhesus matched as there appears to be no risk of anti D immunization.

What is Beriplex®?
Beriplex® is a prothrombin concentrate complex (PCC). It is able to provide a more rapid and complete reversal of warfarin than FFP. It is given IV at 30 units/Kg. Patients should also receive 5mg vitamin K IV at the same time. INR should be checked 10-15 minutes afterwards and if reversal is not complete then discuss with a haematologist.

What does cryoprecipitate contain and when should it be given?
Cryoprecipitate is indicated for bleeding in patients with significant hypofibrinogenemia (plasma levels <1 g per litre). Cryoprecipitate is the only adequate fibrinogen concentrate available for intravenous use. It is prepared from plasma and contains fibrinogen, von Willebrand factor, factor VIII, factor XIII and fibronectin. Each unit provides about 350 mg of fibrinogen.

What are the features of massive blood transfusion?

- Clotting abnormalities:
    - Blood loss results in reduced levels of platelets, coagulation factors and inhibitors. Platelets are unstable in stored blood at 4°C with a rapid fall in platelet count beyond 24 hours of storage. Factor V and Factor VIII in particular lose activity with storage
    - Dilutional coagulopathy: dilutional thrombocytopenia, dilutional coagulopathy
    - DIC: this is seen in approximately 30% of patients and is more a result of hypoperfusion rather than the transfusion itself

Biochemical complications:

- Hyperkaleamia
    - due to potassium leakage from stored red cells
    - this may be compounded by oliguria and the metabolic acidosis associated with shock
- Hypocalcaemia
    - This is the commonest feature of massive blood transfusion and is particularly common in patients with liver impairment as citrate metabolism is slowed
- Metabolic alkalosis
    - Donor blood contains sodium citrate as an anticoagulant
    - Stored blood has a pH of 6.3 but sodium citrate is converted to bicarbonate in the liver with resultant metabolic alkalosis
    - Alkalosis increases the affinity of haemoglobin for oxygen
    - Alkalosis also stimulates production of 2,3-DPG

Other problems

- Fluid overload
    - may lead to acute pulmonary oedema
- Hypothermia
    - Blood is stored at 1 to 6 degrees and then transfused in large volume
    - This may worsen coagulopathy
- Haemoglobin dysfunction
- 2,3-DPG levels fall over time in stored blood thereby increasing the affinity of haemoglobin for oxygen (left shift of oxyhaemoglobin dissociation curve)
- ARDS / TRALI
- Anaphylaxis
- Infectious disease transmission (hepatitis / HIV / CMV / Creutfzfeld-Jacob disease / malaria)

- Immunosuppression: particularly important in the context of surgical oncology with early recurrence demonstrated with the use of blood e.g. renal cell carcinoma. In the early days the immunosuppressive effect was used deliberately to reduce rejection rates after renal transplantation!

What do you understand by the term 'Point of care testing'?

Traditional 'massive transfusion' guidelines use laboratory tests such as prothrombin time (PT) and activated partial thromboplastin time (APTT) to guide blood component replacement. However these tests can be limited by delays between sampling and returning results to the clinical team. Point of care testing (POCT) uses assays of clot formation, clot strength and lysis, such as thromboelastography (TEG), can provide 'real time' laboratory data to guide blood component replacement. It has been used for many years to inform plasma and platelet transfusion in liver transplantation and cardiac surgery. Its value in the management of major haemorrhage is uncertain and is the subject of current research.

What happens to coagulation factors during major haemorrhage?

Dilutional coagulopathy of clotting factors occurs from blood loss and dilution secondary to fluid transfusion. Activation of the coagulation and fibrinolytic systems leads to an 'acute traumatic coagulopathy'. Plasma fibrinogen predictably falls to sub-haemostatic levels (<1.5 g/L) after 1 to 1.5 blood volume replacement. Other factors that further impair coagulation include hypothermia, acidosis and reduced ionised calcium ($Ca2+$) concentration. Although uncommon when liver function is normal, ionised hypocalcaemia may be caused by rapid transfusion of blood components containing citrate anticoagulant.

What is the role of recombinant factor VIIa (NovoSeven™) in major haemorrhage?

Recombinant activated Factor VII has been widely used as a 'last-ditch' measure for patients with major haemorrhage. Studies show no good evidence of improved survival, but life-threatening arterial and venous thromboembolic complications may occur. The latter are particularly more common in older patients with vascular disease. Several national guidelines no longer recommend its use outside research studies.

What is Disseminated Intravascular Coagulation (DIC)?

DIC is a form of consumptive coagulopathy and occurs when free thrombin is released into the circulation leading to widespread microvascular thrombosis. This leads to tissue ischaemia whilst the consumption of coagulation products and activation of fibrinolysis leads to haemorrhagic complications. DIC is primarily a clinical diagnosis with laboratory tests used to confirm the diagnosis and monitor replacement of blood products.

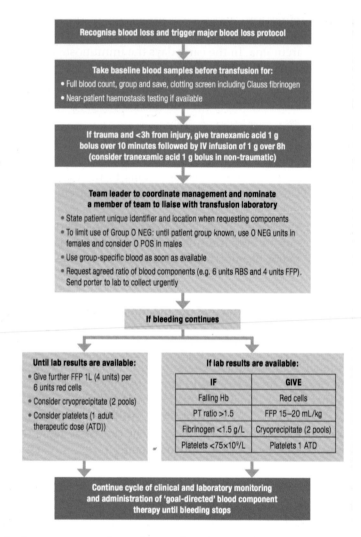

Recognise blood loss and trigger major blood loss protocol

Take baseline blood samples before transfusion for:
- Full blood count, group and save, clotting screen including Clauss fibrinogen
- Near-patient haemostasis testing if available

If trauma and <3h from injury, give tranexamic acid 1 g bolus over 10 minutes followed by IV infusion of 1 g over 8h (consider tranexamic acid 1 g bolus in non-traumatic)

Team leader to coordinate management and nominate a member of team to liaise with transfusion laboratory
- State patient unique identifier and location when requesting components
- To limit use of Group O NEG: until patient group known, use O NEG units in females and consider O POS in males
- Use group-specific blood as soon as available
- Request agreed ratio of blood components (e.g. 6 units RBS and 4 units FFP). Send porter to lab to collect urgently

If bleeding continues

Until lab results are available:
- Give further FFP 1L (4 units) per 6 units red cells
- Consider cryoprecipitate (2 pools)
- Consider platelets (1 adult therapeutic dose (ATD))

If lab results are available:

IF	GIVE
Falling Hb	Red cells
PT ratio >1.5	FFP 15–20 mL/kg
Fibrinogen <1.5 g/L	Cryoprecipitate (2 pools)
Platelets <75×10⁹/L	Platelets 1 ATD

Continue cycle of clinical and laboratory monitoring and administration of 'goal-directed' blood component therapy until bleeding stops

Algorithm for the management of major haemorrhage (adapted from the BCSH Practical Guideline for the Management of Those With, or At Risk of Major Haemorrhage (2014) with permission)

References

http://www.transfusionguidelines.org.uk/transfusion-handbook/7-effective-transfusion-in-surgery-and-critical-care/7-3-transfusion-management-of-major-haemorrhage

CRASH-2 collaborators, Roberts I, Shakur H et al. The importance of early treatment with tranexamic acid in bleeding trauma patients: an exploratory analysis of the CRASH-2 randomised controlled trial. Lancet. 2011 Mar 26;377(9771):1096-101

Nutrition in Critical Care

How common are nutritional problems in critically ill patients?

The majority of surgical patients admitted to ICU will be catabolic, whether from sepsis or surgery by itself. The resting energy expenditure in these patients is usually more than 50% greater than at rest.

The causes for this may be multifactorial - the underlying surgical condition or an inability to manage their own feeding. In some patients who have been hospitalised for a prolonged period the nutritional requirements may have been overlooked.

Why might nutritional requirements be much higher in critically ill patients?

Critical care patients also have an increased susceptibility to infection, which drives up nutritional requirements, due to the underlying disease, impairment of the immune system and the use of invasive monitoring techniques, which can lead to line sepsis.

Many of these patients have been treated with broad-spectrum antimicrobials that can make them prone to infection with resistant organisms. A number of patients on ITU will also have prolonged ventilator requirements, which can increase nutritional requirements.

What is the normal physiological response to starvation?

Initially when there is a disruption to nutritional intake, there is a use of stored calories to provide energy. Adipose tissue becomes the main source of fatty acids to use as an energy substrate once hepatic glycogen stores are used up in the first 24-48 hours.

The majority of cells within the body can use alternatives to glucose for energy metabolism. Skeletal and cardiac muscle may utilize free fatty acids and ketone bodies when glucose is unavailable, and glutamine is used by the gastrointestinal tract.

A small number of cell types (erythrocytes, renal medulla) can only use glucose, and this is provided by protein breakdown. With prolonged starvation, basal metabolic rate decreases and there is a move towards utilisation of fat as the main energy source. Protein and lean body mass are preserved until late in the starvation period. The basal metabolic rate falls by 20%-25% with starvation.

How does this differ in an ITU patient with e.g. sepsis or pancreatitis?

ITU patients may have a hypercatabolic response and thus increased basal metabolic rate and calorie requirement. There is an impaired ability to use carbohydrate and fat as the main energy substrates leading to protein breakdown and subsequent massive nitrogen loss. This catabolic state is not reversed by resumption of adequate nutrition.

What are the problems with glucose as an energy source?

Critical care patients may become glucose intolerant as part of the stress response. Oxidation of excess glucose leads to increased carbon dioxide production and subsequent increase in ventilatory effort, which further increases energy requirements. Fatty infiltration of the liver, hyperinsulinaemia and hypophosphataemia also occur. Lipids can provide 9kcal/g of energy in comparison to 4kcal/g provided by glucose.

What are the normal resting nutritional requirements?

Normal individuals require approximately 30 kcal/kg/day with one third of the intake coming from fats. Other requirements include 0.15/kg/day of nitrogen, as well as vitamins, minerals, electrolytes and trace elements.

What are the approximate nutritional requirements in critically ill patients?

Critically ill patients generally need 30-35 kcal/kg/day, but may require up to 60 kcal/kg/day in sepsis and possibly up to 80 kcal/kg/day for burns patients.

What are the advantages of enteral nutrition?

These include:

- It is a more physiological route

- Prevention of mucosal atrophy as intestinal enterocytes will receive a certain proportion of nutrition directly. This maintains the intestinal barrier. Enteral nutrition also increases splanchnic blood flow and so reduces bacterial translocation which reduces the incidence of sepsis

- Support of the normal gut flora. There is an increase in IgA secretion

- Protection against stress ulcers

- Avoidance of the catheter related problems of TPN

- Fewer metabolic problems than TPN. The presence of nutrients within the small intestine promotes bile flow and so reduces the incidence of cholestasis seen in TPN

- Cheaper than TPN

By what routes can enteral nutrition be administered?

- Orally

- Nasogastric

- Nasojejunal

- Feeding jejunostomy

- Gastrostomy – surgically or radiologically inserted (RIG) tube or endoscope (PEG)

What are the general complications of enteral nutrition?

- Aspiration

- Nausea and vomiting – may require prokinetics such as metoclopramide or erythromycin

- Diarrhoea – high osmotic load induced

- Tube related problems e.g. blocked PEG / jejunostomy tube fallen out

What are the indications for TPN?

These include absolute and relative indications:

Absolute indication: High output enterocutaneous fistula.

Relative indications:

- Patients where enteral nutrition is not possible - e.g prolonged ileus

- Where absorption may be compromised - severe inflammatory bowel disease

- May also be used in patients with intestinal failure/ short gut syndrome as well as in trauma and burns patients

What are the side effects of TPN?

- Line related complication such as infection / blockage. TPN related central line sepsis can lead to septic shock

- TPN may lead to abnormalities in glucose control, liver dysfunction, electrolyte abnormalities, and risk of hepatic steatosis. Bile stasis may lead to acalculous cholecystitis. TPN is also expensive

What are the constituents of a normal bag of TPN?

Parenteral nutrition requires the use of a solution containing amino acids, glucose, fat, electrolytes,trace elements, and vitamins. Specialist additions to parenteral nutrition such as additional fluid or glutamine may be required locally.

Protein is given as mixtures of essential and non-essential synthetic L -amino acids. Ideally, all essential amino acids should be included with a wide variety of non-essential ones to provide sufficient nitrogen together with electrolytes.

Energy is provided in a ratio of 0.6 to 1.1 megajoules (150–250 kcals) per gram of protein nitrogen. Energy requirements must be met if amino acids are to be utilised for tissue maintenance. A mixture of carbohydrate and fat energy sources (usually 30%–50% as fat) gives better utilisation of amino acids than glucose alone.

Glucose is the preferred source of carbohydrate.

In parenteral nutrition regimens, it is necessary to provide adequate phosphate in order to allow phosphorylation of glucose and to prevent hypophosphataemia; between 20 and 30 mmol of phosphate is required daily.

Fat emulsions have the advantages of a high energy to fluid volume ratio, neutral pH, and iso-osmolarity with plasma, and provide essential fatty acids.

What is refeeding syndrome?

This is a potentially serious condition seen when re-feeding malnourished patients whether enterally or parenterally. It occurs due to hormonal and metabolic changes induced by glycaemia from recommencing feed. The cardinal sign of refeeding syndrome is hypophosphataemia, although magnesium and sodium abnormalities also occur.

How does refeeding syndrome develop?

During refeeding there is a surge of insulin in response to glycaemia. The actions of insulin require the presence of phosphate, magnesium and thiamine as a cofactor. This is why patients at risk of refeeding are often given thiamine prior to full feeding being commenced.

Insulin stimulates the absorption of potassium into the cells as well as magnesium and phosphate. This results in a severe sharp fall in serum levels of phosphate, potassium, and magnesium, all of which are already depleted. Whole body depletion of phosphate leads to widespread cellular dysfunction affecting almost every system.

What is the role of phosphate in the body?

Phosphate is predominantly an intracellular mineral and is essential for all intracellular processes, with many enzymes activated by phosphate binding. It is part of the crucial molecule adenosine triphosphate (ATP). Phosphate also influences oxygen delivery as it regulates the affinity of haemoglobin for oxygen. It also has an important role in the renal acid-base buffer system.

Oxygen Delivery

How is oxygen carried in blood?

The majority of oxygen is bound to Hb (99%) and only 1% is dissolved in blood.

Where within a cell is oxygen utilised?

Oxygen is delivered to the mitochondria and is utilised for ATP production by oxidative phosphorylation.

How is oxygen delivery to tissues optimised?

Oxygen delivery is defined by the equation:

$$DO_2 = (O_2 \text{ carried by Hb}) + (O_2 \text{ in solution}) \times CO$$

$$= (1.34 \times Hb \times SpO_2 \times 0.01) + (0.023 \times PaO_2) \times CO$$

where DO_2 = oxygen delivery and CO = cardiac output

The main variables that can be influenced to optimise oxygen delivery are:

- Cardiac output – the main determinants of which are heart rate and stroke volume. This in turn is optimised by venous return and myocardial contractility. Left ventricular end diastolic pressure should be optimised and ideally around 12mmHg. Myocardial contractility can be altered by the use of inotropes.

- Oxygen saturation – supplemental oxygen to increase pO_2 as well as correcting any underlying chest problems such as infections, atelectasis.

- Haemoglobin concentration – this should be optimised through transfusion to ensure an adequate Hb concentration. The aim should be to achieve a haematocrit of 37-40%.

What is the role of pre-optimisation of oxygen delivery in high risk surgical patients?

Although there is some evidence demonstrating reduced morbidity and mortality in high risk surgical patients whose global oxygen delivery is optimised preoperatively, the data to support the routine use of preoperative pre-optimisation is considered somewhat historical.

There are data to suggest that optimising fluid management with the use of cardiac output monitoring intra-operatively may reduce postoperative morbidity and length of stay. These data apply to many types of surgery such as colorectal, urological, orthopaedic.

What is the oxyhaemoglobin dissociation curve and can you draw it?

The curve defines the relationship between oxygen saturation and partial pressure of oxygen. It is a sigmoid shaped curve which reflects the increased affinity of Hb to oxygen as haemoglobin binds more oxygen. The P50 value is the partial pressure of oxygen corresponding to 50% saturation of haemoglobin (usually 3.5kpa).

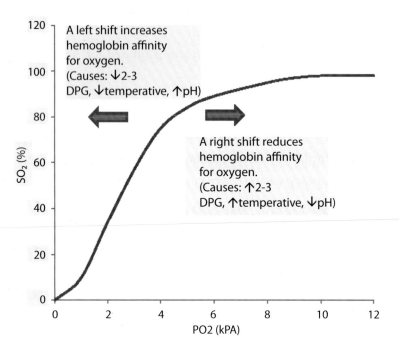

What factors may influence a change in position of the curve?

A shift to the right is associated with increased release of oxygen to tissues i.e a fall in affinity of Hb to oxygen. This can be due to acidosis, pyrexia, anaemia and a fall in 2-3 DPG.

A shift to the left is associated with reduced release of oxygen to tissues i.e. a increased affinity of Hb to oxygen. This can be due to alkalosis, hypothermia and a rise in 2-3 DPG. The curve for foetal Hb is to the left of adult Hb (HbA).

What is the Bohr effect?

This effect refers to the shift of the curve in response to changes in pH. Usually this refers to the right shift which occurs in relation to acidosis, rising pCO_2 and increased 2,3 DPG.

What is 2,3 DPG and what may be its clinical significance?

2,3 DPG is a by-product of the glycolytic pathway which binds to the beta chain of Hb and reduces its affinity to oxygen. In stored blood, levels of 2,3 DPG may fall thereby increasing the affinity of Hb to oxygen and reducing oxygen delivery.

What are the effects of carbon monoxide on the curve?

Carbon monoxide binds to the iron moiety of Hb and increases its affinity to oxygen by 300 times. In doing so it shifts the curve to the left thereby inhibiting oxygen delivery.

What do you understand by the term mixed venous saturation?

The mixed venous oxygen saturation (SvO_2) is a measurement of the balance between oxygen delivery and oxygen consumption, made using a pulmonary artery catheter (the measurements are made from venous blood in the pulmonary artery). The normal SvO_2 is 70%.

$$SvO_2 = \text{Oxygen Delivered} - \text{Oxygen Consumed}$$

A low value may reflect poor oxygen delivery (due to low arterial oxygenation, low haemoglobin or low cardiac output) or increased oxygen extraction. The cellular processes governing oxygen extraction are poorly understood and the measurement of oxygen extraction is not practically possible, therefore assumptions that this is constant must be considered when interpreting this value.

A high value may reflect high oxygen delivery as seen in hyperdynamic states such as septic shock after volume resuscitation. It may also reflect poor oxygen extraction which may occur in sepsis, but again is poorly understood.

Why is it important that the SvO_2 be measured from the pulmonary artery?

The pulmonary artery is the site where adequate mixing of blood from the superior and inferior vena cavae and coronary sinus occurs.

What are the causes of a low SvO_2 and a high SvO_2?

If the SvO_2 value is normal, there is sufficient oxygen supply available to the tissues.

If SvO_2 falls below 60%, a decrease in oxygen delivery and/or an increase in oxygen consumption (e.g. sepsis) should be suspected. Levels below 40% are critical.

If SvO_2 levels are elevated above 80%, an increase in oxygen supply (e.g. increased Fi)2) and/or a decrease in demand (e.g. ventilated or pharmacologically paralysed patient) should be suspected.

Pneumothorax

You are at a trauma call where a 55 year old man has been stabbed in the left upper quadrant of the abdomen and lower chest with a kitchen knife. He is hypotensive, tachycardic and hypoxaemic with oxygen saturations of 79%. On examination you note that he is in respiratory distress and has significantly reduced air entry on the side of the injury.

What is your primary diagnosis and how will you act?

This patient has a tension pneumothorax – this is a clinical diagnosis based on a combination of the history, respiratory distress, cardiovascular instability as well as absent air entry. The patient will need an urgent intercostal chest drain on the affected side as a definitive treatment.

Although there is a role for needle decompression if a chest drain can be inserted swiftly this would be better. You should never wait for a chest X-ray to confirm the diagnosis – only to check that your drain is in the correct position.

There is a delay in setting up for the chest drain. How will you proceed?

Identify the 2nd intercostal space in the mid-clavicular line on the affected side and insert a 14 or 16 gauge cannula into the space entering along the upper border of the rib below. A gush of air will confirm the diagnosis and correct placement. However if this does not work and you still suspect a tension pneumothorax then proceed with the chest drain.

Describe your technique for inserting a chest drain.

- Confirm the correct side for drain insertion

- Prepare the skin with a suitable antiseptic

- Define the triangle of safety – this is bounded by the posterior border of pectoralis major, the anterior border of latissimus dorsi and inferiorly by the chest wall at the 5th intercostal space. It is the area most devoid of muscle

- Infiltrate the skin with local anaesthetic

- Infiltrate the deeper layers down to the parietal pleura – this is the most sensitive layer and should be well infiltrated. Beware of intravascular injection into an intercostal vessel

- Skin incision and blunt dissection straight down to the pleura without tracking (a large clip for this may be required)

- Puncture parietal pleura with clip to enter pleural space. Correct entry will lead to expulsion of some air with an audible sound

- Finger sweep to ensure pleural defect sufficient and no adhesions of lung to chest wall

- Insert and direct tube towards apex with minimal resistance – never use the trocar

- Connect the drain to underwater seal system. If in the correct place the tubing will mist with respiration and the water in the underwater seal will bubble

- Suture in place and obtain a chest X-ray to confirm tube position

What size chest drain would you use and what is French scale?

Generally for a pneumothorax a size 28F drain is sufficient. Trauma teaching tends to recommend use of a 32F drain – this would be suitable for a collection such as a haemothorax.

The French scale (also known as the Charrière scale) describes the size of the tube in relation to the diameter, such that the diameter of the tube in mm is the French size divided by 3. It starts at 1Fr and each increment of French sizing equals 0.33mm. The gauge is a descending scale, opposite the French scale of measurement, which ascends with corresponding size.

How does the underwater seal system work?

The tip of the intercostal drain is placed 2-3 cm below the surface of the water. This then acts as a one way valve system for the drainage of air or fluid preventing flow of air/fluid back into the patient. The underwater seal bottle is filled up to the pre-defined mark ensuring that it is not too shallow (in which case the seal is not adequate and air may entrain back up the tube) or too deep (in which case the pressure created may be too high to expel air from the pleural space).

The nursing staff ask if you would like suction applied to the drain.

A pressure of 10-20 cmH_2O can be applied to increase pleural drainage but is usually not necessary if the drain is correctly positioned and performing its job. If the lung has not fully expanded then suction may be applied.

Can you explain the physiology of a pneumothorax?

In normal respiration a negative transpulmonary pressure exists (-4 to -6 cmH_2O) which prevents the lung from collapsing. When air gains entry into the pleural space the negative transpulmonary pressure is lost and the lung collapses.

What is a sucking chest wound?

This is an open chest wound from trauma and acts as a one way valve leading to air being drawn in with inspiration but trapped during expiration. Ultimately this may lead to a tension pneumothorax as the air flow is unidirectional.

What are the clinical features of a tension pneumothorax?

Mediastinal compression by the expanding mass of air leads to a reduced venous return and fall in cardiac output. This leads to hypotension, tachycardia and may even progress to cardiac arrest. Patients will be tachypnoeic and in respiratory distress. Tracheal deviation may be present. Breath sounds will be reduced on the affected side.

What are the causes of a pneumothorax?

- **Damage to the parietal pleura** may occur most commonly due to penetrating chest trauma. It may also occur from damage to the mediastinal pleura from oesophageal perforation/surgery, tracheostomy, or thoracic spine operations. Gas may also enter the pleural space through defects in the diaphragm during procedures such as laparoscopy – rarely leading to an intra-operative pneumothorax.

- **Damage to the visceral pleura** is usually iatrogenic damage such as CVP line insertion.

- **Damage to the tracheo-bronchial tree** such as during barogenic injury from mechanical ventilation, ruptured bullae, blast injury, and airway trauma. In these cases air dissects and ruptures through the mediastinal pleura.

Post Operative Respiratory Complications

A 79 year old female undergoes a subtotal gastrectomy. She is extubated in theatre and returns to the ward later that evening. You are contacted by the ward sister as the patient is moderately short of breath with SpO_2 of 88%. You instruct her to administer 4 litres of oxygen following which the patient's SpO_2 is 94%. On examination, there are reduced breath sounds at the lung bases. She also reports a pain score of 7/10.

What is the most likely cause of this patient's hypoxemia?

In the immediate postoperative period the most likely cause is atelectasis as a result of a long operation. This affects the most dependent regions of the lung resulting in ventilation-perfusion abnormalities. There may also be a contribution from underventilation due to pain.

Atelectasis comes from the Greek words 'ateles' and 'ektasis' with the literal meaning "incomplete expansion."

What are the consequences of atelectasis?

Atelectasis has two main physiological effects. It increases the work of breathing and leads to ventilation-perfusion mismatch. The latter is due to a lack of ventilation to perfused sections of lung. This type of ventilation/perfusion mismatch is known as a shunt. The increased work of breathing is due to difficulty experienced in reinflating collapsed segments and is akin to trying to inflate a completely collapsed balloon. A ventilation:perfusion mismatch leads to hypoxia and hypercarbia.

Which part of the lung is most prone to atelectasis and why?

The alveoli at the most dependent part of the lung are most vulnerable to atelectasis. These areas are compressed by non-dependent areas and therefore have a lower volume. This favours collapse during expiration. Therefore alveoli in dependent zones are less inflated than those in non-dependent zones and tend to close well before the apical zone.

How should this patient be managed?

Often simple treatment measures are all that is required.

- Supplemental oxygen
- Sit the patient up at 45 degrees wherever possible
- Adequate analgesia e.g. optimising epidural
- Regular chest physiotherapy. Mobilising the patient at an early stage will also be of help

What do you understand by the term functional residual capacity (FRC)?

It is the amount of air that remains at the end of a normal passive expiration i.e. tidal breath. The FRC is the reservoir of gas in the lungs that is continuously available for gas exchange – it is the lung's physiological reserve.

What determines a patient's FRC?

The functional residual capacity is determined by a balance between the compliance of the lung and chest wall. Compliance is the change of lung volume for unit change in pressure. Chest wall compliance may be reduced by factors such as severe obesity or chest trauma. Lung compliance may be reduced by anything that reduces the volume of the lungs such as raised intra-abdominal pressure, pulmonary oedema, fibrosis or consolidation.

What is a ventilation-perfusion mismatch?

Ventilation-perfusion mismatch is where there is an imbalance between ventilation and perfusion. Sections of lung may be relatively poorly perfused or perfusion may be absent, which is termed dead space. Other sections of lung may be relatively poorly ventilated or ventilation may be absent, which is termed shunt.

What is the physiological basis of Positive End Expiratory Pressure (PEEP)?

Alveoli are most vulnerable to collapse at the end of expiration. PEEP acts to splint open the alveoli at the end of expiration – this is known as alveolar recruitment. This will in turn reduce the work of breathing and ventilation:perfusion mismatch. Ultimately this will restore the Functional Residual Capacity (FRC).

Are there any complications associated with the use of PEEP?

Potentially using too much PEEP can cause problems and it is important to give just the correct amount. PEEP may be associated with:

1) Alveolar overdistention particularly affecting the alveoli in non-dependent lung zones. This can potentially lead to barotrauma.

2) Increased dead space through excessive alveolar pressures compressing adjacent blood vessels. This is wasted ventilation and may lead to an increase in the work of breathing.

3) Increased intrathoracic pressure as a result of PEEP may reduce venous return. This may lead to a reduced cardiac output, hypotension and a reduction in end organ perfusion.

What is CPAP? How is it different to PEEP?

CPAP stands for Continous Positive Airway Pressure. It is the application of positive pressure through out the respiratory cycle. Because the pressure is constant, the ventilator does not generate a pressure gradient between the ventilator and the patient. Therefore the patient generates the necessary relative negative pressure to cause gas flow into their lungs and therefore ventilation. Grouping CPAP into Non-invasive Ventilation (NIV) is incorrect. The patient is not ventilated nor is any support to breathing offered.

PEEP refers only to the pressure the ventilator exerts at the end of expiration. By definition a different pressure must occur during inspiration, and this can either be the ventilator giving the patient a breath (mandatory ventilation) or the ventilator supporting a breath that the patient initiates (support ventilation). The ventilator here generates a pressure gradient from the ventilator to the patient and therefore gas flows into the patient's lungs.

Therefore the only difference is in nomenclature. The two have entirely similar physiological effects to prevent atelectasis, increase FRC and improve oxygenation.

What is BIPAP?

BIPAP is biphasic positive airway pressure. It refers to two levels of pressure applied in inspiration and ventilation during mandatory (completely ventilator controlled) ventilation. The higher pressure is applied during inspiration and generates a pressure gradient which results in gas flow into the patient. The lower pressure is the PEEP, which keeps the alveoli open during low volume conditions of expiration. BIPAP is more accurately termed "Mandatory Pressure-controlled Ventilation".

Pre-operative and Peri-operative Care

What are clinical scoring systems? Why are they used?

Scoring systems are objective, evidence-based methods of determining patient risks and outcomes. They allow individual patient risk stratification, which in turn determines, for example, whether a particular treatment is offered (e.g surgery), and if so, the level of peri-operative care that they may require.

The estimation of risk of a particular treatment can also be used to provide the patient with vital information, allowing them to make an informed decision about their care.

Scoring systems are, therefore, a more objective method of quantifying risk than the old-fashioned "end of the bed" test. The ideal scoring system would be easy to use, cheap and accurate in predicting peri- and post-operative risk. However, there is usually a trade-off between these factors, with no current scoring system satisfying all criteria.

What scoring systems are you aware of?

Bedside scoring systems, such as those based on the patient's history and examination findings (eg ASA, Goldman Cardiac Risk Index, Metabolic Equivalents (METS)) are quick and easy to use, but are subject to inter-observer bias and provide only limited information.

Multi-factor scoring systems such as the APACHE are more time-consuming and complicated to calculate, but may provide more comprehensive information regarding risk. Older versions of the APACHE system (APACHE II) may no longer be applicable, as they are based on historical north American datasets and newer versions are costly to healthcare institutions.

A prospectively validated scoring system receiving increasing attention recently is POSSUM (Physiology and Operative Severity Score for the enUmeration of Morbidity and Mortality). It uses 12 "physiological" and 6 "operative" variables and has been found to accurately predict post-operative morbidity and mortality. This has been modified by the Portsmouth group to the P-POSSUM to account for overestimation of morbidity and mortality for "lower risk" procedures (such as laparoscopic appendicectomies in young fit patients).

More recently still, the POSSUM has become "specialty specific," modified with good effect to suit surgical subspecialties, e.g the O-POSSUM for oesophagectomies and the V-POSSUM for some vascular procedures.

What do you understand by cardiopulmonary exercise testing?

Cardiopulmonary exercise testing (CPX- now more commonly CPET) has been used for decades as a lab-based experimental technique to measure the body's physiological response to exercise (i.e a "stress"). However, more recently, a wider availability has led to its use in the pre-operative setting, especially in elderly patients undergoing major surgery.

The CPX variables (including peak oxygen uptake – VO_2 max, anaerobic threshold and ventilatory efficiency) allow measurement of the patient's cardiopulmonary reserve, i.e their ability to respond to the stress of surgery. They are therefore ideally suited to predict outcomes in surgery.

The focus of CPX should not be on using the results to deny surgery to high risk patients, but rather to identify patients preoperatively who will benefit from a higher level of post-operative case in order to optimise their outcomes.

The data pertaining to CPX as a tool for predicting outcome after major surgery are by no means complete but continue to evolve within various surgical specialties.

What do we mean by "pre-optimisation"?

Normal physiological parameters become abnormal (ie insufficient) in the context of a response to stress (eg acute illness, trauma or surgery). Many patients do not have the physiological reserve to deal with this increased demand.

The concept of "pre-optimisation" is therefore the identification of higher risk patients and the use of more intense monitoring (including invasive monitoring) and manipulation of their physiology in order to allow them to deal more effectively with the stress of surgery. This may typically be performed on a critical care unit. Patient parameters that can be optimised include:

- *haemoglobin concentration* (via transfusion) *and arterial oxygen saturation* (oxygen therapy)

- *stroke volume* (restore normovolaemia via fluid resuscitation in patients who are volume-depleted: the use of inotropes)

- *vascular resistance* - the use of vasopressors to tighten the circulation, maintaining blood pressure and therefore organ perfusion pressures.

The concept of pre-optimisation does not pertain to patients with acute instability caused by the surgical insult which will only improve when the surgical pathology has been corrected (such as a perforated viscus).

What methods of haemodynamic monitoring do you know of?

There are a range of methods, both non-invasive and invasive, which reflect the patient's clinical need. Hence methods of monitoring on the ward will be limited to non-invasive, but on the critical care unit may be invasive.

They include:

- *pulse oximetry* - oxygen saturation and heart rate

- *arterial blood pressure* - cuff on ward; arterial line on critical care unit

- *pulmonary artery catheter*

- *pulse contour analysis* (eg PICCO and LiDCO)

- *oesophageal Doppler*

- *mixed venous oxygen saturation*

- *lactate* - simple test that can be performed at the bedside and is a crude indicator of global tissue perfusion.

- *echocardiography*

Should critically ill patients routinely have a pulmonary artery catheter?

No. It was once thought to be the "gold standard" for the measurement of haemodynamic parameters in critically ill patients but recent evidence suggests that patients managed with PAC have no benefit in terms of survival outcomes. Furthermore, PAC can be associated with complications in a significant number of patients (the commonest being arrhythmias on insertion).

Pulmonary Embolism

A 66 year old lady is day 2 following a complicated laparoscopic cholecystectomy and common bile duct exploration. She has no significant past medical history. She becomes acutely short of breath on the ward with SaO_2 of 92% on room air. Chest examination reveals normal bilateral air entry. You are concerned she may have a pulmonary embolism (PE).

How would you investigate her?

The first investigation should be an arterial blood gas. This may confirm hypoxia, which would be suggestive of a PE. The blood gas pattern with a PE can be normal or may show hypoxia with or without a change in pCO_2. A 12 lead ECG should also be done as this may show a sinus tachycardia - the commonest ECG change of a PE. The commonest ECG change is a sinus tachycardia. Other changes include evidence of right heart strain such as right axis deviation, right bundle branch block, S1Q3T3 or T wave inversion in leads V1-4. S1Q3T3 means a large S wave in lead I, large Q wave in V3, T wave inversion in lead III.

The best investigation to confirm the diagnosis would be a CT pulmonary angiogram (CTPA).

The CTPA shows a large embolus close to the bifurcation of the pulmonary arterial bifurcation. She remains haemodynamically stable. What will you do?

Although she is haemodynamically stable she is at major risk of sudden death. I would immediately involve my critical care colleagues, as she should be transferred to a monitored HDU bed, and discuss her case with the on call interventional radiologist to explore the possibility of thrombolysis. I would also discuss her case with the cardiothoracic unit as she may be a candidate for a thrombectomy, which would involve a cardiopulmonary bypass. Anticoagulation with a treatment dose of LMWH must be done.

What is the pathophysiology of a PE?

There is an acute mechanical occlusion by an embolus within a pulmonary artery or one of its branches. The source of the embolus is usually within the deep venous system in the legs (soleus plexus within the calf) or pelvis (external iliac veins/ femoral vein). They may also originate from the IVC or rarely within the heart itself. Hypoxic vasoconstriction then occurs. Furthermore vasoactive mediators such as prostaglandins are released from platelets within the thrombus, leading to increased pulmonary vascular resistance and right ventricular strain. Acute right ventricular pressure overload occurs ultimately leading to right ventricular failure.

The clinical effects of the PE will depend on the size and distribution of the occlusion. A large central PE such as a saddle embolus may lead to sudden collapse or even cardiac arrest. Smaller PEs may not cause much haemodynamic disturbance but may lead to infarction of some lung tissue. Longer term effects include pulmonary hypertension and right heart failure.

What happens to the physiological dead space in a PE?

Arterial occlusion leads to segments of lung that are ventilated but not perfused, leading to a V/Q mismatch. Therefore the physiological dead space increases.

What are the clinical features of a PE?

Symptoms:

- Dyspnoea at rest
- Anxiety
- Pleuritic chest pain and haemoptysis – as a result of pulmonary infarction

Signs:

- Tachypnoea
- Desaturation
- Tachycardia
- Clamminess
- Hypotension
- Evidence of right heart strain e.g. raised JVP or right ventricular heave
- Gallop rhythm on auscultation
- Pleural rub

Many PEs are however asymptomatic.

How would you risk stratify a PE?

Acute PE can be classified into three types: Massive, Submassive or Stable.

- Massive PE is defined by haemodynamic instability (systolic BP<90mmHg) and hypoxia
- Submassive PE is defined as haemodynamically stable but with some evidence of RV dysfunction
- Stable PE occurs in haemodynamically stable patients with no RV dysfunction

How significant are small subsegmental PEs?

These are often picked up on scanning in an asymptomatic patient. Though clinically silent they may herald a much larger PE. Therefore a DVT should be sought and all preventative measures taken to prevent a further PE.

What are the chest X-ray signs of a PE?

The CXR may be normal but otherwise may show:

- Oligaemia of vascular markings beyond the site of occlusion
- Lobar collapse
- Diaphragmatic elevation

Later the following may develop:

- Pleural effusion on ipsilateral side
- Wedge shaped infarct

What are D-dimers?

D-dimer testing measures levels of fibrin-degradation products, which are produced by the action of plasmin on fibrin. D dimers have a sensitivity of 96% for PE. However they have a low specificity, as they can be positive in a range of conditions e.g. cancer patients, infection, injury and inflammatory conditions.

What do you understand by the term 'paradoxical embolisation'?

In a patient with a patent foramen ovale the embolus may pass from the venous circulation direct to systemic, bypassing the lungs. This will present as systemic embolism such as CVA.

What are the national guidelines for VTE prophylaxis for patients who have undergone major abdominal cancer surgery?

Patients undergoing major abdominal surgery for cancer without VTE prophylaxis have a 30% increased risk of VTE compared with those without cancer. Extended venous thromboembolism prophylaxis with low-molecular weight heparin, for 28 days following surgery for cancer, may have a 60% risk reduction for VTE compared with a standard 6-10 day course.

This same patient suddenly develops significant haemodynamic instability with a systolic BP of 80mmHg. Having excluded other causes of her hypotension a diagnosis of massive PE is made. What treatment options are available for her?

Thrombolysis and thrombectomy are treatments reserved for PEs with haemodynamic instability. Approximately 5% of PEs are massive. Thrombolysis is usually given through the peripheral intravenous route although it can also be delivered as catheter directed therapy directly into the pulmonary catheter. Thrombectomy may be performed as an interventional procedure using a special thrombectomy device which can also infuse thrombolytic agents.

What is rivaroxaban?

Rivaroxaban is a direct, highly selective, orally active inhibitor of activated factor X (factor Xa). This means that it blocks factor Xa, an enzyme that is involved in the production of thrombin. It is licensed for the prevention of VTE, prevention of stroke and systemic embolism in adults with non-valvular atrial fibrillation and treatment of deep-vein thrombosis and pulmonary embolism.

Scenario 2

A 57 year old man is admitted with small bowel obstruction and found on CT to have an ileocolic intussusception most likely from a caecal carcinoma. Clinically he has small bowel obstruction. There is no evidence of peritonism. He is haemodynamically stable but clinically and radiologically obstructed.

The CT also showed evidence of an incidentally detected pulmonary embolism in his segmental pulmonary arteries. He needs a right hemicolectomy in the next 24 hours. What are your concerns and how would you address them?

The immediate concern would be of performing a potentially long operation on a patient with a proven PE as well as several underlying risk factors e.g. malignancy. I would be concerned about a serious cardiopulmonary event during or soon after the surgery which would be potentially fatal. Therefore I would discuss his case with my interventional radiology colleagues first to see if he may be a candidate for an IVC filter.

How are IVC filters inserted?

They are performed by interventional radiologists and are either retrievable (temporary) or non retrievable (permanent) filters. These are achieved through either a transfemoral or transjugular route. The patient can then undergo surgery the next day. The filter does not remove the risk of a PE completely as it can be associated with a failure to capture.

What are the problems associated with the use of IVC filters?

Although the overall complication rates are low, problems do exist. Many retrievable IVC filters will become lost to clinical follow up for several reasons e.g. lost to follow up, lack of documentation and lack of haematology clinic review post discharge etc. Retrieval attempts may be unsuccessful in up to 20% of patients. Failure to capture may be associated with pulmonary emboli despite the filter being in place. These filters are also associated with a risk of VTE in the lower limbs including IVC thrombosis and may potentially get infected.

References

Rasmussen MS, Jorgensen LN, Wille-Jorgensen P (2009) Prolonged thromboprophylaxis with low molecular weight heparin for abdominal or pelvic surgery. Cochrane Database of Systematic Reviews issue 1: CD004318

Fulltext: ww.onlinelibrary.wiley.com/doi/10.1002/14651858.CD004318.pub2/full

Pulse Oximetry

What are the principles of the pulse oximeter?

The pulse oximeter utilises the differences in absorption of oxygenated Hb and deoxygenated Hb (DeoxyHb) at different wavelengths of light to measure the saturation of Hb with oxygen.

At 660 nm (red light) wavelength HbO absorbs less than DeoxyHb.

At 940nm (infrared) wavelength HbO absorbs more than DeoxyHb.

The pulse oximeter has two light emitting diodes which transmit red and infra-red light from one side of the probe to the other. The oximeter is able to measure the differences in absorption of the pulsatile component of blood to produce a saturation within arterial blood – SaO_2.

What are the potential sources of error?

Loss of the pulsatile component of blood flow may occur in hypothermia. Vasoconstriction may result in a poor signal. This may also occur with cardiac arrhythmias.

Use of nail varnish or presence of nicotine stain can impede light absorption. Nail varnish should therefore be removed preoperatively.

Jaundiced patient – bilirubin being a pigment has a similar absorption profile to deoxyhaemoglobin, therefore will give abnormally low readings.

Abnormal haemoglobin: Carboxyhaemoglobinaemia will give an abnormally high SaO_2 reading due to its high affinity for O_2. This is seen in CO poisoning or heavy smoking.

Methaemoglobinaemia has an identical absorption at both wavelengths and produces a consistent saturation of approximately 85%.

What does the pulse oximeter not tell you about respiratory status?

It does not measure ventilation, therefore a patient may be in Type II respiratory failure with a high pCO_2 but may have normal SaO_2 despite a rising CO_2 level.

What areas can the pulse oximeter be applied to?

Usually tip of the finger but ear lobes and toes may be used.

Renal Replacement Therapy

What is the difference between dialysis and filtration?

Two fundamental processes underlie continuous renal replacement therapy – diffusion and convection.

Dialysis – blood is pumped through an extracorporeal system that incorporates a dialyser. Within the dialyser solutes diffuse into the dialysate fluid across a semipermeable membrane down a concentration gradient. In order to maintain concentration gradients and enhance efficiency of the system an electrolyte solution runs countercurrent to blood flowing on the other side of the semipermeable filter. Small molecules e.g. urea are removed effectively, but larger molecules are poorly removed. The solute removal is directly proportional to the dialysate flow rate.

Ultrafiltration – Blood is pumped through an extracorporeal system with a semi-permeable membrane. The hydrostatic pressure that is created on the blood-side of the filter drives plasma water across the filter by convection. This process is referred to as *ultrafiltration* – a similar process to the normal kidney. The ultrafiltration rate depends upon the porosity of the membrane and the hydrostatic pressure of the blood, which depends upon blood flow. Larger molecules can also be effectively removed e.g. middle-sized molecules, which are thought to cause uraemia and cytokines of sepsis. The filtered fluid (ultrafiltrate) is discarded and a replacement fluid is added in an adjustable fashion according to the desired fluid balance.

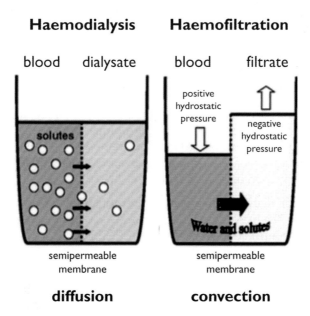

Figure 1: Principles of dialysis (diffusion) and filtration (convection).

What are the indications for dialysis?

- Oliguria (urine output <200 mL/12 h)

- Anuria/extreme oliguria (urine output <50 mL/12 h)

- Hyperkalemia ([K] >7 mmol/L)

- Severe acidemia (pH <7.1)

- Azotemia ([urea] >30 mmol/l or creatinine>300 mmmol/l)

- Pulmonary oedema

Other indications include:

- Uraemic complication e.g. encephalopathy / pericarditis / neuropathy / myopathy

- Temperature control (hyper or hypothermia)

- Drug/toxin overdose

What different modes of dialysis are available?

1) Intermittent haemodilalysis (IH) is considered to be the gold standard method but patients have to be haemodynamically stable. IH has a high flow and clearance rate, and patients only require 3-4 hours of dialysis, two or three times a week. Large amounts of fluid are removed from the intravascular space. Thus electrolyte abnormalities can also be rapidly corrected. The set up is a double lumen catheter, a pump which forces blood into a filter (semi permeable membrane) a dialysate (usually deionized water) which flows in and out, and a return line to the patient. The blood flow rate is 200-400ml/minute. There are huge swings in fluid between the intravascular and extravascular compartments, causing transient hypotension and disequilibrium that is poorly tolerated by ICU patients.

2) Continuous filtration techniques are more physiological for the patient and better tolerated. Continuous techniques lead to more effective urea clearance and more controlled fluid removal. A number of modes are available of which continuous venovenous haemofiltration is the most commonly used in ICU patients – see below.

3) Peritoneal dialysis (PD) has the advantage of being simple and cost effective. The major disadvantages of PD are poor solute clearance, poor uraemic control and a risk of peritoneal infection.

Why is IH not a suitable technique for ICU patients?

In general ICU patients are intravascularly depleted from leaky capillaries. The huge swings in fluid between the intravascular and extravascular compartments cause transient hypotension. The hypotension may worsen the pre-existing renal injury by increasing the ischaemic insult. Many ICU patients cannot tolerate this. 20%-30% of patients with ARF who are being hemodialysed become hypotensive, with huge associated osmotic shifts.

What is the dialysis disequilibrium syndrome?

The dialysis disequilibrium syndrome is a self-limiting condition that is typically seen following dialysis in extremely uraemic patients. As solutes are rapidly cleared from the bloodstream transient hypo-osmolality may occur. This may lead to the rapid movement of water into brain cells. Clinically this presents as nausea, vomiting, headaches, altered consciousness, and rarely seizures or coma.

What is the concept behind continuous RRT?

IHD is an intermittent therapy unlike the normal kidney. Indeed CRRT, by its nature, clears more urea, creatinine and fluid than IHD. The concept behind continuous RRT is to dialyse patients in a more physiologic way, slowly, over 24 hours, just like the kidney. Intensive care patients are particularly suited to these techniques as they are, by definition, bed bound, and, when acutely sick, intolerant of the fluid swings associated with IHD. Most of these modes can remove up to 1 litre per hour of fluid. It is rare that this volume of fluid removal is required in intensive care (critically ill patients rarely tolerate any significant fluid removal).

What techniques of continuous renal replacement therapy do you know of?

The techniques used are:

Continuous Venovenous Haemofiltration (CVVH). It is the commonest form used in critically ill patients. It is a form of convective dialysis. Access is achieved by cannulation of a large central vein with a double lumen catheter. Blood is then drawn through the outflow limb and a roller pump draws blood through the filter to return it via the inflow limb of the cannula. Blood flow is usually between 150 and 200 ml/min and a fluid exchange rate of 35ml/kg/day is recommended. This form of dialysis does not depend on the critically ill patient's blood pressure but does require accessible large veins.

Continuous Venovenous Haemodialysis (CVVHD) – which is continuous diffusive dialysis, the dialysate is driven in a direction countercurrent to the blood. This provides reasonably effective solute clearance, although mostly small molecules are removed.

Continuous Venovenous Haemodiafiltration (CVVHDF), which is the most popular method of dialysis in ICU, combines convective and diffusive dialysis. Both small and middle molecules are cleared, and both dialysate and replacement fluids are required.

Continuous Arteriovenous Haemofiltration/Haemodialysis – are rarely used. This requires cannulation of an artery and vein, hence a higher rate of complications. The arterio-venous pressure gradient drives blood through the circuit.

What are the advantages of continuous RRT?

Continuous RRT is a slower and more gentle and 'physiological' effect on the patient's cardiovascular system. This means that it is suitable for more haemodynamically unstable patients. Large volumes of fluid can still be required by these methods. The larger size of the filter membrane allows removal of cytokines and inflammatory mediators.

What are the disadvantages of continuous RRT?

Anticoagulation – to prevent extracorporeal circuit from clotting

Complications of line insertion and sepsis

Risk of line disconnection

Hypothermia

Severe depletion of electrolytes – particularly K+ and PO4

Why is anticoagulation needed for RRT?

Although anticoagulation is necessary to prevent clotting of the filter as blood comes into contact with it, this may be a problem in patients who are at risk for bleeding (deranged clotting, thrombocytopenia) or recent surgery. No anticoagulation has been used in patients with good venous access as well as deranged clotting.

What are the potential drawbacks of using heparin?

Systemic anticoagulation comes with a risk of bleeding. Many ICU patients have coagulopathy or thrombocytopenia. Heparin requires the presence of antithrombin III, which is often deficient in the ICU population. Heparin also carries the risk of causing Heparin Induced Thrombocytopenia (HIT) syndrome.

Alternative agents that have been used instead of heparin include prostacyclin which has an anti platelet effect, citrate, which binds calcium and inhibits the coagulation cascade, Low molecular weight heparin, hirudin and aprotinin.

What electrolyte disturbances in particular should be monitored for?

Levels of potassium and phosphate can drop very low as the standard dialysate solutions contain neither. Supplementation is often necessary. There is no sodium bicarbonate either in the dialysate, leading to loss of bicarbonate. This is compensated for by the passage of lactate into the blood.

Rhabdomyolysis

An 84 year old lady was found collapsed at home for an undetermined period of time. She was responsive GCS10 but hypotensive 80/50mmHg and noted to have a marked metabolic acidosis pH:7.1, HCO3-= 12 lactate: 5.0mmol/l. Her serum amylase was elevated at 3300u/l and she is in acute renal failure. She is transferred to the intensive care unit for further management.

What do you think may be the cause of her acute renal failure?

The acute renal failure may be pre-renal in origin from hypovolaemia, which may be secondary to the massive fluid loss from her acute pancreatitis. The other potential cause is rhabdomyolysis from a crush injury, as she may have been lying dormant on the floor for a considerable period of time.

What further investigations would you request?

I would request a serum creatine kinase (CK) as well as renal tract ultrasound to exclude any obstructive cause, though the latter would be less likely. Her urine can be dipstick tested for myoglobinuria as well but this is not always accurate as haemoglobin may also react positive – this may be seen if the patient has haemolysis or even a UTI.

What is rhabdomyolysis?

Rhabdomyolysis is a potentially life-threatening complication from the breakdown of skeletal muscle and release of intracellular toxins.

What is the pathophysiology of acute renal failure in this condition?

Myonecrosis is most commonly seen in the postural muscles (thigh, calf and back most commonly involved) and leads to the release of large quantities of potassium, phosphate, CK and LDH. Myoglobin is produced in excess and binds to a protein (Tamm-Horsfall protein) in the thick ascending limb of the loop of Henle leading to the formation of a precipitate, leading to tubular obstruction with subsequent ARF. The risk of ARF correlates with the level of CK. Once CK levels rise above 5000 U/l the risk of ARF is significantly higher.

What is myoglobin?

Myoglobin is an oxygen binding protein found in skeletal and cardiac muscle. It consists of a single globin chain with a single haem component. It acts as a source of oxygen for muscle during times of increased activity. Myoglobinuria produces a characteristic reddish brown "tea-coloured" urine.

How is rhabdomyolysis diagnosed?

The most sensitive marker for muscle injury is CK activity, particularly the CK-MM isoenzyme subtype. CK levels are elevated between 2 to 12 hours of muscle damage.

For chronic rhabdomyolysis muscle biopsy may be required to make the diagnosis e.g. following drug-induced rhabdomyolysis.

What electrolyte disturbances can occur with rhabdomyolysis?

- Hyperkalaemia - often potassium levels rise sharply to dangerous levels which may be associated with risk of cardiac arrhythmias. Haemofiltration may be required.

- Hyperphosphataemia – leads to deposition of calcium phosphate in soft tissue leading to sequestration hypocalcaemia.

- Hypermagnaesaemia.

What are the other causes of rhabdomyolysis?

The other causes are due to either direct muscle injury or excessive muscle contraction:

From direct muscle injury:

- Blunt traumatic crush injury e.g. prolonged compression trapping – fire/earthquake

- Reperfusion injury

- Burns

- Electrocution

- Cold injury

- Compartment syndrome of the extremities

From excessive muscle contraction:

- Status asthmaticus

- Taser gun injuries

Other causes include drug-induced e.g. statins

What measures can be taken to prevent ARF in a patient with rhabdomyolysis?

For the patient at risk, aggressive fluid resuscitation in the patient is the key to preventing myoglobinuric ARF. The use of alkalinisation of the urine by sodium bicarbonate infusion is controversial but has been performed to limit myoglobin induced tubular deposition. The use of osmotic diuretic e.g. mannitol is controversial. There is some evidence to show that the early use of haemodialysis to remove myoglobin may reduce the incidence of ARF.

Sedation

Your registrar is about to do a colonoscopy and administers 3mg of midazolam and 50mcg of fentanyl intravenously to an 84 year old man with COPD and IHD. He desaturates to 77% with a heart rate of 45 bpm, and despite administration of oxygen does not improve his saturation. How would you proceed?

Clearly this patient is having significant cardiorespiratory depression following administration of a high dose of a benzodiazepine. Respiratory depression is more common when an opiate is co-administered. He is not responding to the administration of oxygen. I would reverse the effect of the agent with flumazenil (250mcg up to 500mcg) and naloxone (50mcg up to 400mcg). However this may take several minutes to completely reverse benzodiazepine respiratory depression. The duration of action of both opioids and benzodiazepines is longer than that of their antagonist and reversal may be short-lived, needing repeat administration.

After termination of the procedure assisted ventilation should be given and the critical care team called if deemed necessary. Should the patient improve with these measures I would ensure that he is monitored closely in recovery and kept for an overnight stay.

What recommendations do you give a patient following the use of sedation?

Patients who have been sedated with an intravenous benzodiazepine should not drive a car, operate machinery, sign legal documents or drink alcohol for 24 hours. This is irrespective of whether their sedation has been reversed with flumazenil. Day cases should be accompanied home by a responsible adult who should then stay with them for at least 12 hours if they live alone.

What do you understand by the term conscious sedation?

Conscious sedation has been defined as "a technique in which the use of drug or drugs produces a state of depression of the central nervous system enabling treatment to be carried out, but during which verbal contact with the patient is maintained throughout the period of sedation."

If verbal responsiveness is lost the patient requires a level of care identical to that needed for general anaesthesia.

What patient groups would you consider to be high risk for sedation?

- Elderly patients – particularly with significant co-morbidities
- Respiratory disease – particularly COPD
- Patients with neuromuscular disease and respiratory weakness
- Patients with bulbar dysfunction
- Cardiovascular disease

- Renal failure
- Liver failure
- Morbid obesity
- Patients in shock
- Alcoholics and regular benzodiazepine users can be very difficult to sedate

What are the basic principles for safe conscious sedation?

- Monitor the patient - always with a nurse present. Visual contact with oxygen saturations, heart rate and BP are vital.
- Use sedative drugs in small doses titrated to the desired effect.
- Any patient risk factors such as age or renal impairment should be noted before the start of sedation.
- Dosage of benzodiazepines and opiates should be kept to a minimum to achieve sedation and opioids should, whenever possible, be given before benzodiazepines. This is to allow their effect to be observed before proceeding.
- Sedated patients must have a reliable intravenous cannula in situ throughout the procedure and recovery period.
- Oxygen should be given to all sedated patients throughout the procedure.
- Pulse oximetry monitoring should be used in all sedated patients.

Can you describe the main pharmacological properties of midazolam, fentanyl and pethidine?

Midazolam: has a short half life making it desirable for endoscopy. It can accumulate in hepatic and renal failure with rapid onset. All benzodiazepines are deliriogenic. Generally when given alone benzodiazepines do not cause significant respiratory depression. When administered with opiates they can have a synergistic cardiorespiratory depressive effect.

Fentanyl: this is more potent than morphine. It has a short duration of action and rapid onset. When given as repeated doses it can accumulate and have a prolonged action. All opiates have a respiratory depressive effect. They are in the main negatively inotropic and chronotropic.

Pethidine: myocardial depression can occur with high doses. Accumulates in liver and renal failure.

Shock

A 55 year old HGV driver is hit by a truck leading to a trauma call. He has a history of previous MIs. The patient had to be extricated and resuscitated en route to hospital. On arrival he has a GCS of 15, BP 70/40mmHg, pulse 120 bpm, peripherally shutdown and tachypnoeic. He has significant pain in the left chest with paradoxical movement. Arterial blood gas shows pH 7.21, pCO_2 is 6kPa, PO_2 6 kPa, BE -12 and HCO3 17 mmol/L. He has a large left haemothorax for which a chest drain has been placed and has drained one litre of blood.

Describe the physiological compensatory mechanisms that occur in hypovolaemic shock.

The immediate response is to redistribute the cardiac output to preserve blood supply to essential organs such as the brain and myocardium. This is achieved through sympathetic nervous system stimulation, which in turn leads to peripheral and splanchnic vasoconstriction with subsequent blood redistribution. The reduction in circulating blood volume leads to baroreceptor inhibition (stretch receptors in carotid sinus and aortic arch) and sympathetic activation. In addition the release of circulating stress response hormones such as adrenaline further potentiates vasoconstriction and blood redistribution.

A more delayed response occurs in the hypothalamic-pituitary-adrenal axis. The reduced renal perfusion leads to the conversion of angiotensinogen to angiotensin I which leads to formation of angiotensin II (AII). AII is a highly potent vasoconstrictor that stimulates aldosterone release from the adrenal cortex and the release of ADH from the posterior pituitary. This then leads to water and sodium conservation.

Why does hypovolaemic shock lead to a metabolic acidosis?

Shock is defined as a reduction in tissue perfusion and inadequate delivery of oxygen to meet a tissue's metabolic needs. The reduced perfusion leads to a decline in aerobic metabolism, which ultimately leads to anaerobic metabolism. Hypoxia eventually blocks the citric acid cycle leading to formation of pyruvate, which is converted to lactate. The lactate diffuses out of cells to accumulate as lactic acid, hence a metabolic acidosis (Type A lactic acidosis).

What is the normal blood lactate?

Normal blood lactate is 0.6-1.2mmol/L. Levels >4mmol/L are significant. Levels >9 mmol/L are associated with a 80% mortality.

- Type A lactic acidosis is caused by poor tissue perfusion as seen in shock.
- Type B lactic acidosis is caused by medications (e.g.metformin or adrenaline) or rare metabolic abnormalities.

What are the physiological effects of a metabolic acidosis?

An acidosis leads to a negative inotropic effect as well as arteriolar dilatation. These changes lead to a reduction of cardiac output and blood pressure.

A right shift of the oxygen haemoglobin dissociation curve occurs (Bohr effect) to promote the release of oxygen to tissues.

Explain the physiological basis for the clinical features seen in this patient.

- Cold peripheries, pallor, oliguria and tachycardia are due to redistribution of blood flow from sympathetic activity

- Tachypnoea is due to stimulation of carotid chemoreceptors by pO_2, pH and pCO_2

- Pulse pressure narrows, as a result of a rise in diastolic BP, and is a more reliable indicator than systolic BP, which only falls after significant blood loss. Diastolic BP rises as it is influenced by circulating catecholamines

- Confusion is a result of cerebral hypoperfusion

How does the physiological response differ in fit young patients?

Healthy and fit young patients can demonstrate robust compensatory physiological abilities by preserving systolic pressure despite quite significant blood loss (1.5–2.0 L). A narrow pulse pressure is often the earliest sign.

In stark contrast an elderly patient may demonstrate hypotension at an early stage of blood loss. The reduced physiological reserve means that they are less able to respond to sympathetic release of catecholamines with a tachycardia. Such early hypotension may lead to rapid onset of organ failure.

In the context of hypovolaemic shock what is the physiological significance of this patient's past medical history of ischaemic heart disease?

Patients with IHD may develop myocardial insufficiency much earlier and exhibit hypotension at an earlier stage. Such patients may also be on medications that can alter their response to hypovolaemia such as beta-blockers that prevent their ability to mount an appropriate sympathetic response and may also become hypotensive after moderate blood loss.

During the course of resuscitation the patient's core temperature falls to 34°C. What are the sources of hypothermia in such a patient?

Hypothermia (core temperature less than 35°C) is a serious complication and may be due to exposure of the patient, hypoperfusion and infusion of inadequately warmed IV fluids. Hypothermia is an independent predictor of survival in trauma patient.

What are the effects of hypothermia?

- Hypothermia contributes to coagulopathy

- Left shift of the oxyhaemoglobin dissociation curve, thereby increasing the affinity of Hb for oxygen which impairs its release i.e. reduced oxygen delivery

- Shivering may compound the lactic acidosis which typically accompanies hypovolaemia

- Increased propensity to cardiac arrhythmias

- Hyperglycaemia and increased incidence of wound infection

What ratio of blood products (packed cells, FFP and platelets) should be given to those with massive blood loss from hypovolaemic shock?

Conventional teaching suggested transfusing one FFP for every six units of packed cells. Studies in military trauma (and latterly in civilian populations) have indicated that transfusion in a 1:1:1 ratio is associated with improved outcomes. This is because massive blood loss is associated with dilution, consumption of clotting factors, hypothermia and acidosis, which leads to coagulopathy. Timely early transfusion of all blood products helps to minimize this problem.

The Joint United Kingdom Blood Transfusion and Tissue Transplantation Services Professional Advisory Committee (JPAC) have produced guidelines and an algorithm for managing major haemorrhage. This suggests an initial 6 units of red blood cells to 4 units of FFP and if bleeding is ongoing a further 4 units of FFP to 6 units of red cells and consideration of 2 pools of cryoprecipitate and an adult therapeutic dose of platelets.

There is good evidence that tranexamic acid (1 gram over 10 minutes given within 3 hours of the injury, and then an infusion of 1 gram 8 hourly) reduces mortality from bleeding in trauma patients (CRASH 2 study).

What is the role of recombinant factor VII in haemorrhagic shock?

The initial enthusiasm for using this agent has reduced over time based on a multicentre, randomised, placebo-controlled phase III trial that failed to show benefit for this agent in severely injured trauma patients with bleeding refractory to standard treatment.

If coagulopathy persists then the use of recombinant factor VII may still be considered.

What is the classification of haemorrhagic shock?

Hypovolaemic shock is classified according to the degree of blood loss.

	Class I	Class II	Class III	Class IV
Blood loss:				
Percentage	<15	15–30	30–40	>40
Volume (mL)	750	750–1500	1500–2000	>2000
Blood pressure:				
Systolic	Unchanged	Normal	Reduced	Very low
Diastolic	Unchanged	Raised	Reduced	Very low or unrecordable
Pulse (beats/ min)	Slight tachycardia	100–120	120 (thready)	>120 (very thready)
Capillary refill	Normal	Slow (>2 sec)	Slow (>2 sec)	Undetectable
Respiratory rate	Normal	Tachypnoea	Tachypnoea (>20/min)	Tachypnoea (>20/min)
Urinary flow rate (mL/h)	>30	20–30	10–20	0–10
Extremities	Normal	Pale	Pale	Pale, clammy and cold
Complexion	Normal	Pale	Pale	Ashen
Mental state	Alert	Anxious or aggressive	Anxious, aggressive or drowsy	Drowsy, confused or unconscious

Based on the clinical findings of hypoxia and paradoxical movement you suspect that this patient has a flail segment. What do you understand by the term flail segment?

A flail segment occurs when a segment of the chest wall does not have continuity with the rest of the chest wall. This leads to paradoxical movement of the flail segment. Clinically the segment may be palpable and associated with crepitus.

What are the causes of hypoxia in this patient?

This patient has severe chest trauma leading to a flail segment. This results in significant pain and limits tidal ventilation. Flail segments are associated with pulmonary contusions which cause hypoxia as well.

References

ATLS manual

ABC of Major Trauma, 4th Edition. Hypovolaemic Shock; BMJ 2014; 348

Joint United Kingdom Blood Transfusion and Tissue Transplantation Services Professional Advisory Committee (JPAC) http://www.transfusionguidelines.org.uk

SIRS/Sepsis

What is the definition of SIRS?

The systemic inflammatory response syndrome (SIRS) is defined as a standardised response of the body to a wide variety of clinical insults, both infective (e.g pneumonia, urinary sepsis, surgical site infection) and non-infective (including acute pancreatitis, trauma or surgery).

It is manifested by two or more of the following:

- Temperature >38°C or < 36°C

- Heart rate > 90 beats/minute

- Respiratory rate > 20 breaths/minute or $PaCO_2$ less than 4.3 kPa

- White cell count of >12 or <4 (or with more than 10% immature forms)

SIRS therefore comprises an inflammatory response in the absence of an identifiable pathogen or need for circulatory support making it distinct from sepsis and its variants.

How do you define "sepsis"?

Sepsis is defined as the presence of the systemic inflammatory response syndrome (SIRS) with evidence of infection.

Sepsis is defined according to the criteria originally established by the American College of Chest Physicians (ACCP) and the Society of Critical Care Medicine in 1992 (led by Dellinger and colleagues). Their aim was to create broad and universal definitions using specific physiological parameters so that sepsis could be identified and treated quickly.

What is the definition of severe sepsis?

Other terms were defined in the original paper:

Severe sepsis: sepsis with organ dysfunction or failure.

Septic shock: sepsis with persistent hypotension despite fluid resuscitation.

Multi-organ dysfunction syndrome (MODS): organ dysfunction in an acutely unwell patient that requires intervention to prevent irreversible organ damage. Dysfunction is the inability of the organ to maintain homeostasis.

What is the Surviving Sepsis Campaign?

The Surviving Sepsis Campaign is a quality improvement initiative introduced in 2002 spearheaded by Dellinger and colleagues. As sepsis is a leading cause of death on critical care units and surgical wards, this collaborative aimed to improve the early identification and treatment of sepsis, which has been shown to significantly decrease mortality. The campaign has developed a number of guidelines and has a dedicated website (*www.survivingsepsis.org*). The third edition of the Surviving Sepsis Guidelines have recently been published. The Surviving Sepsis Campaign also publishes a manual and conducts regular training courses.

What are the Surviving Sepsis Campaign bundles?

"Bundles" are simplified protocols distilled from evidence-based guidelines, which involve early diagnosis and management of patients with sepsis. They suggest the following:

To be completed within 3 hours:

- Measurement of serum lactate

- Blood cultures prior to administration of broad spectrum antibiotics

- Volume resuscitation with boluses of crystalloid (up to 30ml/kg) if lactate > 4 or hypotensive

To be completed within 6 hours:

- repeat lactate if original lactate > 4

- with persistent hypotension despite initial resuscitative measures above, measure central venous pressure and central venous oxygen saturation (therefore needing a central line)

- for hypotension unresponsive to initial volume resuscitation, consider vasopressors to maintain mean arterial blood pressure > 65 mmHg

Using principles of goal-directed therapy, aim for a central venous pressure of > 8 mmHg, central venous oxygen saturations of > 70% and normalisation of serum lactate. The use of CVP-guided fluid therapy and lactate as a physiological endpoint have been challenged on the basis of recent physiological and clinical studies, and the beneficial effects of protocol-guided resuscitation seen in early studies has not been replicated by a more recent randomised controlled trial.

What are the "Sepsis Six"?

The Sepsis Six refers to six basic interventions which can be administered by junior doctors on suspecting the presence of sepsis; ideally they should be administered within an hour of identification of sepsis to optimise outcomes and maximise patient survival (Give 3, take 3).

They are:

1) administer high-flow oxygen

2) take blood cultures

3) start broad spectrum antibiotics

4) give intravenous fluid challenges

5) measure serum lactate and haemoglobin

6) measure accurate hourly urine output

What is meant by "early goal-directed therapy"?

Early goal-directed therapy is a concept that has emerged in parallel with the sepsis guidelines over the past decade. Its principles are the invasive monitoring of oxygenation and haemodynamic parameters in acutely unwell patients in order to maintain physiological parameters within strict pre-determined ranges, tailored to the individual patient's physiological reserve.

Typical physiological goals include:

- urine output > 0.5ml/kg/hr

- central venous oxygen saturations (SvO_2) > 70% (or *mixed* SvO_2 > 65%)

- mean arterial blood pressure > 65mmHg

- central venous pressure > 8mmHg

Goal-directed therapy has more recently been successfully used during the peri-operative period.

There is now evidence that intra-operative cardiac output monitoring coupled with post-operative monitoring on the critical care unit can reduce the onset of subsequent complications on the ward and reduce the length of hospital stay following major surgery. Optimising oxygen and fluid delivery in theatre and on the critical care unit in this way allows the patient's "oxygen debt" (created by the stress response of surgery) to be adequately repaid prior to being transferred to the ward. The onset of a "second hit" to the patient's already stressed physiological reserve on the ward following surgery is therefore avoided. Ideally, patients who benefit most from such a post-operative period on the critical care unit should be identified pre-operatively, for example, by the use of cardiopulmonary exercise testing and physiological scoring systems.

What other methods may be used in the management of sepsis?

- Early iv antimicrobials and source control (eg drainage of abscess)

- Haemodynamic support and optimisation of oxygen delivery (including use of fluid resuscitation, vasopressors, inotropes, respiratory support; and invasive monitoring - central lines, arterial lines, and cardiac output monitoring)

Does "early goal directed therapy" for sepsis lead to improved outcomes?

A study by Rivers et al looked at the effect of goal directed therapy (GDT) prior to admission to intensive care. Most outcome studies of GDT had looked at outcome following intervention after ICU admission. In a prospective RCT of 263 patients to either standard care or GDT prior to ICU admission, they showed reduced mortality in the GDT group (30.5% vs 46.5% p<0.009). The main benefit was believed to be due to early aggressive fluid resuscitation.

References

Dellinger RP *et al.* Surviving Sepsis Campaign: International Guidelines for Management of Severe Sepsis and Septic Shock: 2012. *Crit Care Med* 2013; 41:580–637

Rivers E, Nguyen B, Havstad S, et al. Early goal-directed therapy in the treatment of severe sepsis and septic shock. N Engl J Med. 2001;345:1368-1377.

Cecconi M, Corredor C, Arulkumaran N, Abuella G, Ball J, Grounds RM, Hamilton M, Rhodes A. Clinical review: Goal-directed therapy-what is the evidence in surgical patients? The effect on different risk groups. Crit Care. 2013 Mar 5; 17(2):209.

Stress Response to Surgery

How do you define the stress response to surgery?

The stress response to surgery is defined as the profound and widespread metabolic and hormonal changes in response to surgery or major trauma. It is important to understand, as the morbidity and mortality from surgery can to some extent be influenced by our ability to control the response.

What are the main components of the stress response?

The main components of the response are a neuroendocrine response and an acute inflammatory response. The neuroendocrine response consists of:

- Sympathetic stimulation due to release of adrenal medullary catecholamines mediated via the hypothalamus. This leads to stimulation of the renal angiotensin system and vasoconstriction.

- Hypothalamic pituitary axis – stimulation of the anterior pituitary by the hypothalamus leads to ACTH release and subsequent release of adrenal glucocorticoids. The posterior pituitary releases ADH.

- The neuroendocrine response results in the release of catabolic hormones such as catecholamines, cortisol and pituitary hormones whereas anabolic hormones such as insulin and testosterone are suppressed. Cortisol released from the adrenal cortex is the main hormone that drives intense catabolism (protein breakdown, gluconeogenesis and lipolysis) and antagonises the effects of insulin through insulin resistance. Insulin is an anabolic hormone but the catabolic effects of cortisol override it.

The acute inflammatory response consists of cytokine release and increases in pro-inflammatory cells (e.g.macrophages). Cytokines are the principal mediators of an acute inflammatory response that occurs in response to tissue injury. A variety of cytokines are involved, which may act in a paracrine (local) manner or systemic manner. For example interleukin 1 (IL-1) mediates fever and interleukin 6 mediates the acute phase protein response. There is much individual variation in the systemic inflammatory response to surgery, which can influence the general condition of the patient.

IL-6 is the most important cytokine associated with surgery. Peak circulating levels are found 12–24 hours after surgery. The magnitude of the IL-6 response is a reflection of the degree of tissue damage.

What factors may modify the extent of the stress response in a patient?

The magnitude of the response may be influenced by a number of factors:

Patient-related factors are important such as a genetic pre-disposition to inflammatory mediators, immune status of the patient, medications e.g. steroids / immunosuppressants and nutritional status.

Surgical factors are important such as the severity of surgery/trauma. The greater the extent of tissue damage the greater the response e.g. major burns. The presence of co-existing infection may result in an exaggerated response. The use of minimally invasive surgery may result in lesser surgical trauma and faster recovery.

Anaesthetic factors can modulate the response. Regional anaesthetic techniques (epidural or spinal anaesthesia) may reduce the release of cortisol, adrenaline and other pro-inflammatory hormones. Opioids are known to suppress the endocrine response e.g. high doses of fentanyl can markedly reduce the hormonal response to pelvic and abdominal surgery. Maintenance of normothermia is highly beneficial in reducing the extent of the metabolic response to surgery.

Why do patients develop a reduced urine output following surgery?

The neuroendocrine response results in the activation of the renin angiotensin aldosterone system (RAAS), which acts to conserve body water as a direct effect of aldosterone on the collecting ducts and by stimulating the release of ADH. ADH release results in water retention, concentrated urine, and potassium loss, and may continue for 3–5 days after surgery.

Can you describe the steps involved in activation of RAAS?

Renin is secreted from the juxtaglomerular cells of the kidney secondary to sympathetic activation. Plasma renin then carries out the conversion of angiotensinogen released by the liver to angiotensin I. Angiotensin I is subsequently converted to angiotensin II by the enzyme angiotensin-converting enzyme (ACE) - an enzyme found in the lungs. Angiotensin II is not only a potent vasoconstrictor but also releases aldosterone from the adrenal cortex promoting sodium and water retention from the distal convoluted tubule. This increases the volume of fluid in the body, which also increases blood pressure.

What are the metabolic effects of the stress response on carbohydrate, lipid and protein metabolism?

Hyperglycaemia is a major feature of the metabolic response to surgery and results from an increase in glucose production at the same time as a reduction in glucose utilization. This is mainly due to increased glycogenolysis and gluconeogenesis driven by catecholamines, cortisol and glucagon. Peripheral insulin resistance and reduced insulin production also play an important part. Glucose concentrations >12 mmol/l can adversely affect wound healing and infection rates.

Protein catabolism is driven by cytokine release. Major abdominal surgery may result in loss of up to 0.5-1 kg/day–1 of lean body mass, which can cause significant muscle wasting and weight loss of upto 0.5-1kg/day of lean body mass. Skeletal muscle protein is mainly affected. Amino acids are also used for gluconeogenesis to maintain circulating blood glucose.

Lipolysis is promoted by the increased catecholamine, cortisol and glucagon secretion. Triglycerides are metabolized to fatty acids and glycerol. Glycerol is used in gluconeogenesis and free fatty acids are converted in the liver to ketone bodies through acetyl coenzyme A. These ketone bodies (β-hydroxybutyrate, acetoacetate and acetone) are an important energy source for the brain and myocardium.

Temperature Regulation

What is a normal core body temperature?

Core body temperature is maintained at between 36.5°C and 37.5°C

Why is maintenance of body temperature important?

Temperature homeostasis is important for optimal enzymatic function. Denaturation of proteins occur below 32°C, with loss of consciousness below 30°C. Hypothermia may be classified as mild, moderate or severe.

Why is peri-operative heat loss important to the surgeon?

Inadvertent peri-operative hypothermia is a common but preventable complication associated with poor outcomes for patients. There is good evidence that prevention of peri-operative heat loss may reduce infection rates and decrease hospital stay.

What are the mechanisms of heat loss?

There are five mechanisms of heat loss in the surgical patient:

Radiation: The body is a very efficient radiator and accounts for 40% or more of heat loss and is the main mechanism. Radiation is the process by which heat is transferred from a hot to a cooler object.

Convection: Convection currents remove air in the layer that is warmed by conduction. This accounts for 30% of heat loss.

Evaporation: Particularly important during exposure of a large moist surface area e.g. intra-abdominal surgery – moisture on the body evaporates, accounting for 25% of heat loss.

Conduction: Not a significant cause of heat loss and only so if the patient is in unprotected contact with a cool surface e.g. metal table, surgeon pouring in cold fluids during washout etc..

Respiration: Heat loss through heating of inspired air. This accounts for 10% of total heat loss.

What are the clinical effects of hypothermia?

Oxygen consumption can increase by 500% during shivering as a patient rewarms. The oxen-Hb dissociation curve left shifts, thereby reducing oxygen delivery.

Cardiac output falls with hypothermia

Cardiac arrhythmias are more common

Metabolic acidosis is more common and renal and hepatic function suppressed

Wound infection rates are increased

What measures can be taken to prevent inadvertent hypothermia?

All patients who are having anaesthesia for longer than 30 minutes should be warmed intra-operatively from induction of anaesthesia using a forced air warming device.

Induction of anaesthesia should not begin unless the patient's temperature is 36°C or above unless surgery is for bleeding or ischaemia.

Forced air warming should be maintained throughout the intraoperative phase and the patient's temperature should be measured and documented before induction of anaesthesia and then every 30 minutes until the end of surgery.

Intravenous fluids (500 ml or more) and blood products should be warmed to 37°C using a fluid warming device.

Post-operatively ward transfer should not be arranged unless the patient's temperature is 36°C or above. If the patient's temperature is below 36°C, they should be actively warmed using forced air warming until they are discharged from the recovery room or until they are comfortably warm.

Tracheostomy

You are looking after surgical HDU where a 57 year old man is recovering from a laparotomy for blunt abdominal and chest trauma. He has a laparostomy. He had a percutaneous tracheostomy performed one week ago. He has a single lumen cuffed tracheostomy in situ, which has not been changed. He is in respiratory distress with a respiratory rate of 40/min, heart rate 120/min, SpO$_2$ 81%.

How will you approach this scenario?

I would approach this patient by assessing and managing their Airway, Breathing and Circulation as a priority. Specifically in terms of his airway it is vital to ensure he has a patent tracheostomy. I would immediately call for critical care/anaesthetic help as a matter of urgency. I would then administer 100% O$_2$ via a facemask as well as via the tracheostomy as the upper airway may still be patent. The patency of the tracheostomy can be checked with a suction catheter which may not pass if the tracheostomy is blocked. If the tracheostomy is blocked I may be able to remove the inner tube. If the patient continues to deteriorate then he may need to be intubated per orally and ventilated.

How could the tracheostomy have been prevented from occluding?

Meticulous tracheostomy care is absolutely essential with regular suction by healthcare staff competent to look after the tracheostomy, the use of humidification and a double lumen tracheostomy with a cleanable inner tube.

The NAP 4 audit project highlighted critical care as a high risk area for critical incidents pertaining to airway management with a high mortality and morbidity when such incidents occur. Many of these incidents were related to tracheostomies. A subsequent NCEPOD report has found deficiencies in tracheostomy care and made recommendations to improve patient safety.

What are the advantages and disadvantages of using a double cannula tracheostomy tube?

Advantages:

- Able to remove inner tube and clean easily
- Less likely to obstruct
- Vocalisation can be facilitated by the use of a fenestrated tube

Disadvantages:

- Increased breathing resistance compared to a similar external diameter single lumen tube

- Often need an inner tube (which may have been misplaced) to connect to a breathing circuit in an emergency

- Still need replacing after 30 days (10-14 days for simple single lumen tracheostomies)

How easy would it be to replace a percutaneous tracheostomy once removed?

A percutaneous tracheostomy will be difficult to change within the first 7-10 days as the tract will occlude quickly. Therefore it may be necessary to re-fashion a new tracheostomy. A surgical tracheostomy is more likely to have a well defined track.

What are the indications for a tracheostomy?

The indications include:

- Prolonged mechanical ventilation

- Chronic respiratory insufficiency

- Failure of airway protective reflexes

- To facilitate the removal of pulmonary secretions

- To protect the airway, as the patient was at high risk of aspiration

- Laryngectomy

What may be the benefits of using a tracheostomy?

- include improved patient comfort

- reduced sedative drug use

- faster weaning from mechanical ventilation

- reduced incidence of nosocomial pneumonia

- shorter hospitalization

There is no evidence to support early tracheostomy formation when compared to later tracheostomy formation. A large multi centre RCT involving patients receiving mechanical ventilation treated in adult critical care departments in the UK found that tracheostomy within 4 days of admission to the critical care unit was not associated with an improvement in 30-day mortality. (TrachMan randomised trial). Serious complications may arise from a tracheostomy, and it important that it is not necessarily regarded as being a safer alternative to an endotracheal tube.

Are there any advantages to performing a percutaneous tracheostomy over surgical tracheostomy?

Percutaneous tracheostomy (PCT) at the bedside in ICU is increasingly popular. Studies have shown that use of PCT is associated with a reduced incidence of wound infection, major peri-procedural and long term complication. These results suggest that PCT, performed electively in the ICU, should be the method of choice for performing tracheostomies in critically ill adult patients.

Why is it necessary to humidify the inspired gases used for a tracheostomy?

Compressed air and oxygen used for ventilation in hospitals is both cold and dry. Since a tracheostomy tube bypasses the upper airway which normally provides heat and humidification to inspired gases, a replacement mechanism is important, in order to assist with clearance of thick and/or infected secretions. As discussed, the use of an inner cannula is recommended as a standard part of tracheostomy tube design and care and is used alongside good humidification to prevent blockage with secretions. Patency is ensured by regular cleaning.

The most common method used is hot water humidification which may be seen by many as the 'gold standard'. However, there is no apparent consensus - whilst hot water humidification is used in about two thirds of cases it is not universal, and the next most common method is a heat and moisture exchanger, which though relatively cheap and simple will not provide such a high level of humidification.

What are the basic steps to performing a percutaneous tracheostomy?

A percutaneous tracheostomy is less invasive, and usually performed under general anaesthesia or deep sedation. It is often performed in a critical care unit. The technique requires a small skin incision in the midline of the neck and a tract is then created down to the trachea. Under fibreoptic airway endoscopic observation a needle and guide wire are inserted into the tracheal lumen. The tract is then dilated, and a tracheostomy tube inserted over the dilator. The diameter and length of the tube used should be appropriate for the size and anatomy of the individual patient.

What are the basic steps to performing a surgical tracheostomy?

Usually this is performed under general anaesthesia. A skin incision is made of about 3-6cm in length, between the cricoid cartilage and the sternal notch, and blunt dissection is employed to identify the trachea under direct vision. Any blood vessels can be tied or coagulated during the dissection. A scalpel is used to make an opening on the tracheal wall. Either a vertical slit opening, removal of a piece of cartilage to create a window, or Björk flap are created. The tracheostomy tube is then inserted into the tracheal lumen under direct vision. The endotracheal tube is carefully partially withdrawn. Once the position of the tracheostomy tube is confirmed the inserted endotracheal tube is fully removed. The diameter and length of the tube used should be appropriate for the size and anatomy of the individual patient.

References

NAP4 Report and findings of the 4th National Audit Project of The Royal College of Anaesthetists. http://www.rcoa.ac.uk/nap4

Young D, Harrison DA, Cuthbertson BH, Rowan K; TracMan Collaborators. Effect of early vs late tracheostomy placement on survival in patients receiving mechanical ventilation: the TracMan randomized trial. JAMA. 2013 May 22;309(20):2121-9.

Ventilator Associated Pneumonia (VAP)

An 81-year-old man underwent an emergency laparotomy for a perforated segment of ischaemic jejunum. He is a heavy smoker with a history of COPD. He is day 4 post op, on the ICU, and making poor progress on the ventilator. He is pyrexial at 38.5°C and raised WCC 21 with a CRP 350.

How common and significant is ventilator associated pneumonia (VAP)?

VAP is the most common cause of HAI in the ICU. The incidence of VAP increases by as much as 20-fold in mechanically ventilated patients. VAP is associated with a significant increase in length of mechanical ventilation, length of hospital stay and cost of hospital admission. The 2004 ATS guidelines highlighted that crude mortality rate for HAP may be as high as 30% to 70%, but many of these critically ill patients with HAP die of their underlying disease rather than pneumonia. Estimates for VAP-related mortality are higher, with a range of 20% to 60% depending on the patient, severity of disease, specific pathogen isolated, and management.

What is the pathogenesis of VAP?

Aspiration is the most important factor in the pathogenesis of VAP. Delayed gastric emptying and impaired consciousness secondary to sedation also contribute. Leakage around the endotracheal tube leads to local colonisation with oropharyngeal flora. A bacterial biofilm, which is impervious to systemic antibiotics, gradually forms on the inner surface of the endotracheal tube. This, in turn, may progress to ventilator-associated tracheobronchitis (VAT), which is a precursor to VAP. In addition, ventilated patients have neutrophil dysfunction and impaired phagocytosis.

Early onset pneumonia occurs within four days of intubation and mechanical ventilation. It is generally caused by antibiotic-susceptible bacteria. Late onset pneumonia develops after four days and is commonly caused by multidrug resistant pathogens. However, patients who have been in hospital for two or more days before intubation will probably harbour organisms more commonly associated with late onset pneumonia, regardless of the duration of ventilation.

What causative organisms are implicated in VAP?

As with HAP, the dominant organisms in VAP are aerobic Gram-negative bacilli. These organisms are commonly multi-drug resistant (MDR), and may include extended-spectrum beta-lactamase (ESBL) – producing *Klebsiella pneumoniae*, *Acinetobacter baumannii* and *Pseudomonas aeruginosa*. The latter is the most common MDR gram-negative pathogen implicated in VAP.

Below is a table giving the distribution of organisms isolated from cases of ventilator associated pneumonia by bronchoscopic techniques in 24 studies (1989-2000) including 1689 episodes and 2490 pathogens.

Pathogen	Frequency (%)
Pseudomonas aeruginosa	24.4
Acinetobacter spp	7.9
Stenotrophomonas maltophilia	1.7
Enterobacteriaceae (esp. *Klebsiella*)	14.1
Haemophilus spp	9.8
Staphylococcus aureus	20.4
Streptococcus spp	8.0
Streptococcus pneumonia	4.1
Coagulase negative staphylococci	1.4
Neisseria spp	2.6
Anaerobes	0.9
Fungi	0.9
Other (<1% each)	3.8

What measures do you know of that may help reduce the incidence of VAP?

Numerous modifiable risk factors are important in the pathogenesis of VAP. In recognition of the importance of these factors, six of which have been adopted in the Department of Health's "high impact intervention" bundles:

1) Elevation of the head of the bed

   a) Elevation of 30-45 degrees (rather than supine)

2) Sedation level assessment

   a) Daily assessment of sedation, in combination with protocols to accelerate weaning from the ventilator, is important

3) Oral hygiene

   a) Mouthwash with chlorhexidine gluconate (≥1-2% gel or liquid) QDS

   b) Teeth are brushed 12 hourly with standard toothpaste

4) Subglottic aspiration

   a) Suction of subglottic secretions can reduce the risk of VAP

5) Tracheal tube cuff pressure

   a) Endotracheal tube cuff pressure should be maintained to prevent leakage of bacteria

6) Stress ulcer prophylaxis

   a) For high-risk patients, to be reviewed daily

In addition to the factors listed above, other modifiable risk factors should be kept in mind with a view to preventing future cases of VAP:

- Standard infection control measures (Universal Precautions)
    - Staff education and compliance with Universal Precautions
- Surveillance of ICU infections
    - Useful in the detection of MDR pathogens, informing infection control practices and guiding appropriate antimicrobial therapy
- Intubation and mechanical ventilation
    - Intubation and reintubation should be avoided, if possible
    - Noninvasive ventilation should be used whenever appropriate
    - Inspired gas should be humidified as clinically indicated
- Enteral nutrition with a post-pyloric feeding tube
    - Enteral feeding via a nasogastric tube may cause reflux of gastric contents and increase the risk of aspiration
- Modulation of colonisation
    - In addition to correct oral hygiene, selective decontamination of the digestive tract (also known as SDD), with or without systemic antibiotics, may be considered

How do you make a diagnosis of VAP?

VAP is a HAP that occurs 48 hours or more after tracheal intubation. Despite the lack of a universally agreed definition, ICU physicians generally agree that pneumonia should be suspected when there are new or persistent infiltrates on chest radiography *plus* two or more of the following:

- Purulent tracheal secretions
- Blood leucocytosis ($>12\times10^9$ white blood cells/L) or leucopenia ($<4\times10^9$ white blood cells/L)
- Temperature greater than 38.3°C

Lack of a "gold standard" definition leads to both underdiagnosis and overdiagnosis. Postmortem studies of patients suspected of having VAP suggest that using clinical criteria alone for diagnosis produces 30%-35% false negative results and 20%-25% false positive results. The diagnosis of VAP is challenging and controversial. General signs of infection are neither highly sensitive nor specific in the critically ill population. Numerous disease processes, including pulmonary oedema, pulmonary haemorrhage, and acute respiratory distress syndrome, can mimic the signs and symptoms of pneumonia.

How is VAP treated?

A high clinical suspicion of pneumonia in a ventilated patient should prompt the immediate administration of an appropriate broad spectrum antibiotic. Although no optimal regimen has been identified, the chosen drug(s) should have a high degree of activity against aerobic Gram negative bacilli. Late onset pneumonia is more commonly associated with drug resistant bacteria, particularly *Pseudomonas aeruginosa*.

It is advisable to discuss suspicious cases with the clinical microbiology service to select the most appropriate antimicrobial therapy. Local patterns of resistance will dictate the drug of choice pending the culture results of appropriate specimens.

Prevention is the best cure: the three main ways of preventing pneumonia are to reduce colonisation of the aerodigestive tract with pathogenic bacteria, prevent aspiration, and limit the duration of mechanical ventilation. Prevention of VAP is possibly one of the most cost-effective interventions currently attainable in the ICU. There is now substantial data suggesting that using a preventative, bundle-based approach in this setting is highly effective in reducing VAP.

References

Choudhuri AH. Ventilator-Associated Pneumonia: When to hold the breath? Int J Crit Illn Inj Sci. 2013 Jul;3(3):169-74.

American Thoracic Society, 2005. Guidelines for the management of adults with hospital-acquired, ventilator-associated, and healthcare-associated pneumonia. *American journal of respiratory and critical care medicine*, 171(4), pp.388–416. Available at: http://www.ncbi.nlm.nih.gov/pubmed/15699079 [Accessed July 10, 2014].

Berton, D.C., Kalil, A.C. & Teixeira, P.J.Z., 2012. Quantitative versus qualitative cultures of respiratory secretions for clinical outcomes in patients with ventilator-associated pneumonia. *The Cochrane database of systematic reviews*, 1, p.CD006482. Available at: http://www.ncbi.nlm.nih.gov/pubmed/22258968 [Accessed October 15, 2014].

Craven, D.E. & Chroneou, A., 2009. Nosocomial pneumonia. In G. L. Mandell, J. E. Bennett, & R. Dolin, eds. *Mandell, Douglas, and Bennett's principles and practice of infectious diseases, 7th Edition*. Philadelphia: Elsevier, p. 3717.

Department of Health, 2011. High Impact Intervention Care bundle to reduce ventilation-association pneumonia. , pp.1–6.

Hunter, J.D., 2012. Ventilator associated pneumonia. *BMJ (Clinical research ed.)*, 344, p.e3325. Available at: http://www.ncbi.nlm.nih.gov/pubmed/22645207 [Accessed October 15, 2014].

Pugin, J., 2002. Clinical signs and scores for the diagnosis of ventilator-associated pneumonia. , 68, pp.261–265.

EMERGENCY SURGERY

Jacub Kadlec Bhaskar Kumar Michael Lewis
Saeed Mirsadraee Alexander Phillips Nicola Phillips
Ali Robb Loveena Sreedharan Filip Van Tornout
Daniel Weiand Robert Winterton

Contents

Acute Acalculous Cholecystitis

You are asked to see a 57 year old man being treated on neurosurgical ICU for a subdural haemorrhage. He has developed a fever and vague upper abdominal pain. A portable USS of the abdomen shows a grossly distended gallbladder with wall thickening and pericholecystic fluid but no stones. A provisional diagnosis of acalculous cholecystitis is made.

How would you manage this patient?

Although the mainstay for treating AAC is cholecystectomy, given his high risk for surgery I would treat this patient with appropriate broad spectrum antibiotics and a percutaneous cholecystostomy. If percutaneous cholecystostomy does not result in improvement within 24 hours, operative intervention may be required.

Although the most common bacteria isolated from bile in acute cholecystitis are E. coli, Klebsiella, and Enterococcus faecalis, in critically ill patients resistant or opportunistic pathogens may be encountered. Pseudomonas, staphylococci (including methicillin-resistant strains), Enterobacter and related species, anaerobic organisms (Clostridium, Bacteroides), and fungi may be involved.

The cholecystostomy has resulted in a significant improvement. At what stage would you think of removing the catheter?

The catheter should be left in situ for approximately 6 weeks to form a tract. A cholangiogram should be performed through the catheter first to exclude any distal obstruction prior to removal. Premature removal before 6 weeks may result in biliary peritonitis.

In what groups of patients is this condition most commonly seen?

Acute acalculous cholecystitis (AAC) most often occurs in critically ill patients especially after trauma, shock, burns, sepsis, major surgery or total parenteral nutrition. AAC accounts for about 10% of all cases of cholecystitis, and is associated with a high mortality of approx 30% in critically ill patients. This high mortality is mainly due to late diagnosis in a group of patients who are very sick.

What conditions are associated with AAC?

Commonly associated risk factors for AAC are trauma, recent surgery (often extra-abdominal), shock, burns, sepsis, critical illness, TPN as well as diabetes and vasculitis. It is associated with vasculitic diseases such as SLE, PAN and antiphospholipid syndrome.

What is the pathogenesis of AAC?

This is not completely understood, but microvascular ischaemia of the gallbladder and biliary stasis are important factors.

Gallbladder ischaemia/reperfusion injury is a critical factor in the pathogenesis of AAC. Bacterial invasion of ischaemic tissue is believed to be a secondary phenomenon. Bile stasis is also believed to be an important factor particularly with TPN.

How is AAC diagnosed?

Often the diagnosis is difficult since it occurs mainly in critically ill patients in whom the clinical features may be overshadowed by other problems and inability to give a history. A high index of suspicion is required in the critically ill patient with abdominal pain, deranged LFTs or sepsis of unknown origin.

Radiological diagnosis is also difficult and USS may not always be diagnostic. Alternative investigations such as cholescintigraphy may be required but have limited value in critically ill or injured patients.

Rapid and accurate diagnosis is essential, as ischaemia can progress rapidly to gangrene and perforation. AAC is sufficiently common that the diagnosis should be considered in every critically ill patient with sepsis of unknown origin.

What is the natural history of this condition?

Gallbladder necrosis and perforation are not uncommon due to late diagnosis and inherent severity of the condition. Rates of perforation may be in the order of 15-20%.

Reference

Huffman JL, Schenker S. Acute Acalculous Cholecystitis: A Review. Clinical Gastroenterology and Hepatology; 2010; 8:15-22.

Acute Appendicitis in Pregnancy

You are asked to see a 24 year old lady on the delivery suite who is 32 weeks pregnant and has presented with a history of generalised abdominal and fever. Her temperature is 38°C and she is tachycardic 100bpm. On examination she is tender generally across her abdomen but this is not localised.

USS of the abdomen by the obstetrics team showed normal gallbladder, liver, spleen and kidneys, and no free fluid with the appendix not visualised. A foetal scan performed by obstetricians showed a viable foetus. WCC is $20 \times 10^9/l$ and CRP 200. Urine analysis showed trace leucocytes only.

The patient's obstetrician is concerned but you are not convinced that she has appendicitis.

What further imaging may be considered?

Diagnostic accuracy is of utmost importance during pregnancy because a missed diagnosis of appendicitis may lead to perforation with subsequent foetal loss / maternal harm. It would be sensible to start with a departmental USS performed by the radiologist on call. Their scanning abilities and equipment will be more sensitive than what is available on the delivery suite.

A departmental USS shows a small amount of free fluid in Morison's pouch, and a thin walled gallbladder containing a solitary stone but no appendix visualised. How would you proceed?

Since the clinical suspicion of appendicitis is not high it may be wise to consider further imaging or a watch and wait approach. The risk with the latter is that of missing a perforated appendix, which can place the unborn baby at risk as well as risking maternal welfare. Therefore a proactive approach is important particularly with respect to the obstetrician's concerns. A discussion can be made with the radiology consultant on call to get a CT scan or MRI. The main concern with CT is that of radiation induced childhood neoplasia. Concerns exist regarding the safety of MRI with no data to support its safety, and it lacks the sensitivity of a CT scan in this context. For the CT to be approved the patient will need to be fully informed by the surgical and obstetric team of any possible long term implications.

A CT scan is performed without iv contrast and this shows evidence of a 11mm faecolith in the vicinity of the appendix and moderate volume of free fluid. You decide to go ahead with an appendicectomy. What would be your approach and why?

	Pros	Cons
Open appendicectomy	Less risk of uterine trauma as umbilical port insertion avoided. No exposure of foetus to physiological effects of pneumoperitoneum	Position of appendix can be highly variable therefore incision must be placed accurately. If appendix normal may be difficult to find alternative cause
Laparoscopic appendicectomy	Risk of uterine trauma and manipulation at port insertion.	If appendix normal easier to find cause of pain e.g. ovarian cyst Effect of exposing foetus to pneumoperitoneum

What are the commonest non-obstetric causes of abdominal pain in pregnancy? What is the incidence of appendicitis in pregnancy?

The commonest causes are acute appendicitis and acute cholecystitis. Appendicitis occurs in approximately 1 of every 1,500 pregnancies and most commonly develops in the second trimester.

What are the physiological changes during pregnancy that can complicate the diagnosis?

Nausea and vomiting, and anorexia are common in pregnancy. Tachycardia may be normal in the later stages of pregnancy, as circulating blood volume is higher. Leukocytosis is a common physiological change of pregnancy. The appendix may be in an atypical position as it moves with gravid uterus.

In addition to the standard consent for an appendicectomy what additional risks need to be discussed with the patient?

The risk of miscarriage needs to be discussed as well as risk of inducing early labour. It needs to be emphasised that a similar risk may be faced if the appendix perforates. Therefore the overall balance favours surgery.

The patient would like to know what the risk of miscarriage is with appendicitis – what will you tell her?

Though the incidence of appendicitis is the same in non-pregnant women as pregnant women the risk of ruptured appendicitis is 2 or 3 times higher. A perforated appendix is associated with a foetal mortality rate which can be as high as 20% to 35%. In uncomplicated appendicitis this rate is as low as 0% to 1.5%.

You decide to perform an open appendicectomy – how can you judge where to make your incision?

As the position of the appendix is even more variable in pregnancy it is useful to mark the area of maximal tenderness pre-operatively and target the skin incision accordingly. It would also be useful to carefully study the preoperative imaging for further guidance.

The patient underwent an uneventful open appendicectomy. There was a perforation at the tip of the appendix with moderate contamination with purulent fluid. How would you manage this patient post-operatively?

In addition to a course of intravenous antibiotics specific complications are higher in pregnancy such as VTE. The patient will need to be managed jointly with the obstetrics team. As the appendix was perforated then special attention needs to be made to foetal well-being.

Further reading

Bakker OJ. Systematic review and meta-analysis of safety of laparoscopic versus open appendicectomy for suspected appendicitis in pregnancy Br J Surg 2012; 99: 1470-1478.

Pear J, Price R, Richardson W, Fanelli R. Guidelines for diagnosis, treatment, and use of laparoscopy for surgical problems during pregnancy Surg Endosc 2011 25:3479–3492

Acute Diverticulitis

A 58 year old man presents with severe sudden onset of left sided lower abdominal pain, temperature 38°C. He is usually fit and well. He has significant localized peritonism and a CRP of 350. A CT scan is obtained and is shown below.

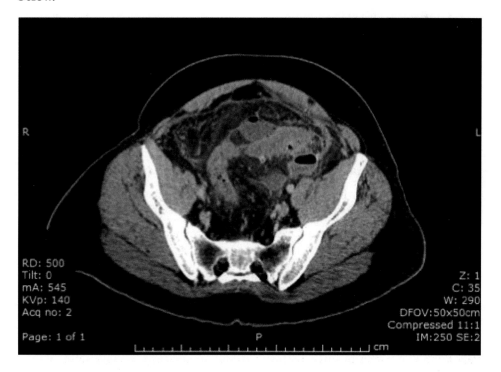

What are the findings and how would you manage him?

The scan shows thickening of the sigmoid colon, which contains multiple diverticula and surrounding mesenteric fat stranding. There is a discrete collection within the pelvis containing locules of gas and inseparable from the sigmoid colon. These findings are consistent with perforated diverticular disease of the sigmoid colon with a secondary abscess.

He needs intravenous fluid resuscitation as well as intravenous broad spectrum antibiotics. Blood cultures should also be obtained prior to antibiotics. Appropriate VTE prophylaxis should be given. Given his young age and in the absence of generalized peritonitis every effort should be made to avoid operative intervention resulting in a stoma. Therefore I would obtain radiological drainage of the collections first and reassess him clinically. Young patients with severe diverticulitis are best managed by a colorectal surgeon as the patient may well require elective resection.

How do you stage the diverticulitis?

Hinchey's Staging

- Stage 1: Localised pericolic or mesenteric abscess
- Stage 2: Pelvic or retroperitoneal abscess away from inflamed phlegmon
- Stage 3: Purulent peritonitis
- Stage 4: Faecal peritonitis

Are you aware of any controversies in the use of antibiotics for treating diverticulitis?

In 2012, a multi centre randomised trial reported that in uncomplicated diverticulitis antibiotics do not accelerate the recovery from the acute episode. This study included 623 patients with CT-scan-proven uncomplicated diverticulitis. There was no difference in complication rates between the groups.

What is the non operative management of acute diverticulitis?

Antibiotics – generally broad spectrum antibiotics are given although some may avoid using them in selected uncomplicated mild diverticulitis.

Percutaneous drainage - almost 80% of abscess/collections can be radiologically drained. Generally collections that are 3cm or less in size can be treated with antibiotics alone. If symptoms do not improve in 24-48 hours then further evaluation is performed with a view to surgical intervention.

If symptoms do improve, the drain can be removed and further assessment is performed in the future to decide if elective surgical intervention is required.

Once the acute episode is over it is conventional to evaluate the colon with endoscopy. A retrospective cohort study comparing complicated versus uncomplicated diverticulitis reported that the odds of harbouring cancer were 4 times higher when there was diverticulitis and localised perforation, 6.7 times higher in patients with diverticulitis and abscesses, and 18 times higher when there was evidence of fistula formation. By contrast some authors report that CT scan is the gold standard and high quality imaging should obviate the need for colonoscopy. A recent study reported low yield of cancers in routine colonoscopy after an episode of uncomplicated diverticulitis.

What are the emergency operative options for diverticulitis?

Emergency indications are: failed medical management, peritonitis, failed radiological drainage of a large abscess, enterocutaneous fistula formation, and bowel obstruction.

Options are:

1) Laparoscopic lavage

2) Laparoscopic or open Hartmann's resection

3) Resection of diverticular segment and primary anastomosis +/- proximal stoma

4) Rarely laparotomy, washout and proximal stoma (only when there is a risk of major organ damage)

What is the role of laparoscopic lavage?

In purulent peritonitis, some authors report laparoscopic lavage and drainage obviate the need of laparotomy and stoma formation. A systematic review reported less than 2% risk of mortality.

The results of a multi centre randomised trial from the Netherlands are awaited. In this study the patient either had laparoscopic lavage and drainage or Hartmann's resection in 2:1 ratio. No results have yet been made public.

References

Wieghard N, Geltzeiler C B, Tsikitis V L. Trends in the surgical management of diverticulitis. Ann Gastroenterol, 2015 Jan-Mar; 28(1); 25-30.

Chabok A, Påhlman L, Hjern F, Haapaniemi S, Smedh K, AVOD Study Group Br J Surg. 2012 Apr;99(4):532-9. Randomized clinical trial of antibiotics in acute uncomplicated diverticulitis.

Westwood DA, Eglinton TW, Frizelle FA.Routine colonoscopy following acute uncomplicated diverticulitis. Br J Surg. 2011 Nov;98(11):1630-4.

Toorenvliet BR, Swank H, Schoones JW, Hamming JF, Bemelman WA, Laparoscopic peritoneal lavage for perforated colonic diverticulitis: a systematic review.Colorectal Dis. 2010 Sep;12(9):862-7..

Acute Large Bowel Obstruction

You are on the post take round reviewing an 81 year old man who has been admitted with abdominal pain and distension, two episodes of vomiting and absolute constipation. He has a CRP of 100, other bloods are normal. Plain abdominal x-ray shows loops of dilated colon with a few prominent small bowel loops. He has been kept nil by mouth overnight and given iv fluids. What investigation would you request?

This patient has clinical features of large bowel obstruction. A CT scan with iv contrast would be the investigation of choice as it can confirm the presence of large bowel obstruction (LBO) as well as provide information on the possible aetiology such as neoplasia. A CT would also provide staging information in the context of neoplasia.

A retrograde water soluble enema can be done to demonstrate the level of cut-off but this has largely been superseded by cross imaging modalities.

The CT confirms the presence of a sigmoid obstruction suggestive of a colonic cancer. There is no evidence of distant disease. What are your treatment options?

There are essentially two options - emergency surgery or consideration of a colonic stent. The operation of choice would be a Hartmann's procedure with end colostomy and rectal stump. This would form part of a two stage procedure if the stoma is reversed at a later date. However up to a third of patients will never have their stoma reversed and of those who do undergo stoma reversal, mortality may approach 10%. I would be reluctant to consider a primary anastomosis in an elderly obstructed patient.

An alternative option would be to use a self-expanding metallic stent. This would then act as a bridge to elective surgery at a later stage. The role of stents in acute obstruction is currently the subject matter of a randomised study (CREST study) in the UK.

In your opinion, with this patient, what are the advantages and disadvantages of a colonic stent in the acute setting of large bowel obstruction?

The advantages of stents are threefold. First, the use of a stent allows colonic decompression in someone who is physiologically ill and allows conversion of an acute patient into an elective one. This might reduce his morbidity from emergency surgery. A stent also allows patients with locally advanced disease to receive neoadjuvant treatment. By definition, those patients with obstructed tumours have a poorer prognosis and decompression allows them to participate in trials (FOXTROT study) where surgery can be done after tumour downstaging. Last, in patients with successful stent decompression, permanent stoma rates may be lower because primary anastomosis is more likely to be considered in an elective setting rather than in the acute. Having said that, the latest trials on the subject matter have not demonstrated a reduction in stoma rate formation.

The disadvantages of a stent are to do with technical and practical aspects of the procedure. Stent insertion requires a joint effort between endoscopy and radiology. Not all lesions can be transversed. Lesions on the left are easier to get to. Lesions on the right are less so. Lesions in the rectum, if low - cannot be stented because the lower edge of the stent can lead to intractable tenesmus. Failure to decompress with or without stent deployment requires expedient surgery. There is a risk of perforation either at the caecum from insufflation (thereby necessitating more extensive acute surgery) or at the site of the tumour fracture from stent deployment (where the long-term oncological outcome from this remains unknown).

You do not have stenting facilities so you decide to take the patient to theatre. At surgery you find no liver or peritoneal metastases but a very dilated caecum with serosal tears. How would you proceed?

In my opinion there are two options, and these would depend on how ill the patient is. The unstable and ill patient requires a quick operation, so I would resect the caecum and bring out an end ileostomy and a mucous fistula. The mucous fistula will decompress the obstruction and the tumour can be dealt with at a later time. The stable patient who is physiologically intact should have a subtotal colectomy (including resection of the tumour) and an end ileostomy. The rectal stump is left as long as possible and consideration towards restoration of intestinal continuity is made at a later date.

At laparotomy you find the obstructing tumour is much lower down than you expected. In fact, it is below the peritoneal reflection and not the sigmoid (you curse your radiologist!). What would you do intraoperatively?

This is bad news. You do not want to be doing pelvic surgery when you do not know the extent of disease within the pelvis. Even if you can get below the cancer with both a clear circumferential and longitudinal margin, most surgeons would not be happy to consider primary anastomosis in this setting. The anal stump disappears after cross stapling and the prospects of restorative surgery in the future are minimal. Hence, for those patients with a tenuous caecum, I would do as earlier with limited resection and exteriorisation of both ends. In those with a viable caecum, I would decompress with a loop sigmoid colostomy in the left iliac fossa. This is more acceptable than a loop transverse colostomy with a lower prolapse, and has higher patient acceptability rates. The patient is decompressed and can then complete the necessary staging work up as an elective patient.

Just before you close the abdomen, your very keen eyed registrar notices a tiny nodule in the abdominal wall and another in segment two of the liver. Does this alter what you would do intra and postoperatively?

In short - yes. If the nodule in the abdominal wall is discreet, I would resect it with clear margins and send it off for histology. The margins of the resection will be marked with some metallic clips to facilitate the use of radiotherapy in the future. The liver nodule if tiny and easily accessible can also be removed. If it is too large but outside my comfort zone for removal, I will consider a Tru-cut biopsy of any readily accessible lesion for purposes of staging. The long term prognosis of this patient is even more guarded now and postoperative staging scans of the liver with MRI and PET-CT become necessary.

References

Finan PJ, Campbell S, Verma R, et al. The management of malignant large bowel obstruction: ACPGBI Position Statement. Colorectal Disease 2007;9(Suppl. 4):1e17.

CREST study website

http://www.birmingham.ac.uk/research/activity/mds/trials/bctu/trials/coloproctology/crest/index.aspx

Acute Lower Limb Ischaemia

An 80 year old lady from a residential home was admitted. She was known to be in AF and was admitted after the carer had noticed that she had been complaining of pain in her right leg for the last 2 days and had since been unable to walk.

How would you assess the lower limbs?

Due to the recent onset (<2 weeks), this patient by definition has acute lower limb ischaemia. Patients typically present with the clinical features of pain, paraesthesia, pallor, perishingly cold, pulselessness and paralysis (6 Ps). The history taking and examination should focus on presence of prior symptoms of claudication to differentiate between acute on chronic ischaemia (due to thrombosis of underlying stenosis) and acute limb ischaemia (due to an embolic event). Patients with lower limb ischaemia due to thrombosis often have less pronounced symptoms and signs due to the collaterals. As diseases in lower limbs tend to mirror each other, the presence of pulses in the contralateral lower limbs would suggest that the affected limb may have normal pulses prior to the current episode and therefore is most likely due to an acute embolic event. It is important to ascertain if the vascular compromise is reversible (blanches with pressure even with mottling), viable (no altered sensation or weakness), threatened (altered sensation or weakness) or non-salvageable (fixed mottling, insensate, fixed plantar flexion with no Doppler signal).

What are your immediate management plans?

The viability of the lower limb will determine the course of action. A viable limb will allow for extra time to investigate the vasculature. A threatened limb will require immediate surgical intervention, and a non-salvageable limb will require consideration if the patient is fit for major lower limb amputation or palliative care. Patients will require adequate resuscitation with administration of oxygen and rehydration with intravenous (IV) fluids. Patients requiring surgical intervention should also be given 5000 u IV bolus of heparin with IV heparin infusion (according to weight), analgesia and urinary catheter to monitor the urine output.

What investigations would you arrange?

I would arrange baseline blood tests (full blood count, urea and electrolytes, blood glucose, INR if she was already on warfarin, group and save, and electrocardiogram) and imaging depending on local availability (duplex, CT angiogram or MR angiogram). CTA and MRA will delineate the site of thrombosis and potential underlying stenosis which may not have been appreciated. In patients without AF, CTA will help rule out underlying mural thrombus or aortic aneurysm which may be the source of peripheral embolism. A transoesophageal echocardiogram may be indicated to ascertain the source of embolus if there are no other discernible causes.

What treatment options are appropriate in her case?

As her lower limb is viable, I would consider offering her an embolectomy. An embolus classically obstructs at the level of vessel bifurcations. If clinically or radiologically, the embolus is at the level of the iliac or common femoral artery (CFA) bifurcation, the patient should be offered the option of femoral embolectomy. This is approached via a longitudinal incision in the groin to allow control of common femoral, superficial femoral (SFA) and profunda femoris (PFA) arteries. A transverse arteriotomy is then made at the common femoral artery (CFA). A size 4F or 5F Fogarty balloon is passed proximally if there is a weak femoral pulse. If the proximal femoral pulse is good, a 3F balloon could then be passed as distally as possible down the SFA and PFA. The balloon is inflated to an appropriate level to avoid excessive intimal friction as the catheter is withdrawn. The clot is then sent for microbiology to rule out cardiac vegetation and histology (atrial myxoma). The arteriotomy is closed with 5/0 prolene. Both groins should be prepped and draped in the event that the inflow could not be established and the patient will then require a femoro-femoral crossover. If the embolus is at the below knee popliteal level, a longitudinal incision is made at the upper medial calf to access the below knee popliteal, tibioperoneal trunk and anterior tibial artery. A transverse arteriotomy is made at the popliteal artery and a size 3F or 2F Fogarty catheter is then passed distally and the arteriotomy is closed with 6/0 prolene.

The patient is not keen to undergo surgery. Are there any other treatment alternatives?

As her limb is viable, the alternative treatment would be catheter directed thrombolysis. This will depend on the availability of an interventional radiologist. This has the advantage of angioplasty in the event of underlying stenosis. There are contraindications to thrombolysis (active bleeding, stroke within the last two months, recent gastrointestinal bleeding, pregnancy, cranial surgery within the last two months, vascular or abdominal surgery within two weeks, bleeding disorder or extensive trauma), which would need to be considered.

Percutaneous mechanical thrombectomy devices use various techniques such as simple aspiration and a device that macerates thrombus to resolve the obstruction. The majority of devices are expensive with little consensus for their use.

What is the evidence base with regards to treatment?

A recent meta-analysis does not recommend universal initial treatment with either surgery or thrombolysis (2013). There is no overall difference in limb salvage or death at 30 days, six months or one year between initial surgery or initial thrombolysis. Thrombolysis may be associated with a higher risk of ongoing limb ischaemia and bleeding complications including stroke (Berridge 2013). The decision should therefore be based upon local expertise and weighing the risk benefit ratio of each modality in individual patients.

What are the potential complications post-operatively?

Apart from bleeding, two other main complications are compartment syndrome and rhabdomyolysis. The former presents with acute pain in the calf associated with inability to dorsiflex the foot and swelling. If compartment syndrome is suspected, an emergency four compartment (anterior, lateral, superficial and deep posterior) fasciotomy of the calf is performed. In patients who are on ITU and ventilated, a compartment pressure of more than 20 mmHg would also mandate fasciotomy. Rhabdomyolysis can result in acute tubular necrosis leading to renal failure. Patients often present with dark urine, elevated serum creatine kinase and myoglobinuria. Treatment will involve rehydration and alkalinising urine to remove the myoglobin and occasionally haemofiltration or dialysis.

What are the long term strategies to prevent further embolic events?

This patient has most likely presented with an embolic event secondary to AF. In the absence of AF, patients will require further imaging of the whole aorta and trans-oesophageal echocardiogram to ascertain the source. The CHA_2DS_2-VASc [**C**ongestive heart failure, **H**ypertension, **A**ge (scores 2), **D**iabetes, **S**troke (scores 2), **Va**scular disease, **S**ex **c**ategory] scoring system is used to determine if AF patients will benefit from long term anticoagulation and this is balanced against the HAS-BLED (**H**ypertension, **A**bnormal renal or liver function, **S**troke, **B**leeding, **L**abile INRs, **E**lderly, **D**rug therapy and Alcohol usage) score for the risk of bleeding. As a general guide, if the former score is higher than the latter, the patient will benefit from long term anticoagulation.

Further reading

Berridge DC, Kessel DO, Robertson I. Surgery versus thrombolysis for initial management of acute limb ischaemia. Cochrane Database Syst Rev. 2013; 6: CD002784.

LaHaye SA, Gibbens SL, Ball DG, Day AG, Olesen JB, Skanes AC. A clinical decision aid for the selection of antithrombotic therapy for the prevention of stroke due to atrial fibrillation. Eur Heart J. 2012; 33(17): 2163-71.

Acute Pseudo-obstruction

The orthopaedic team have referred a 75 year old gentleman with a distended abdomen four days after total hip replacement. How would you assess this patient?

My assessment would involve a history and examination aimed at establishing the diagnosis and excluding a mechanical bowel obstruction. From the history, I would like to know if there is abdominal pain. Pain indicates a mechanical component to the obstruction or excessive distention to an extent where there is a risk of ischaemia and/or perforation.

On examination I would look for signs of sepsis such as tachycardia and pyrexia. It is important to determine the extent of tenderness/peritonism over the caecal region. A rectal examination is mandatory.

What investigations would you request for him?

This gentleman needs an abdominal film and routine blood tests particularly FBC and urea and electrolytes. A mechanical obstruction needs to be excluded - this can be difficult even in the best radiological hands. A CT scan (with rectal contrast) of the abdomen/pelvis is the best test to exclude a mechanical obstruction.

The CT scan reveals no mechanical obstruction. There is distended colon throughout with no transition point - this is consistent with a colonic pseudo-obstruction. What are the principles of management?

Treatment of the underlying cause is the key. Sometimes simple correction of electrolyte disturbances and reduction in the use of opiates is all that is necessary. When patients become uncomfortable from the physical effects of distension, flatus tube and/or endoscopic decompression can be considered. There is no need for bowel preparation, minimal insufflation should be utilised, the scope is passed as far proximal as possible and a flatus tube inserted after successful decompression.

Reassessment is a vital part of safely managing the patient. Clinical examination should focus carefully on the degree of tenderness over the caecum as this may indicate impending perforation. Radiological reassessment is also necessary with plain X-ray to check for the caecal diameter. In the majority (80%) of cases, there is an obvious precipitant to the pseudo obstruction. These include:

- Orthopaedic trauma or surgery
- Pneumonia or sepsis
- Acute renal failure
- Medications e.g. narcotics
- Retroperitoneal malignancy - rarely

What endoscopic features at the time of decompression would worry you?

The vast majority of patients have a capacious and tortuous colon full of gas and semi liquid faeces. It can be a challenge to get into the splenic flexure and beyond. One must not see blood within the lumen. Worse is the presence of dark mucosal patches. If you see either of these, then either the diagnosis is wrong or there is ischaemic colon and surgery must be considered.

When should operative intervention be considered in patients?

Patients with worrying endoscopic features or progressive caecal enlargement (greater than 12cms on abdominal X-ray) and focal tenderness that cannot be decompressed safely should be considered for surgery. Needless to say, those with frank peritonitis also require a laparotomy.

Are you aware of any medications to facilitate colonic decompression in those with pseudo obstruction?

There are two. The first is neostigmine, the second is alvimopan. Neostigmine is an anticholinesterase and thereby increases the parasympathetic activity of the colon. It is given intravenously and usually results in prompt decompression of the colon. Caution should be employed when using neostigmine and patients should have cardiac monitoring with availability of atropine in case of extreme bradycardia. Other side effects include salivation, vomiting, hypotension and bronchospasm. It is rarely used in the UK.

Alvimopan is increasingly used in the USA for ileus and pseudo-obstruction postoperatively. It is an opiate derivative with partial agonist/antagonist properties and does not cross the blood brain barrier. It therefore does not interfere with the centrally acting analgesic properties of standard opiates, but it helps reduce the unwanted side effects of colonic inertia which are not centrally mediated. In randomised trials, alvimopan improves the return of gut function by a median of 24 hours. This drug is not routinely used in the UK.

Appendix Abscess

A 51 year old man presents with a two week history of right sided abdominal pain and 14lbs/6kgs weight loss. He experiences diarrhoea after meals. On examination he was apyrexial and well. He has a soft mass felt in the right iliac fossa with a CRP 230, WCC 18 × 10^9/l. A CT scan of his abdomen and pelvis was requested.

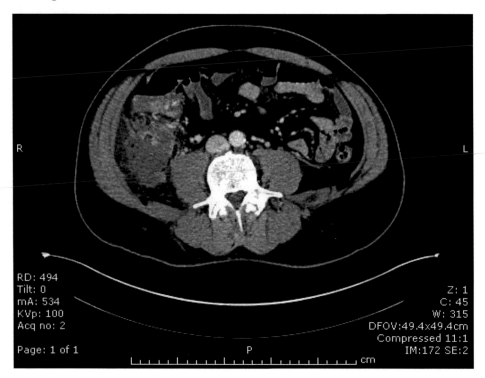

What does the CT image show?

A retrocaecal appendix leads into a 5cm x 5cm ill-defined fluid collection in the right flank which contains several small locules of gas. There is thickening of the peritoneal reflection but no free fluid. The appearances are in keeping with appendicitis and a localised abscess.

How would you manage this patient?

He is systemically well and not showing any signs of sepsis. I would approach the radiologists to see if the collection can be drained percutaneously first. If this is successful I would continue antibiotics as per sensitivities and leave the drain in for at least one to two weeks.

The patient underwent percutaneous insertion with a 10 french pigtail catheter under CT guidance. The collection was aspirated to dryness with approximately 100 mL of pus obtained. Over the course of the next few days he was discharged with the drain in and continued a course of antibiotics.

You see him back in your clinic in 3 weeks. He is very well and asymptomatic. How would you manage him at this stage?

I would certainly remove the pigtail drain. There are two options at this stage. One is to simply adopt a watch and wait policy, but accepting that there is a risk of appendicitis flaring up again at any time. On the other hand he may remain symptom free. The alternative is to consider an interval appendicectomy, but this is more than likely going to be an open procedure with associated risks, and disruption off work etc.. In the meantime it would be wise to obtain a colonoscopy, to exclude any underlying right sided colonic lesion.

There is good evidence in the literature that routine interval appendicectomy is not justified after treatment of an appendix mass/abscess. The incidence of recurrent appendicitis is low, therefore it has been suggested that the majority of patients with appendiceal abscesses can successfully be treated without an operation. Patients who develop recurrent appendicitis have been shown to have a milder clinical presentation compared with their initial presentation.

Reference

Tannoury Jl, Abboud B. Treatment options of inflammatory appendiceal masses in adults. World J Gastroenterol. 2013 Jul 7;19(25):3942-50.

Bile Leak Post Lap Cholecystectomy

Scenario 1

A 61 year old lady underwent an elective laparoscopic cholecystectomy one week ago. It was an uncomplicated procedure and she was discharged the same day. She now presents with severe upper abdominal pain and temperature of 39°C. She is mildly icteric. Blood tests show a WCC of $18 \times 10^9/l$ and bilirubin 45μmol/L and a CRP of 342. How would you manage her?

The main concern here is a bile leak following the cholecystectomy. She needs to be resuscitated and given intravenous antibiotics and analgesia. I would obtain the operation notes to see if a cholangiogram was performed, and if available examine it. I would obtain a CT scan of her abdomen and pelvis rather than an USS as the CT will provide more information on the presence of free fluid and characterise any collections which are usually either a biloma, haematoma or abscess.

CT scan shows presence of free fluid around the liver and pelvis and no evidence of CBD stones. What are the commonest sources of bile leak after a laparoscopic cholecystectomy?

Bile leak is a well recognised complication of laparoscopic cholecystectomy and occurs in approximately 1%-2% of cases. It is usually evident in the first week post surgery. The commonest source is leaking from a cystic duct stump followed by an accessory duct such as a duct of Luschka or intrahepatic duct. The least likely is a bile duct injury.

You decide to perform a laparoscopy and washout the abdomen as well as pelvis. On examining the gallbladder bed you notice a continuous but slow trickle of bile which fails to stop despite applying pressure. How would you proceed?

In the presence of an ongoing bile leak measures must be taken to definitively stop the leak. The most effective way would be to suture the area of the leak with an absorbable suture such as vicryl. Usually a few interrupted sutures would be sufficient and would require advanced laparoscopic skills with intracorporeal suturing. Once the leak is controlled a large drain should be left in the vicinity of the gallbladder bed.

Scenario 2

An 85 year old diabetic lady is admitted with severe acute cholecystitis and acute kidney injury. You decide to perform an urgent cholecystectomy. At laparoscopy you find that the gallbladder has perforated into the liver parenchyma. As a result progress could not be achieved laparoscopically, therefore a decision is made to convert to an open procedure, where you struggle to clearly identity Calot's triangle. How would you proceed?

The priority here is to drain the sepsis and not to injure the vital structures within Calot's triangle. If dissection around Calot's triangle is treacherous I cannot afford to risk damage to the CBD and other major structures in its vicinity. Therefore I would proceed to a subtotal cholecystectomy. I would retrograde dissect as much of the gallbladder as possible, then open the fundus to drain any sepsis and remove stones. The gallbladder is then divided usually at the level of the GB neck to leave a stump well above Calot's. If possible a cholangiogram can be performed through the gallbladder stump. The stump then needs to be closed watertight using a suture such as 2.0 vicryl in one or two layers. A large drain is then left in the vicinity of the gallbladder remnant.

Two days post op she is systemically very well but has approximately 1 litre of bile in 24 hours in the drain. She is not complaining of abdominal pain and is apyrexial. How would you proceed?

She has a high volume bile leak but in the absence of peritonitis and abdominal pain she does not require surgical intervention as yet. However if the leak is ongoing in the next couple of days and not showing any signs of slowing down an ERCP will be required.

How would an ERCP help in this situation?

ERCP is able to detect the site of bile leak in the majority of cases and is both diagnostic and therapeutic. An ERCP would help to exclude any other source of bile leak such as a bile duct injury, as well as allow placement of a CBD stent to promote antegrade bile flow, through reducing the pressure gradient across the sphincter of Oddi, which in turn may reduce any leak from the GB remnant. A removable plastic stent is usually placed which can be removed endoscopically in the next 4-6 weeks. An alternative is to perform a sphincterotomy but it is generally accepted that a stent provides a more rapid result. An ongoing bile leak even after ERCP would suggest leak from an accessory duct such as a duct of Luschka and may require surgical intervention.

Reference

Kim KH, Kim TN. Endoscopic management of bile leakage after cholecystectomy: a single-center experience for 12 years. Clin Endosc. 2014 May;47(3):248-53.

Biliary Sepsis

You are reviewing a frail 80 year old lady on the post take ward round admitted with ultrasound-proven acute cholecystitis with no intra/extra-hepatic ductal dilatation. She is pyrexial 38°C but haemodynamically stable. She has a history of atrial fibrillation for which she is on warfarin with an INR of 2.7 as well as COPD and previous MIs. LFTs are within normal range, WCC 18 × 10⁹/l and CRP 210.

How would you manage this patient?

Further management will depend, in part, on the severity of her illness.

This patient has proven acute cholecystitis. She is a high-risk patient given her advanced age and need for anticoagulation. I would fully resuscitate this patient with intravenous fluids, taking into account recommendations in the Surviving Sepsis Campaign Guidelines. Considering her high-risk status, I would have a low threshold to transfer her to HDU, if she becomes systemically unstable.

Whilst antimicrobials are clearly indicated for patients with complications of cholecystitis, the role of antimicrobials in the treatment of uncomplicated cholecystitis is less certain. Many cases of acute cholecystitis remit spontaneously. In uncomplicated cholecystitis, rates of pericolic abscess or perforation are not affected by the administration of antimicrobial therapy.

- The Tokyo Guidelines provide some guidance on the issue of antimicrobial therapy in the management of acute cholangitis and cholecystitis: in early and non-severe cases, it is not obvious that bacteria play a significant role in the pathology encountered. In these patients, antimicrobial therapy is at best prophylactic, preventing progression to infection.

- With clinical findings of a systemic inflammatory response, antimicrobial therapy is therapeutic, and treatment may be required until the gallbladder is removed.

Although the patient is haemodynamically stable, there are some signs of a systemic inflammatory response. Therefore, according to the Tokyo Guidelines, antimicrobial therapy is clinically indicated. Antimicrobial agents appropriate for initial therapy (empirical therapy or presumptive therapy) for various grades of severity of biliary tract infections have been developed (see "antimicrobial therapy" section, later in this chapter).

Once she is stabilized and resuscitated, the options are to treat her conservatively or to proceed directly to intervention, which may be surgical or radiological. In my opinion, given her high risk and non-diabetic status she may be best initially managed conservatively, with intervention reserved if she doesn't settle.

What types of pathogens are responsible for acute cholecystitis?

- Initially, the inflammation of acute cholecystitis may be sterile. Infection is not thought to precipitate acute cholecystitis, but it may complicate 20% to 50% of cases.

- Over time, bacterial colonisation of the obstructed bile and inflamed tissue occurs and may result in an empyema of the gallbladder. With severe inflammation, ischaemic necrosis of the gallbladder occurs, leading to perforation, the incidence of which is much higher in diabetic patients. Pyogenic liver abscess and bacteraemia may also complicate the disease course.

  Although the initial inflammation is usually sterile, secondary infection with constituents of the normal bowel flora may occur. The most common bacterial isolates from patients with acute cholecystitis are members of the *Enterobacteriaceae* (which are Gram negative bacilli), including *E. coli*, *Klebsiella* species and *Enterobacter* species. *Enterococcus* species (which are Gram positive cocci) and anaerobes (including *Bacteroides* spp., *Fusobacterium* spp., and *Clostridium* spp.) may also be isolated.

From Tokyo Guidelines 2013:

Common microorganisms isolated from bile cultures among patients with acute biliary infections

Isolated microorganisms from bile cultures	Proportions of isolated organisms (%)
Gram-negative organisms	
Escherichia coli	31–44
Klebsiella spp.	9–20
Pseudomonas spp.	0.5–19
Enterobacter spp.	5–9
Acinetobacter spp.	–
Citrobacter spp.	–
Gram-positive organisms	
Enterococcus spp.	3–34
Streptococcus spp.	2–10
Staphylococcus spp.	0[a]
Anaerobes	4–20
Others	–

Antimicrobial therapy: What are your first-line antimicrobials for treating this patient and why?

Antimicrobial therapy should be directed against the usual enteric flora implicated in acute cholecystitis:

- Prescribe antimicrobials in line with your local Trust's antimicrobial guidelines
- Take into account relevant microbiological-, antimicrobial- and patient-related factors (see appendix 1)

Empirical antimicrobial therapy may include:

- A beta-lactam/beta-lactamase inhibitor combination
    - E.g. amoxicillin/clavulanate (also known as Augmentin) or piperacillin/tazobactam
- dihydrofolate reductase inhibitors.
    - E.g. Trimethoprim/sulphamethoxazole (also known as co-trimoxazole and Septrin)
- Cephalosporins
    - E.g. cefuroxime (a second-generation Cephalosporin)
- Fluoroquinolones
    - E.g. ciprofloxacin, levofloxacin or moxifloxacin

NB: Cephalosporins, co-trimoxazole and ciprofloxacin/levofloxacin are not active against *Enterococcus* spp. or anaerobes. To cover for anaerobes, metronidazole is often added in combination with these antimicrobials.

NB: Beta lactam-beta lactamase inhibitor combinations (e.g. co-amoxiclav, also known as Augmentin) have activity against *Enterococcus faecalis* but not *Enterococcus faecium*. Therefore, additional cover with an agent that has increased enterococcal activity may be required.

Other alternatives exist, but clinicians are advised to discuss complex cases with an infection specialist.

The Tokyo Guidelines provide some recommendations on antimicrobial therapy, which are dependent on the nature of infection: (i) community-acquired disease, including the severity of disease (Grades I, II and III); (ii) healthcare-associated infection:

Antimicrobial recommendations for acute biliary infections

Severity	Community-acquired biliary infections			Grade III[c]	Healthcare-associated biliary infections[e]
	Grade I		Grade II		
Antimicrobial agents	Cholangitis	Cholecystitis	Cholangitis and cholecystitis	Cholangitis and cholecystitis	Healthcare-associated cholangitis and cholecystitis
Penicillin-based therapy	Ampicillin/sulbactam[b] is not recommended without an aminoglycoside	Ampicillin/sulbactam[b] is not recommended without an aminoglycoside	Piperacillin/tazobactam	Piperacillin/tazobactam	Piperacillin/tazobactam
Cephalosporin-based therapy	Cefazolin[a], or cefotiam[a], or cefuroxime[a], or ceftriaxone, or cefotaxime ± metronidazole[d] Cefmetazole,[a] Cefoxitin,[a] Flomoxef,[a] Cefoperazone/sulbactam	Cefazolin[a], or cefotiam[a], or cefuroxime[a], or ceftriaxone, or cefotaxime ± metronidazole[d] Cefmetazole,[a] Cefoxitin,[a] Flomoxef,[a] Cefoperazone/sulbactam	Ceftriaxone, or cefotaxime, or cefepime, or cefozopran, or ceftazidime ± metronidazole[d] Cefoperazone/sulbactam	Cefepime, or ceftazidime, or cefozopran ± metronidazole[d]	Cefepime, or ceftazidime, or cefozopran ± metronidazole[d]
Carbapenem-based therapy	Ertapenem	Ertapenem	Ertapenem	Imipenem/cilastatin, meropenem, doripenem, ertapenem	Imipenem/cilastatin, meropenem, doripenem, ertapenem
Monobactam-based therapy	–	–	–	Aztreonam ± metronidazole[d]	Aztreonam ± metronidazole[d]
Fluoroquinolone-based therapy[c]	Ciprofloxacin, or levofloxacin, or pazufloxacin ± metronidazole[d] Moxifloxacin	Ciprofloxacin, or levofloxacin, or pazufloxacin ± metronidazole[d] Moxifloxacin	Ciprofloxacin, or levofloxacin, or pazufloxacin ± metronidazole[c] Moxifloxacin	–	–

[a] Local antimicrobial susceptibility patterns (antibiogram) should be considered for use

[b] Ampicillin/sulbactam has little activity left against *Escherichia coli*. It is removed from the North American guidelines

[c] Fluoroquinolone use is recommended if the susceptibility of cultured isolates is known or for patients with β-lactam allergies. Many extended-spectrum β-lactamase (ESBL)-producing Gram-negative isolates are fluoroquinolone-resistant

[d] Anti-anaerobic therapy, including use of metronidazole, tinidazole, or clindamycin, is warranted if a biliary-enteric anastomosis is present. The carbapenems, piperacillin/tazobactam, ampicillin/sulbactam, cefmetazole, cefoxitin, flomoxef, and cefoperazone/sulbactam have sufficient anti-anaerobic activity for this situation

[e] Vancomycin is recommended to cover *Enterococcus* spp. for grade III community-acquired acute cholangitis and cholecystitis, and healthcare-associated acute biliary infections. Linezolid or daptomycin is recommended if vancomycin-resistant *Enterococcus* (VRE) is known to be colonizing the patient, if previous treatment included vancomycin, and/or if the organism is common in the community

48 hours into the admission the patient remains pyrexial with a rising CRP (350). She is systemically well though tender, localized to the right upper quadrant. Her anticoagulation is fully reversed.

How would you proceed?

Given that she is failing conservative management I would proceed to intervention. As she is a high risk surgical candidate I would pursue an urgent percutaneous cholecystostomy. The cholecystostomy tube may be left in situ permanently for patients with a limited life expectancy or act as a bridge to surgery at a later stage if the clinical condition improves.

How is a percutaneous cholecystostomy performed?

Ultrasound guided cholecystostomy can be performed under local anaesthetic either by a transhepatic or transperitoneal approach. The transhepatic approach is preferred due to earlier maturation of the track and lower risk of biliary peritonitis.

Transcystic cholangiography may be performed, which may identify additional stones in the common bile duct. These can be managed by pushing the stones into the duodenum via the cystostomy access, sparing them surgical exploration.

What are the possible specific complications of this procedure?

Specific complications include bile leak and visceral injury. A tubogram should be performed to demonstrate patency of the cystic duct and CBD. Complications are fewer following the use of a locking drain compared to non locking drains.

What is the role of emergency laparoscopic cholecystectomy versus interval laparoscopic cholecystectomy?

There is emerging evidence that acute laparoscopic cholecystectomy is superior to the interval approach. However local resources and culture of practice will determine which approach is followed. Within the NHS theatre resources are scarce preventing 'hot gallbladder' surgery from being widespread through the UK. In other countries such as Australia there is a general move to perform LC as an acute procedure.

There have been several studies to look at this issue. One of the latest studies was an RCT and it showed acute LC to be associated with a lower morbidity rate than interval LC (11.8% vs 34.4%). Mean length of hospital stay (5.4 days vs 10.0 days; P < 0.001) and total hospital costs (€2,919 vs €4,262; P < 0.001) were significantly lower in the interval cholecystectomy group.

Choosing appropriate antimicrobial therapy

Choice of antimicrobial therapy requires consideration of multiple factors:

1) The nature of the infecting organism(s) must be known, or at the very least one must be aware of the likely causative pathogens. This requires knowledge of the normal flora at the site of infection.

2) Antimicrobial therapy should be tailored to cover the likely causative pathogens, and should take into account recent and past culture results, including antimicrobial susceptibility test results. In particular, one should enquire about a history of colonisation or infection with multi-drug resistant organisms (e.g. multi-drug resistant Enterobacteriaceae; methicillin-resistant *S. aureus* [MRSA]; Vancomycin-resistant enterococci [VRE])

3) Antimicrobial-related factors include issues of drug absorption, distribution, metabolism, and excretion.

   a) Patient-related factors must be considered to arrive at the optimal choice of antimicrobial agent for each patient. These include:

   b) History of Previous Adverse Reactions to Antimicrobial Agents

   c) Age

   d) Genetic or Metabolic Abnormalities

   e) Pregnancy

   f) Renal and Hepatic Function

   g) Site of Infection

References

Gomi, H. et al., 2013. TG13 antimicrobial therapy for acute cholangitis and cholecystitis. *Journal of hepato-biliary-pancreatic sciences*, 20(1), pp.60–70. Available at: http://www.ncbi.nlm.nih.gov/pubmed/23340954 [Accessed October 12, 2014].

Sifri, C.D. & Madoff, L.C., 2009. Infections of the Liver and Biliary System. In G. L. Mandell, J. E. Bennett, & R. Dolin, eds. *Mandell, Douglas, and Bennett's principles and practice of infectious diseases, 7th Edition*. Philadelphia: Elsevier, p. 1035.

Kortram K, van Ramshorst B, Bollen TL, Besselink MG, Gouma DJ, Karsten T, Kruyt PM, Nieuwenhuijzen GA, Kelder JC, Tromp E, Boerma D. Acute cholecystitis in high risk surgical patients: percutaneous cholecystostomy versus laparoscopic cholecystectomy (CHOCOLATE trial): study protocol for a randomized controlled trial. Trials. 2012 Jan 12;13:7. doi: 10.1186/1745-6215-13-7.

Rodríguez-Sanjuán JC, Arruabarrena A, Sánchez-Moreno L, González-Sánchez F, Herrera LA, Gómez-Fleitas M. Acute cholecystitis in high surgical risk patients: percutaneous cholecystostomy or emergency cholecystectomy? Am J Surg. 2012 Jul;204(1):54-9. doi: 10.1016/j.amjsurg.2011.05.013. Epub 2011 Oct 13.

Gutt CN1, Encke J, Köninger J, Harnoss JC, Weigand K, Kipfmüller K, Schunter O, Götze T, Golling MT, Menges M, Klar E, Feilhauer K, Zoller WG, Ridwelski K, Ackmann S, Baron A, Schön MR, Seitz HK, Daniel D, Stremmel W, Büchler MW. Acute cholecystitis: early versus delayed cholecystectomy, a multicenter randomized trial (ACDC study, NCT00447304). Ann Surg. 2013 Sep;258(3):385-93. doi: 10.1097/SLA.0b013e3182a1599b.

Gurusamy KS1, Davidson C, Gluud C, Davidson BR. Early versus delayed laparoscopic cholecystectomy for people with acute cholecystitis. Cochrane Database Syst Rev. 2013 Jun 30;6:CD005440. doi: 10.1002/14651858.CD005440. pub3.

Capacity and Consent to Treatment

A 25 year old lady presents to A & E with her carer. She has a mild learning disability. She is able to point to her abdomen and tell you that it hurts. Her carer reports that she has had a two day history of abdominal pain, nausea and fever. After taking a thorough history and undertaking an examination, she appears clinically to have acute appendicitis, with localised signs of peritonism in the right iliac fossa. You are concerned about whether she has capacity to consent to the procedure. What considerations need to be made when assessing capacity?

Assessment of Capacity is outlined within the Mental Capacity Act 2005. It should be assumed that a person has capacity unless it has been shown otherwise. An assessment of capacity is decision specific. Even if someone makes an unwise decision it does not mean that they lack capacity. All possible measures must have been undertaken to assist the person to be able to make their own decision.

You explain to the patient that they have appendicitis and that they need an urgent operation or they will become more unwell. What are the important factors involved in being able to give consent?

A person is deemed to be able to make a decision if they are able:

- To understand the information relevant to the decision
- To retain the information
- To use or weigh up that information as part of the process of making the decision
- To communicate their decision

It is very important to consider the four components of capacity and to clearly document whether the person does or does not have the capacity to make the specified decision but also to clearly write your reasons for your decision.

If you deem the patient has capacity - are they able to refuse treatment?

If she has capacity, she has the right to make any decision about her treatment. This would include being able to refuse treatments even if this could mean that her presentation would worsen as a result of this. If someone treats a person who has capacity to consent to the treatment and has refused the treatment then they could be liable to legal challenge and the patient could make a claim for compensation against the treating doctor.

If you feel the patient lacks capacity what are your options?

If she lacks capacity to consent to her treatment, then all subsequent decisions made must be done so in her best interests. Any intervention or action which is needed must be the least restrictive option. It would be the job of the surgeon carrying out the operation to assess her capacity. If the decision is a difficult or contentious one then the surgeon could ask for a consultant psychiatrist's opinion.

How do you make a "best interest" decision?

The person making the decision must not make it due to a person's age or appearance, or a condition of theirs, or an aspect of their behaviour which might lead others to make unjustified assumptions about what might be in their best interests i.e. an unprejudiced decision.

It is crucial to consider:

Whether the person will at some point in time have capacity to make the decision. If it is possible that she will, *when* would this occur?

The treating doctor must, as much as is possible, encourage the patient to be involved in the decision making process and improve her ability to be able to participate as much as is possible in making any decisions which affect them.

They must consider, so far as is possible: -

- The person's past and present wishes and feelings including any written statement made by the patient when she had capacity

- The beliefs and values that would be likely to influence their decision if they had capacity

- The other factors that they would be likely to consider if she were able to do so

They must also take into account, if it is possible, the views of :-

- Anyone named by the person as someone to be consulted on the matter in question or on matters of that kind

- Anyone engaged in caring for the person or interested in their welfare

- Any donee of a lasting power of attorney granted by the person, and

- Any deputy appointed for the person by the court, as to what would be in the person's best interests

In this case, if she was found to lack capacity to consent to having an operation, would she have capacity after she has received some analgesia and antiemetics? If a best interests decision were required, it would be important to include her carers and her next of kin in any decisions.

Further reading

Mental Capacity Act 2005: http://www.legislation.gov.uk/ukpga/2005/9/contents

Clostridium difficile Infection

An 81 year old diabetic lady underwent a laparoscopic cholecystectomy for a gangrenous gallbladder. She has been on antibiotics for biliary sepsis. She has a history of IBD from many years ago. On day 5 following her surgery she has profuse watery diarrhoea and colicky lower abdominal pain and a temperature of 38.6°C. Her stool frequency is six times per day and it is reported as foul smelling.

What is the differential diagnosis?

- *Clostridium difficile* (*C. difficile*)
- Diverticulitis
- Crohn's disease
- Ulcerative colitis
- Intra-abdominal sepsis
- Malabsorption
- Gastroenteritis, viral

Infections (Salmonellosis, shigellosis and Vibrio) are less likely because of the patient's chronology of symptoms. Infections with these organisms would normally present with symptoms earlier in the course of an admission. For this reason, many laboratories only routinely test stool specimens collected >48-72 hours after admission for *C. difficile* toxins.

You send a stool specimen to the laboratory. Her stool specimen is positive for GDH, PCR for *C. difficile* toxin gene and *C. difficile* toxin A/B.

How would you assess the severity of this patient's *C. difficile* infection?

C. difficile infection is associated with considerable morbidity and risk of mortality:

- Supportive care should be given, including attention to hydration, electrolytes and nutrition.
- The precipitating antibiotic should be stopped wherever possible; agents with less risk of inducing CDI can be substituted if an underlying infection still requires treatment.
- Acid suppression drugs, especially proton pump inhibitors [PPIs], may be over-prescribed and their continued use should be reviewed.

To choose the most appropriate antibiotic therapy, one needs to assess the patient's severity of disease:

- Mild-moderate *C. difficile* infection:

- WCC <15 x 10^9 cells/L

- ≤ 5 stools per day

- Severe *C. difficile* infection:

  - WCC >15 x 10^9 cells/L

  - Acute rising serum creatinine (i.e. >50% increase above baseline)

  - Temperature of >38.5°C

  - Evidence of severe colitis (abdominal or radiological signs)

  - The number of stools may be a less reliable indicator of severity

How would you treat this patient's *C. difficile* infection?

Mild-moderate disease:

- Oral metronidazole is recommended (dose: 400–500 mg tds for 10–14 days)

Severe disease:

- Oral vancomycin is preferred (dose: 125 mg qds for 10–14 days).

In this case, the lady has symptoms that may suggest active infective colitis, and she is pyrexial. This puts her into the severe category of *C. difficile* infection. Therefore, she should be treated with oral vancomycin.

Close liaison with the infection control and microbiology team is important. The patient will need to be nursed in a side room and an accurate stool chart kept. I would ensure that she is clinically reassessed on at least a daily basis, as she is at high risk of developing fulminant colitis.

In 2012, oral fidaxomicin was approved for the treatment of C. difficile infection in Europe. Fidaxomicin should be considered for patients with severe CDI who are considered at high risk for recurrence; these include elderly patients with multiple comorbidities who are receiving concomitant antibiotics. Fidaxomicin is more expensive than vancomycin, and should only be prescribed for patients in close discussion with an infection specialist.

What are the disadvantages of using vancomycin instead of metronidazole?

Oral vancomycin is only minimally absorbed into the systemic circulation from the gut. Although oral vancomycin is used in the treatment of *C. difficile*, it has the same potential as any other systemically administered antibiotic to impact on patients' normal bowel flora. Patients' normal bowel flora include, amongst many other bacteria, the enterococci. In particular, oral administration can select for vancomycin-resistant enterococci (VRE).

What features of this patient place her at high risk of developing *C. difficile* infection?

Hospitalised elderly patients with multiple comorbidities are at highest risk of *C. difficile* infection, and more likely to require specific treatment. *C. difficile* infection is not only more prevalent in elderly patients but can also be more severe. The strongest risk factor for the development of *C. difficile* infection is antimicrobial exposure.

Any antibiotic – even a single dose of prophylaxis – can predispose patients to C. difficile infection. In 2008, guidelines published by the Health Protection Agency [now Public Health England] recommended avoiding the use of clindamycin and second- and third-generation cephalosporins [e.g. cefuroxime and cefotaxime] (especially in the elderly). They also recommended minimising the use of fluoroquinolones [e.g. ciprofloxacin], carbapenems [e.g. meropenem] and prolonged courses of amoxicillin-based therapy. One should seek to reduce the use of repeated courses of antibiotics in hospitals.

How would you classify *C. difficile* as an organism?

C. difficile is a bacterium. It is an anaerobic, Gram-positive, spore-forming bacillus that produces toxins that are cytotoxic to the colonic mucosa and are capable of causing a marked systemic inflammatory response.

Explain the pathophysiology of *C. difficile* infection?

The symptoms and signs of *C. difficile* infection (as opposed to colonisation) are mediated through the production of *C. difficile* enterotoxin (toxin A) and the cytotoxin (toxin B) which are encoded by the pathogenicity locus (PaLoc). Only strains producing *either* toxin A or toxin B cause *C. difficile* infection. *Both* toxins A and B lead to a breakdown of cellular cytoskeleton, which results in cell apoptosis.

Symptomatic infection is due to transformation of resting *C. difficile* spores into active vegetative bacteria, which is more likely to occur following antibiotic exposure. Morbidity from infection is due to a direct cytotoxic effect on the colonic mucosa.

Bloodstream infections with *C. difficile* are extremely rare.

What is the epidemiology of *C. difficile* infection?

C. difficile is the most frequently identified cause of hospital-acquired diarrhoea, with significant associated costs to the NHS.

C. difficile may colonise 3%-5% of the healthy population and 30% of healthy neonates. In 2006, Sunenshine et al. suggested that between 20%-30% of sedentary patients may have *C. difficile* isolated from the faeces. Meanwhile, in 1989, MacFarland et al. suggested that the majority of hospitalised patients who become colonised with *C. difficile* throughout their inpatient admissions remain asymptomatic.

Recurrent disease occurs in about 20% of patients treated initially with either metronidazole or vancomycin.

Outbreaks of *C. difficile* infection may be traced back to specific environmental sources, including mattresses and curtains.

What percentage of *C. difficile* cases result in fulminant disease?

Fulminant disease may manifest as pseudomembranous colitis, toxic megacolon, perforation or shock, and can be seen in 3% to 5% of patients. Consequential mortality has been estimated at between 34% to 80%.

What is the role of endoscopy for diagnosing *C Diff* colitis?

Due to the potential risk of perforation, endoscopy should be reserved for cases where there is ongoing diagnostic uncertainty.

A CT scan on this lady shows a grossly thickened colon in keeping with a pancolitis with large amounts of free fluid, but no intramural gas. She is now distended and is tachycardic and hypotensive.

She has been on oral vancomycin 125mg QDS. In line with 2008 Department of Health Guidance, following a surgical review, IV metronidazole 500mg TDS is added to her oral vancomycin.

In which patient groups would you consider urgent surgical intervention? Are there any markers that may help to identify patients associated with a higher mortality?

From the 2008 guidelines:

- "Colectomy is required in some patients with megacolon (dilatation >10cm), perforation or septic shock, and should be done before the blood lactate rises above 5 mmol/L (Lipsett et al., 1994; Longo et al., 2004; Koss et al., 2006)..."

Urgent surgical intervention should be considered in elderly patients, those with haemodynamic collapse, and patients with organ failure. In addition leukocytosis >50x10^9 cells/L, lactate≥5 mmol/L, and hypoalbuminemia, may identify patients who have a higher mortality. An urgent colectomy should be considered in these patients.

Even with early intervention, the mortality rate from surgery for fulminant colitis remains 30%-40%.

What is the operation of choice in these patients?

From the 2008 guidelines:

- "…Patients should have a total or subtotal colectomy rather than a hemicolectomy or a caecostomy. It may be preferable to preserve the rectal stump for subsequent ileo-rectal anastomosis. The rectocolonic stoma can then be perfused with vancomycin liquid if necessary."

Due to the pancolonic distribution of the process a subtotal colectomy with end ileostomy is the procedure of choice. An open approach is the preferred approach in unstable patients. Although the rectal stump may harbour residual disease these patients are too sick to undergo extensive pelvic dissection.

Segmental resection, ileostomy alone, and colostomy have all been shown to be associated with an increased mortality.

What specific postoperative complications may the patient experience?

These patients may require ICU management. A prolonged ileus is to be expected and feeding via TPN may need to be addressed.

Antibiotic therapy targeted against *C. difficile* should be continued for at least 10-14 days, with regular clinical review thereafter to decide on further management, in discussion with an infection specialist.

References

Medscape. Clostridium Difficile Colitis Differential Diagnoses [Internet]. 2014 [cited 2014 Oct 30]. Available from: http://emedicine.medscape.com/article/186458-differential

PHE. Updated guidance on the management and treatment of Clostridium difficile infection [Internet]. 2013 [cited 2014 Oct 30]. Available from: https://www.gov.uk/government/uploads/system/uploads/attachment_data/file/321891/Clostridium_difficile_management_and_treatment.pdf

Stevens DL, Bryant AE, Berger A, Von Eichel-Streiber C. Clostridium. Manual of clinical microbiology. 2011. p. 834–57.

Sunenshine RH, McDonald LC. Clostridium difficile-associated disease: new challenges from an established pathogen. Cleve Clin J Med [Internet]. 2006 Mar [cited 2014 Oct 30];73(2):187–97. Available from: http://www.ncbi.nlm.nih.gov/pubmed/16478043

McFarland L V, Mulligan ME, Kwok RY, Stamm WE. Nosocomial acquisition of Clostridium difficile infection. N Engl J Med [Internet]. 1989 Jan 26 [cited 2014 Oct 30];320(4):204–10. Available from: http://www.ncbi.nlm.nih.gov/pubmed/2911306

DH and HPA. Clostridium difficile infection : How to deal with the problem [Internet]. 2008. Available from: http://www.hpa.org.uk/webc/HPAwebFile/HPAweb_C/1232006607827

Seltman AK. Surgical Management of *Clostridium* difficile Colitis. Clin Colon Rectal Surg. 2012 Dec;25(4):204-9.

Colonic Volvulus

Scenario 1

A 51 year old man is admitted with a history of severe central abdominal pain and vomiting. On examination he had fullness in the left upper quadrant but no peritonism. A plain abdominal x-ray was requested (see below image).

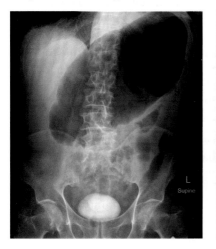 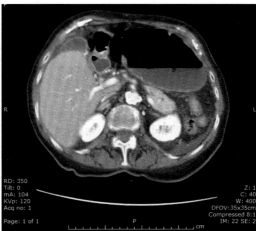

Describe the appearances of the plain axr and the CT abdomen

On the plain axr there is a dilated loop of large bowel in the left upper quadrant with no large bowel identified in the right iliac fossa. These appearances are suggestive of a caecal volvulus.

On the CT scan the caecum is rotated and displaced into the left upper quadrant. *Additional CT signs that may be seen indicative of a caecal volvulus include swirling and twisting of the mesenteric vessels around the ileocolic artery - this is pathognomic of caecal volvulus. The mesentery may also appear oedematous. There is no evidence of perforation.*

Overall, radiographic studies confirm the diagnosis of caecal volvulus 90% of the time. The remainder are diagnosed at surgery.

How would you manage this patient?

Surgery is the treatment of choice. After full resuscitation this patient will need a laparotomy and right hemicolectomy. The incidence of perforation and mortality with a caecal volvulus is higher than with a sigmoid volvulus.

In the absence of caecal compromise other approaches include caecopexy and caecostomy but are generally limited to the very frail. Caecopexy consists of securing the caecum to the parietal peritoneum to reduce the risk of recurrence by reducing its mobility. It may be performed laparoscopically. Caecopexy is a safe procedure with a low mortality rate but has the disadvantage of a recurrence rate up to 40%. Caecostomy should be reserved for the very frail who cannot undergo laparotomy. It consists of placing a tube in a small hole in the caecal wall, often through the lumen via an appendectomy. The caecum is then fixed to the anterior abdominal wall. This can be done through a small incision and even under local anaesthesia. Serious complications may occur such as gangrene, caecal necrosis, and intraperitoneal leakage of faeces. The recurrence rate is less than with caecopexy – up to 15%. Attempts at reduction by colonoscopy or barium enema should not be made and may result in a dangerous delay before surgery.

You perform a right hemicolectomy on this patient with a primary anastomosis using a linear stapler. Post operatively the patient is complaining of per rectal bleeding of moderate amounts and has dropped his Hb to 57g/l. He is haemodynamically stable but with borderline urine output. How would you manage him?

The main concern here is bleeding from the anastomotic staple line, which is a rare complication of a stapled anastomosis. He is haemodynamically stable at present but needs to be transfused and urine output optimised. If he is actively bleeding then a CT angiogram may help to confirm that bleeding is from the anastomosis and if he becomes unstable may require laparotomy. In the meantime blood should be crossmatched and coagulation checked. The majority of staple line bleeding should stop over time with conservative measures.

What are the other associations of a caecal volvulus?

They are associated with pregnancy, Hirschsprungs disease and occur in a younger age group in comparison with sigmoid volvulus. In approximately 10% of cases, the caecum and ascending colon bend in the cephalic direction – this is known as a caecal bascule. This does not produce ischaemia from twisting of the mesentery but from swelling of the caecum.

Scenario 2

You have been called to see an 85 year old man from a nursing home who has been getting progressively more unwell over the last three days, with vomiting and a distended abdomen. A plain axr has been performed. What is your diagnosis?

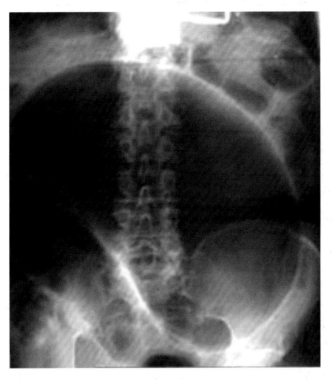

The plain axr shows the characteristic coffee bean sign that is pathognomic of a sigmoid volvulus. There is a markedly distended sigmoid loop, which assumes a bent inner tube or inverted U-shaped appearance, with the limbs of the sigmoid loop directed toward the pelvis. The dilated loop usually lies in the right side of the abdomen, and the limbs taper inferiorly. The colonic haustra are lost, and progressive distention elevates the sigmoid loop under one side of the diaphragm. The involved bowel walls are oedematous, and the contiguous walls form a dense white line. This line is surrounded by the curved and dilated gas-filled lumen, resulting in a coffee bean-shaped structure; this is the coffee bean sign. There is no gas in the rectum.

What other conditions may cause diagnostic confusion on the plain x-ray?

Other forms of large-bowel obstruction, especially those due to sigmoid colon carcinoma, pseudo-obstruction, caecal volvulus, and an ileosigmoid knot, may mimic or be confused with a sigmoid volvulus.

The CT confirms a sigmoid volvulus with no evidence of complications. How should this patient be managed?

All patients will need resuscitation and optimization of fluid and electrolyte balance. These are often elderly frail patients with significant co-morbidities. If the patient has obvious signs of peritonitis then a laparotomy may be indicated depending on the patient's comorbidities and quality of life. In the absence of peritonitis non-operative detorsion is advocated as the primary treatment. Decompression should be performed either by flatus tube insertion or via flexible sigmoidoscopy. Drainage of blood via the rectal tube is a worrying sign and may indicate strangulation. Late recurrence rate following non-operative treatment in elderly patients is high (90%). Decompression through flexible sigmoidoscopy has the advantage of allowing visualization of the colonic mucosa for evidence of ischaemia.

You decide to perform a flexible sigmoidoscopy and this confirms gross ischaemia of the descending colon and sigmoid colon. After discussion with the patient a decision is made to proceed to emergency laparotomy. At laparotomy you find gross perforation of the sigmoid colon with generalized contamination. What operation would you perform and why?

I would perform a Hartmann's procedure with an end colostomy. I would not perform a primary anastomosis in this patient due to the extent of contamination as well as his frail condition, as he may not survive an anastomotic leak.

Under what circumstances might you perform a primary anastomosis?

I would only perform a primary anastomosis if surgery is performed in a stable patient who has minimal contamination and insists on avoiding a stoma. Such an operation should only be performed by a specialist colorectal surgeon.

Are you aware of any percutaneous endoscopic treatments for sigmoid volvulus?

Although sigmoid colectomy remains the gold standard treatment, PEC provides an alternative for those who are too unfit for surgery. Percutaneous endoscopic colostomy (PEC) is an alternative for option in selected patients with recurrent sigmoid volvulus. It allows fixing, venting and irrigation of the colon.

What is the pathophysiology of a sigmoid volvulus?

A long redundant mesentery predisposes to volvulus formation particularly if there is narrowing of the mesentery, which provides an axis for rotation. The sigmoid colon rotates through 180-720 degrees clockwise or anticlockwise. The result is a closed loop obstruction. Predisposing factors to sigmoid volvulus include congenital factors such as a mobile long mesentery or acquired factors such as chronic constipation that thins out the sigmoid but with a relatively narrow mesentery. Hirschsprung's disease and Chagas disease are associated with sigmoid volvulus. Interestingly a sigmoid volvulus is the commonest cause of bowel obstruction in pregnancy!

Compartment Syndrome

A 69 year old man is day 2 following an elective pan-proctocolectomy for UC. It's 2am and he is complaining of severe pain in his left foot. He has no history of peripheral vascular disease. On examination he has severe pain on calf extension along with marked tenderness on calf compression. You suspect he may have compartment syndrome.

Which is the most commonly affected leg compartment?

The anterior compartment is the most commonly affected followed by the lateral, deep posterior and superficial posterior compartments. Although the leg is most commonly affected, the thigh may be affected in some cases – the anterior quadriceps being the most frequently involved.

What is the pathogenesis of compartment syndrome?

The initiating stimulus is always injury, leading to oedema and swelling. As muscles are contained within a non-expansile osseofascial compartment a vicious cycle of swelling and worsening venous compression occurs. This will eventually affect the arterial inflow leading to ischaemia.

What are the typical clinical features of compartment syndrome?

Pain out of proportion to clinical findings is typical. The affected limb may be swollen, tense and tender within the muscle compartment. Pain with passive stretching is a cardinal feature (pain is due to muscle ischaemia). Neurological signs are a late feature and are suggestive of neural ischaemia.

Peripheral nerves and muscle can survive 4 hours of ischaemia. At 6 hours ischaemia is partially reversible but at 8 hours irreversible damage occurs.

How would you diagnose compartment syndrome in this patient?

The diagnosis of compartment syndrome is usually a clinical diagnosis. Although intracompartmental pressure can be measured it can be difficult to interpret. A Stryker needle is the most commonly used instrument, but other instruments are available if the correct equipment is usually not available within a department. If intra-compartmental pressure is >30mmHg (normal is 0-8mmHg) then this is highly suggestive of compartment syndrome.

How would you perform a lower limb fasciotomy?

There are 4 compartments to release: Anterior
                                     Lateral (peroneal)
                                     Posterior: superficial
                                                       Deep

A lateral incision is centered between the fibular shaft and the crest of the tibia. This incision overlies the intermuscular septum between the anterior and lateral compartments. Skin and subcutaneous flaps are developed medially and laterally to expose the fascia of the intermuscular septum and the fascia of the anterior and lateral compartments. The anterior compartment fascia is incised and extended proximally and distally using scissors. Once the anterior compartment is decompressed, the procedure is performed on the lateral compartment. The proximal extent of fasciotomy should end 4cm to 5cm distal to the fibular head, minimizing the risk of a nerve injury (see figure below).

LATERAL INCISION

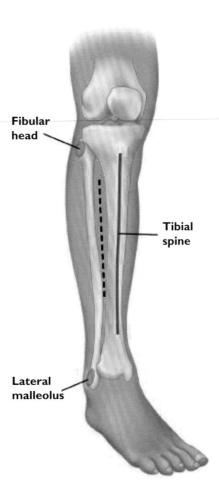

Damage Control Laparotomy

A 55 year old male is admitted to the resuscitation room following multiple stab injuries to his abdomen. He has peritonitis and evisceration of small bowel. A decision is made to proceed to a laparotomy. He is haemodynamically unstable. He has a past medical history of previous MIs and chronic renal impairment.

At laparotomy he has extensive contamination from multiple small bowel injuries, colonic injuries as well as a significant liver laceration with haemoperitoneum. He is on escalating doses of inotropes and the anaesthetist expresses concerns about the patient's stability.

What are the principles of a damage control laparotomy?

The principles of a damage control laparotomy (DCL) are to perform an abbreviated laparotomy to rapidly achieve control of haemorrhage, sepsis and source control through shorter operating times, to allow the patient to be transferred for ongoing resuscitation and stabilisation. DCL usually involves temporary abdominal closure to allow control / prevention of IAH and a second look laparotomy for definitive treatment and closure.

What factors help you decide when an abdomen is ready for closure?

The following factors can help to decide whether the abdomen is ready for closure or not:

- IAP < 15mmHg
- Fascia can be closed without excess tension
- Sepsis is controlled
- No further intra-abdominal surgical procedures are planned
- Other physiological factors such as acidosis, hypothermia and coagulopathy need to be kept in mind as they may aggravate IAH. However these factors tend to be more of a concern in the acute phase.

What are the risks involved in leaving a patient with a laparostomy?

Loss of domain and retraction of the fascia laterally occur from an early stage and over the course of time may prevent definitive closure. This can lead to a high rate of significant ventral herniation. Also there is a risk of fistula formation with prolonged use of negative pressure therapy, but this is a contentious issue.

You are about to perform a laparostomy and ask the theatre staff to provide you with a commercial temporary closure system such as a Vacuum Assisted Closure (VAC). However this is not available. What are your other options for temporary closure?

A polyethylene sheet is perforated multiple times with a scalpel blade. It is then placed over the peritoneal viscera and beneath the peritoneum of the abdominal wall. A moist sterile surgical towel(s) is folded to fit the abdominal wall defect and is placed over the polyethylene sheet. The edges of the towel are positioned below the skin edges. Two 10-French flat silicone drains are placed on top of the towel exit 3cm to 5 cm away from the superior part of the wound. The benzoin-painted skin is kept dry until covered with a plastic polyester drape backed with iodophor-impregnated adhesive. Each drain tube is connected to a bulb suction with Y adapter which is then connected to a suction source at 100 to 150 mm Hg continuous negative pressure. This technique involves materials that are available from standard stock in most operating rooms.

There are in fact a number of similar methods (e.g. Opsite sandwich) to achieving TAC. Be sure you can explain the one you are most familiar with.

ERCP Perforation

An 80 year old woman is admitted from endoscopy following a therapeutic ERCP for choledocholithiasis. The procedure was difficult. A sphincterotomy was performed. She develops severe back pain, tachycardia, fever and tachypnoea post procedure.

What is your initial treatment?

Firstly the patient requires analgesia, oxygen, an intravenous line and iv fluids. In line with suspected sepsis, management blood culture, broad spectrum antibiotics and a catheter. Baseline bloods including lactate and arterial blood gas should be performed.

What investigations are you going to carry out?

The likeliest scenario is a duodenal perforation. Ascending cholangitis and pancreatitis may also be possible. On top of baseline blood tests, cultures and ABGs mentioned above, the patient requires an urgent abdominal CT with iv contrast.

A CT scan reveals retroperitoneal stranding, fluid and air collections. What treatment should be initiated?

Initiation of sepsis bundle should be carried out. The patient should be moved to a level 2 bed, with consideration of CVP and arterial lines. Most ERCP-induced perforations are retroperitoneal and can be treated with initial antibiotic therapy, nil by mouth with nasoduodenal or nasogastric drainage and percutaneous drainage of any large collections.

What types of perforation may be seen with ERCP?

There are three types of post ERCP perforation:

1) The commonest is a retroperitoneal perforation, which can vary from a relatively asymptomatic mild form to severe sepsis.

2) Free bowel perforation with intraperitoneal contamination.

3) Direct bile duct perforation.

When would you consider surgery?

Surgery should usually be considered if there is any intraperitoneal or free oesophageal perforation. Peritonitis and the presence of free air within the peritoneal cavity will usually indicate a need for urgent surgery. Surgery should follow resuscitation and initiation of antibiotics. Successful outcome from surgery is improved with early surgery, though duodenal perforations can often heal poorly.

What are the risk factors for ERCP perforation?

Therapeutic procedures are far more commonly associated with perforation: sphincterotomy, especially performed with a pre-cut papillotome is especially at risk

Other risk factors include:

- Periampullary diverticulum
- Ampullectomy
- Small calibre bile duct
- Intramural injection of contrast
- Longer duration of the procedure
- Biliary dilation

Haematemesis

A 56 year old man presents following large bouts of haematemesis. You are called to A&E to see the patient urgently. Resuscitation has commenced. He has a pulse rate of 104 and a blood pressure of 100/70mmHg. A week ago he had been endoscoped as part of investigations for anaemia and found to have an ulcer in the duodenal cap. He is fit and well and on omeprazole but no other medications.

What are the priorities in managing this patient?

My main priority in this patient is to fully resuscitate him based on ABC principles prior to any intervention. A patent airway is secured, high flow oxygen given, large bore intravenous cannulae placed and crossmatched blood requested. I would involve the critical care team for additional support. In the presence of significant haematemesis the airway may particularly be at risk during an endoscopy, therefore the anaesthetist may choose to intubate and ventilate this patient.

A definitive diagnosis needs to be obtained by urgent upper GI endoscopy, which may also allow therapy to be performed as well.

What do you think is the aetiology of this bleed?

Given the recent history of a newly diagnosed duodenal ulcer then this is the most likely source of bleeding. However, one needs to keep an open mind towards other causes that may have been overlooked at the time of endoscopy such as varices or bleeding tumours.

At endoscopy you find a bleeding duodenal ulcer in D1. What treatment modalities are available endoscopically to control the bleed?

I would inject adrenaline (1 in 10,000) in four quadrants around the bleeding point, which acts by volume tamponade, and has a local vasoconstrictor effect. I would also perform thermocoagulation using either a gold probe or argon plasma coagulation.

Endoscopic treatment modalities may be classified into injection, thermocoagulation and mechanical. The main injection modality used is adrenaline. Other injection modalities include sclerosants such as sodium tetradecyl sulphate or ethanolamine, but these are discouraged from use and may even cause perforation. Mechanical methods use haemoclips but these can be difficult to apply, particularly for awkwardly sited ulcers such as those on the lesser curve.

How is endoscopic treatment best delivered?

Current evidence suggests a more successful outcome of dual therapy rather than single modality e.g. combining adrenaline injection with gold probe. Numerous meta-analyses indicate that adding a second procedure, such as a second injectate (for example, alcohol, thrombin, or fibrin glue), thermal contact, or clips, is superior to adrenaline injection alone in significantly reduced re-bleeding, surgery and mortality compared with adrenaline monotherapy.

Several recent meta-analyses have better quantified the efficacy of endoscopic therapies. Although monotherapy with adrenaline injection is more effective than medical therapy in patients with high-risk stigmata, it is inferior to other monotherapies or to combination therapy that uses two or more methods.

How endoscopically can you judge if the patient is at risk of re-bleeding?

The Forrest classification is used to describe endoscopic appearances of bleeding ulcers. The highest risk of re-bleeding is seen with active bleeding ulcers or a non-bleeding visible vessel in an ulcer bed.

If there is active bleeding during endoscopy there is a 90% chance of recurrence, if there is a visible vessel there is a 50% chance of re-bleeding, with adherent clot there is a 30% chance of re-bleeding. Recent evidence suggests that removing clot to treat the underlying ulcer can reduce the re-bleeding risk.

Forrest Ia = spurting active bleeding; Ib = oozing active bleeding; IIa = visible vessel; IIB = adherent clot; IIc = flat pigmented spot; III = ulcer with clean base. Patients with low risk stigmata (III or IIc) do not need endoscopic therapy.

Following combination therapy using adrenaline and gold probe, treatment control was achieved and the patient haemodynamically stable. Would you plan a second look endoscopy for this patient?

The use of scheduled second look endoscopy in these situations is controversial. In patients at very high risk (eg, active bleeding), high risk stigmata (Forrest Ia-IIb) and/or unsatisfactory initial endostasis, routine second-look endoscopy may be more sensible. If primary endostasis has been optimum there is no need for a second look.

There is certainly an argument for a second look endoscopy in patients with smaller ulcers as the success rate with further endostasis is high. However large chronic ulcers that were difficult to control at the original endoscopy and those in shock from re-bleeding are best managed by surgery. Another option if available at the time of the re-bleed is transcatheter embolisation by an interventional radiologist.

What pharmacotherapy is indicated for this patient and why?

Administration of PPIs have been shown to reduce re-bleeding risk. The majority of studies used iv omeprazole but other PPIs are also suitable. Several meta-analyses support the use of an intravenous bolus followed by continuous-infusion PPI therapy for 72 hours, to decrease re-bleeding and mortality in patients with high-risk stigmata who have undergone endoscopic treatment.

What are the Glasgow-Blatchford score and Rockall score?

The Glasgow-Blatchford Bleeding Score stratifies upper GI bleeding patients who are 'low-risk' and therefore candidates for outpatient management. It is based on urea, haemoglobin, systolic blood pressure, pulse, presence of melaena, presence of syncope, cardiac failure and liver failure. A score of 0 is the cut-off with any patient scoring >0 being at risk of requiring intervention. UK Guidelines suggest patients with a score of zero can be considered for safe early discharge.

The Rockall score is used to determine the mortality rather than the need for intervention (see table below). It involves age, systolic BP, scoring for co-morbidities, underlying diagnosis, and evidence of bleeding at gastroscopy.

Initial Score Criteria (prior to gastroscopy)	
Age	Age <60 – 0 points Age 60-79 - 1 point Age ≥80 - 2 points
Shock	"No shock" = (SBP ≥100 mm Hg, pulse <100/min) - 0 points "Tachycardia" = (SBP ≥100 mm Hg, pulse ≥100/min) - 1 point "Hypotension" = (SBP <100 mm Hg)
Co-morbidity	No major comorbidity - 0 points Cardiac failure, IHD or any major comorbidity - 2 points Renal or liver failure, disseminated malignancy - 3 points
	Initial Rockall Score = /7
Additional Criteria for Full Score (after gastroscopy)	
Diagnosis	Mallory-Weiss tear, no lesion seen nor SRH - 0 points All other diagnoses - 1 point Malignancy of upper GI tract - 2 points
Major stigmata of recent haemorrhage (SRH)?	None or dark spot only - 0 points Blood in the upper GI tract, adherent clot, visible or spurting vessel - 2 points
	Full Rockall Score /11

Original tables in Rockall TA, Logan RF, Devlin HB, et al; Risk assessment after acute upper gastrointestinal haemorrhage. Gut. 1996 Mar; 38(3):316-21. ©1996 BMJ Publishing Group Limited.

Score	Mortality	Mortality with re-bleed
Score 1	Nil	Nil
Score 2	Nil	Nil
Score 3	5%	5-10%
Score 4	5-10%	15-25%
Score 5	5-10%	15-25%
Score 6	5-10%	15-25%
Score 7+	10-35%	25-50%

Rockall score and corresponding risk of mortality

Despite initial stabilisation this patient has further massive haematemesis. A second endoscopy proves to be difficult due to the presence of a large volume of blood and inadequate views. You are asked to perform a laparotomy. Describe your surgical approach to a bleeding duodenal ulcer.

Bleeding duodenal ulcers are usually found in the first part of the duodenum on the posterior wall, the bleeding being due to erosion into the gastroduodenal artery. My approach would be to carry out an upper midline incision. The duodenum may need to be Kocherised and a transverse duodenotomy made. Sutures should then be placed above to provide traction and visualisation. Once the ulcer has been identified it can be under-run using a small but heavy round-bodied needle (absorbable or non absorbable suitable). The duodenotomy should then be closed in a vertical fashion (Heineke-Mikulicz pyloroplasty). If it is not possible to control bleeding from within the ulcer the gastroduodenal artery may be ligated superior to the duodenum.

References

http://www.sign.ac.uk/pdf/sign105.pdf Management of acute upper and lower gastrointestinal bleeding. The BSG guidelines for acute non-variceal haemorrhage were written several years ago and have become dated. BSG have adopted the Scottish Inter-collegiate Guideline Network (SIGN) guidelines as the standard of care.

Barkun AN, Bardou M, Kuipers EJ, Sung J, Hunt RH, Martel M, Sinclair P; International Consensus Upper Gastrointestinal Bleeding Conference Group. International consensus recommendations on the management of patients with nonvariceal upper gastrointestinal bleeding. Ann Intern Med. 2010 Jan 19;152(2):101-13.

Head Injury

What is primary and secondary brain injury?

Primary brain injury is sustained at the time of the impact and may result in:

- Fractures, as a result of a direct blow, with or without underlying brain injury

- A spectrum of injury ranging from concussion to diffuse axonal injury as a result of inertial forces

- Contre coup injury, ie damage away from the site of impact

- Extradural / subdural / intracerebral haematoma / subarachnoid haemorrhage

Secondary brain injury occurs as a result of damage after the primary brain injury and can be accentuated by:

- Hypoxia (pO2 <10 kPa)

- Hypotension (systolic BP <90 mmHg)

- Hypercarbia

- Hypoglycaemia

- Delay in diagnosis

- Delay in definitive treatment

- Seizures: hypoxia and hypercarbia may develop

- Raised ICP

- Suboptimal management of other injuries

Many of these factors are easily preventable, recognisable and treatable. Management should be directed at identifying and treating the factors that cause secondary brain injury.

When is permissive hypercapnia used following a head injury?

Hyperventilation is generally reserved for those patients in danger of imminent coning and should only be used after discussion with a neurosurgeon or with the aid of close monitoring in a neurosurgical unit.

Following intubation hyperventilation may be used to reduce PaCO2 to 4.5kPa. This causes vasoconstriction of cerebral arterioles, thereby reducing the volume of arterial blood in the head. However, if excessive it can severely reduce blood flow to already compromised areas, and exacerbate any injury.

How is intubation of a head injured patient performed?

Manual inline stabilisation is used to maintain stability whilst intubation is being carried out. Leaving the semi-rigid collar in place limits mouth opening and makes intubation much more difficult. Once intubation has been completed, the airway team must ensure that the collar, tape and sandbags are reapplied. It is vital to ensure the collar fits adequately and the head is maintained in a neutral position, as constriction of the neck veins from too tight a collar or tube tie, or poor positioning, can elevate the ICP from venous congestion.

How does the cardiovascular system respond in a head injury?

Hypertension is a sign that the body is trying to maintain cerebral perfusion in the face of raised ICP. Hypovolaemic shock is never due to a head injury unless there is a profound amount of blood loss from a scalp wound. In the presence of shock a systolic pressure >110mmHg should be aimed for in order to maintain cerebral perfusion pressure (CPP).

Why are dextrose containing fluids avoided in a head injury?

In cases of head trauma, dextrose-containing fluids (5% dextrose, 4% dextrose plus 0.18% saline) are avoided because they reduce plasma sodium, thereby lowering the plasma osmolality and exacerbating cerebral oedema. They also may cause hyperglycaemia, which is associated with a worse neurological outcome.

What neurological assessment is made for head injured patients?

A detailed examination needs to be performed including a repeat of the GCS, pupillary responses, and detection of any lateralising (focal) signs that may indicate intracranial injury.

What is the aim of using the GCS?

The aim is to detect any change in neurological state that may indicate injury or worsening of the patient's condition, and so it is helpful to have the same person assessing these parameters each time.

What are the common pitfalls in using GCS?

Inability to open the eyes due to swelling does not automatically mean "no eye-opening". Simply record that the assessment cannot be made. A response to pain is best elicited by applying pressure on the supratrochlear nerve in the supraorbital ridge. A peripheral stimulus may not be sensed in the presence of a spinal cord injury. Localising to pain means that a hand reaches above the clavicle following the supraorbital stimulus. Limb movements confined to below the clavicle represent "withdraws from pain". Splints and painful fractures limit limb movement. This may cause differences between sides. Record the best side and indicate if there is disparity. A verbal response cannot be assessed in an intubated patient. Record "patient intubated".

What lateralizing signs may occur in a head injury?

Lateralising signs are a strong indicator of intracranial pathology. These are most often a unilateral weakness or asymmetry of motor or pupillary responses, and strongly suggest the presence of focal injury. In a conscious patient, upper-arm drift is a sensitive test of partial hemiplegia. The patient is asked to close their eyes and hold their arms out in front of them, palms facing upwards. Rotation of the arm, so the palm faces downwards, is an early and sensitive sign and should be a cause for concern.

What are the signs of a base of skull fracture?

The base of the skull lies along a line joining the landmarks of the mastoid process, tympanic membrane and orbits, and a fracture.

Early:

- Haemotympanum
- Bloody CSF from the ear or nose
- Scleral haemorrhages with no posterior margin

Late (occurring up to 12-24 hours after injury):

- Bruising over the mastoid - Battle's sign
- Orbital bruising "raccoon" eyes

How do you distinguish blood from cerebrospinal fluid (CSF)?

Blood dripping from the nose or ear can be tested for CSF by dropping some of the fluid onto an absorbent sheet e.g. paper towel. If CSF is mixed with the blood, a double ring pattern will develop.

How would you drain the stomach of an unconscious head injured patient with a base of skull fracture?

A nasogastric tube should not be used if there is a fractured base of skull, as the tube may be pushed up into the skull vault. As a general rule, it is safer to use the orogastric route for gastric drainage in an unconscious head injured patient.

How would you deal with a fitting patient with a head injury?

An initial convulsion can be treated with a slow intravenous bolus of diazepam to a maximum dose of 5-10 mg depending on age and size. If this does not terminate seizures phenytoin is considered.

What are the indications for head CT scanning after head injury?

NICE indications for immediate CT scanning after cranial trauma:

- GCS less than 13 at any time since injury

- GCS equal to 13 or 14 at 2 hours after injury

- Suspected open or depressed skull fracture

- Any sign of a basal skull fracture (haemotympanum, "panda eyes", Battle's sign, CSF otorrhoea

- Post-traumatic seizure

- Focal neurological deficit

- More than one episode of vomiting (use clinical judgement if less than 12 years of age)

- Amnesia for more than 30 minutes of events before impact (not possible in very young children)

Also in patients with the following risk factors providing they have experienced some loss of consciousness or amnesia:

- Age equal to or greater than 65 years

- Coagulopathy (history of bleeding, known clotting disorder, warfarin therapy) Dangerous mechanism of injury (e.g. pedestrian hit by car, fall more than 1m or down 5 steps). Use a lower threshold for height of fall in young children.

What sort of agents may be advised by neurosurgeons to reduce ICP?

Mannitol

This is an osmotic diuretic agent that has a dual effect in reducing ICP. Its early effect is due to an improvement in cerebral blood flow by altering red cell deformability and size. It also reduces interstitial brain water by establishing an osmotic gradient and movement of water between brain tissue and blood. Initially, 0.5g/kg, of 20% mannitol (175 ml in 70 kg adult), is administered and the patient reassessed, e.g. for a reduction in pupil size. A urinary catheter is always required if not already in place. Repeated doses can cause hypovolaemia or electrolyte disturbances.

Furosemide

This is a potent diuretic that also reduces ICP by reducing brain water and the rate of CSF production. It can be used instead of mannitol at a dose of 0.5 mg/kg. The effect of furosemide can be extremely potent if used in conjunction with mannitol, and will cause hypovolaemia, hypotension and biochemical derangement.

Currently no neuroprotective drugs exist. The use of steroids should be avoided because of the risk of hyperglycaemia that is associated with a worse outcome.

What is cerebral blood flow?

Cerebral blood flow is 750ml/minute, which is approximately 15% of the cardiac output. Cerebral autoregulation functions between systolic blood pressures of 50-150 mmHg.

What is the Monro-Kellie doctrine?

The Monro-Kellie doctrine states that the volume of intracranial contents must stay constant as the cranium is non-expansile.

$$CPP = MAP - ICP$$

To compensate for an intra-cranial haematoma (subdural/epidural) or cerebral oedema, CSF and venous blood are squeezed out so as to limit ICP. However once the limits of compensation are superseded then there is an exponential rise of ICP for even a small additional increase in volume of haematoma:

Pressure – volume curve

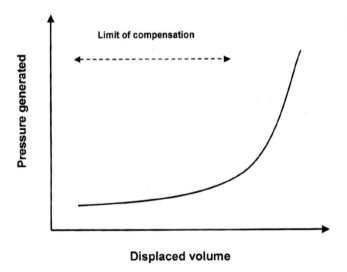

What is the normal ICP?

Normal ICP is usually around 10 mmHg. ICP greater than 20mmHg (particularly if sustained) is associated with poor outcome.

What is the significance of a skull fracture?

The significance of a skull fracture should not be underestimated as it takes a considerable amount of force to fracture the skull. The likelihood of an intracranial haematoma is significantly higher in the presence of a skull fracture.

Which is the commonest form of focal brain injury?

Subdural haematomas are more common than extradural haematomas and occur due to tearing of the bridging veins from the cerebral surface. Subdural haematomas normally cover the entire surface of the hemisphere, and the brain damage from a subdural haematoma is much more severe than from an extradural. Extradural haematomas are relatively uncommon. They are located outside the dura and are typically biconvex shaped. They are located in the temporoparietal region and are usually due to tearing of the anterior branch of the middle meningeal artery secondary to a fracture.

What is the volume of CSF?

140-150 mls of CSF. 70% of CSF is produced by the choroid plexus of the lateral, third and fourth ventricles. 30% comes from the vessels lining the ventricular walls. 80% of the CSF is absorbed at the arachnoid villi and 20% is absorbed at the spinal nerve roots.

What is the blood brain barrier?

This is a barrier formed between blood and CSF and is composed of:

- Tight junctions between the epithelial cells of the capillary
- Astrocytic foot processes applied to the basal membrane of cerebral capillaries

The blood brain barrier is soluble to lipids, lipid soluble agents e.g. GA, drugs e.g. opiates, and glucose.

What is Cushing's response?

This is a response to raised ICP and is a mixed vagal and sympathetic response leading to hypertension and bradycardia.

Ischaemic Colitis

A 59 year old man presents with a history of severe left lower abdominal pain associated with passage of blood and mucus per rectally. He is a smoker and takes medication for hypertension. On examination he is tachycardic (110bpm) has a temperature of 38°C and mild left lower quadrant peritonism.

What are the main differential diagnoses to consider?

Diverticulitis

Ischaemic colitis (IC): fits with the story, risk factors (hypertension/smoker) and blood per rectum

Inflammatory bowel disease

Infective colitis

Other rarer causes include radiation enteritis, microscopic colitis, neutropenic enterocolitis. Although ischaemic colitis is typically seen in elderly patients it can still occur in younger patients with risk factors.

What is the typical distribution of ischaemic colitis? What is the anatomical basis for this?

The splenic flexure, descending colon and sigmoid colon are the most frequently affected, most commonly at "watershed" areas – these are between the junction of the superior mesenteric artery (SMA) and inferior mesenteric arteries (IMA). Griffiths' point is located at the splenic flexure and represents a watershed area between the distribution of the SMA and IMA. Sudeck's point is another watershed area located at the rectosigmoid junction between the inferior mesenteric and superior haemorrhoidal arteries. Although these are the commonest areas to be affected, in reality any portion of the colon and rectum may be affected.

What are the causes of ischaemic colitis?

IC is due to occlusive or non-occlusive causes. Occlusive causes include small vessel disease (atherosclerosis/ vasculitis / radiation). Non-occlusive causes include myocardial infarction / sepsis / hypovolaemia. There are two pathological forms of IC. The commonest form (80%) is a transient non-gangrenous form and reversible form characterized by mucosal and submucosal ischaemia. This form is usually seen in arteriopaths with small vessel disease. The more severe form is rare. This is characterized by transmural colonic ischaemia and may lead to multi organ failure.

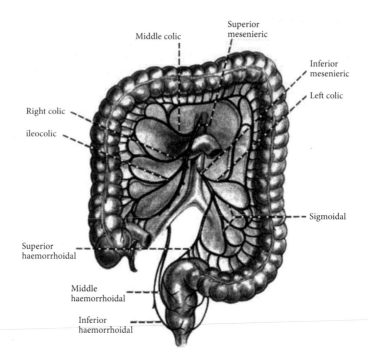

What are the indications for surgery in ischaemic colitis?

Although it is unusual for patients to progress to fulminant colitis with perforation this would be one indication for an emergency laparotomy. In the absence of frank perforation an aggressive surgical approach seems justified in patients with multiple organ failure and findings of severe form of ischaemia at endoscopy. In the chronic phase some patients may develop a fibrotic stricture and need a resection.

Why do some patients develop ischaemic colitis following abdominal aortic aneurysm (AAA) surgery?

If the IMA is ligated during repair of an AAA then there is a chance of developing ischaemic colitis. This is particularly higher if the patient has a stenotic and diseased SMA. In addition other factors such as hypotension or cross clamping may contribute to ischaemia. The incidence of this complication is higher following emergency than elective AAA repair and may become evident in the first few days after surgery.

Ischaemic colitis following AAA repair can be transient and self-limiting but, when severe, is associated with mortality even as high as 80%. In the elective setting careful preoperative assessment can help to anticipate the need for the IMA reimplantation. Some patients lack sufficient collateral blood supply to the colon and can benefit from IMA reimplantation. This not only reduces the risk of postoperative ischaemic colitis but can be lifesaving.

What is the role of endoscopy in IC?

Colonoscopy is considered by many to be the gold standard for diagnosing IC. It should be performed if the diagnosis is in doubt or the patient is deteriorating. The first part of the colon to become affected by ischaemia is the mucosa on the antimesenteric side. A single linear ulcer running longitudinally along the antimesenteric colonic wall (colonic single stripe sign) may be seen. Oedema, ulceration, friability and pseudomembranes may also be seen. In more severe ischaemia with transmural infarction, the mucosa may appear grey-green or even black.

Do you know of any unusual aetiologies when IC occurs in younger patients without arterial risk factors?

When IC occurs in young patients an association with vasculitis (e.g. polyarteritis nodosa), medications, sickle cell disease and extremes of exercise have been implicated.

Reference

Washington C, Carmichael JC. Management of ischemic colitis. Clin Colon Rectal Surg. 2012 Dec;25(4):228-35.

Laparoscopic Injuries

Scenario 1

Your new registrar is performing a laparoscopic cholecystectomy with a junior doctor. He has established pneumoperitoneum via Veress needle insertion. You are called to theatre urgently as the patient is significantly hypotensive 60/40mmHg. Upon inspection of the operating field you notice an expanding retroperitoneal haematoma.

How will you proceed?

My main concern here is that the patient may have had a major vascular injury from the use of the Veress needle. Therefore my priority would be to control haemorrhage and stabilise the bleed. I would immediately inform the anaesthetist and summon the help of a vascular surgeon. I would tell the theatre staff to get the laparotomy tray opened immediately and get a vascular set ready as well. The patient will need to be crossmatched ten units of blood straight away. The abdomen has to be opened through a generous midline incision and immediately packed in all 4 quadrants to establish control. I would gain entry into the abdomen, using the knife all the way down to the rectus sheath, and then using heavy scissors, as this would be the quickest method.

If I am able to get control of haemorrhage through packing and there is a vascular surgeon on site immediately available then I would let the anaesthetist 'catch up' with resuscitation as the vascular repair may be best performed by a vascular surgeon.

Scenario 2

You are called to theatre recovery to see a 28 year old patient on whom you performed a straightforward laparoscopic appendicectomy a couple of hours ago. She has been kept in recovery as she has been in significant pain requiring high doses of fentanyl. On examination she looks lethargic but is haemodynamically stable. She does not allow you to fully examine her abdomen as it is so tender. What are your general thoughts on how to proceed?

Although the operation was uneventful and straightforward I am concerned for her degree of abdominal pain in recovery. I would not be expecting her to require so much analgesia at this stage from a straightforward operation. My main concerns are whether she has an underlying vascular or visceral injury - given her young age the haemodynamic status may be misleading. It would be a good idea in the meantime to check her Hb as well as ensuring a group and save is available. Personally I would have a very low decision threshold to re-laparoscope this patient, rather than to watch and wait.

What may you expect to find at laparoscopy?

There is a good chance it may be a negative examination, but the laparoscopy would at this stage help to exclude a major problem within the abdomen such as an unrecognised vascular or visceral injury.

You decide to re-laparoscope the patient. At laparoscopy you find 1.5 litres of fresh dark red blood in the pelvis. You perform a thorough washout and suspect the bleeding is coming from the appendicular artery. You proceed to clip this vessel and the bleeding is under control.

Why do you think this bleeding was not seen at the first operation?

Although it is possible that it was a simple error of judgement in the first operation it is possible that the bleeding vessel had retracted and not become evident due to the pressure from the pneumoperitoneum and any hypotension under GA. Such a phenomenon is typical of venous bleeding. This should always be kept in mind during laparoscopic surgery.

Scenario 3

You are called urgently to the urology theatre where a laparoscopic radical prostatectomy is being performed and the urologist is concerned that the rectum has been inadvertently injured during the pelvic dissection. The procedure is converted to an open operation. You scrub in and find a 1cm defect in the anterior rectal wall. How would you proceed?

I would first ascertain whether this is a full thickness tear. A 1cm tear, even if full thickness, can be primarily repaired. I would like to know whether the pelvis has been irradiated or not. If it has then it would be safer to bring out a defunctioning loop colostomy proximal to the injury. In either case it would be sensible to leave a drain in situ near the rectal injury.

Liver Trauma

A 32 year old lady is admitted to the emergency department following a kick to the lower right chest / upper abdomen by a horse. She is complaining of severe right sided abdominal pain. On admission she is haemodynamically stable. Hb:135g/l and liver function tests are normal. She is normally fit and well. A CT scan of the chest, abdomen and pelvis is performed.

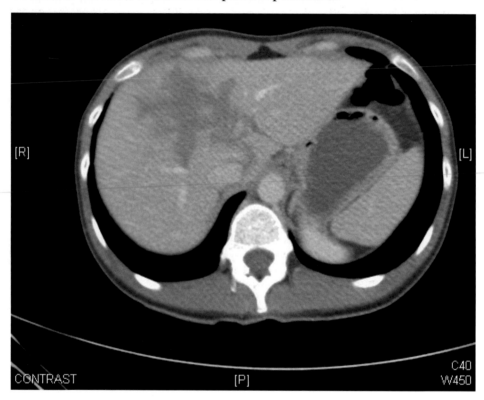

What are the main findings of this CT?

There is an area of low attenuation within the liver, involving segment 8. This extends along the right and middle hepatic veins with an appearance consistent with haemorrhage. No focal extravastation of contrast is seen. No portal venous or biliary gas is seen. No evidence of free fluid is seen on this section of the scan.

How would you manage this patient's liver injury?

Following full resuscitation and stabilisation of the patient, specific management of the liver lesion is applied. The vast majority of haemodynamically stable patients with blunt hepatic trauma may be treated conservatively. This would involve admission to a high dependency unit, close observation of haemodynamic parameters, strict bed rest and daily bloods to look for a significant drop in haemoglobin. Early involvement of the regional hepatobiliary unit should be sought for such complex and high grade injuries.

With availability of high-resolution CT the manner in which blunt hepatic trauma is managed has shifted from operative to non-operative management. 85% of patients with blunt liver trauma are haemodynamically stable and can be managed conservatively. The degree of haemodynamic stability is the most important factor that determines the suitability for non-operative management. If non-operative management is selected then haemodynamic instability is the main indication for intervention. Delayed haemorrhage from liver trauma is rare unlike following splenic injury – but it does occur. Although mortality following blunt hepatic trauma is low, in modern days there is still a considerable morbidity associated with it. Successful management of injuries of grade III and higher often entails a combined angiographic and surgical approach.

What strategies are available in the event of a sudden haemodynamic deterioration?

There is a small failure rate of non-operative management which may be due to liver related complications such as further bleeding or biliary complications. Therefore strict vigilance is essential in these patients. In the event of haemodynamic deterioration, treatment strategies include surgical intervention or radiological intervention.

The patient is now 48 hours into admission and remains stable. Her LFTs show some derangement in the transaminase levels. Are there any further radiological investigations you may wish to consider?

An MRI scan may be useful to assess the laceration in more anatomical detail as well as study the vasculature and biliary tree. The size of the laceration may also be compared to the admission scan. Information on hepatic artery as well as portal vein involvement may be obtained. Bile leak from ductal injury may manifest at a later stage and may require specific treatments such as ERCP and stenting.

The MRI shows an extensive liver laceration through segment 8 of the liver which was stable in size with no surrounding collection (Grade IV AAST). The laceration was found to extend adjacent to the middle hepatic vein without evidence of extravasation. There was no extension into the right or left hepatic arteries. The common bile duct was assessed and found to be normal. On day 5 she deteriorates rapidly and becomes haemodynamically unstable. There is no interventional radiology service available in your unit, therefore you urgently take this patient to theatre.

Describe your technique for dealing with this liver injury.

The falciform ligament is divided and a square bowel bag is placed over the liver as far posteriorly as possible. The bag is also folded under the liver. Abdominal packs are then placed around the liver from the posterior hepatic space starting from 6 or 7 o'clock and working in a clockwise manner to 5 o'clock. Once stable, the patient should be transferred to the regional HPB centre.

What interventional radiological options are available for liver trauma?

Arterial embolisation (AE) has an important role in the modern day management of high-grade liver injuries. The two main indications for AE are 1. CT evidence of active arterial bleeding in a haemodynamically stable patient. 2. Adjunctive haemostatic control in patients with uncontrolled arterial bleeding despite emergency laparotomy.

What are the potiential complications of angioembolisation in these patients?

Awareness of the ischaemic complications due to angioembolisation is important. Liver related complications of AE include biliary leak, hepatic necrosis and gallbladder infarction. Though less common major hepatic necrosis is a particularly significant complication.

What are the mechanisms of blunt liver trauma?

Blunt trauma can be deceleration (shearing) trauma and crush trauma. Deceleration occurs following a fall from a height or RTA and produces shearing stresses on the liver. Movement of the liver occurs relative to its diaphragmatic attachments. Deceleration or shearing injuries produce lacerations in the hepatic parenchyma typically between right anterior and right posterior segments. Injury to the hepatic veins and juxtahepatic IVC can also occur. Crush injury is caused by direct trauma to the liver which can lead to rupture of Glisson's capsule leading to subcapsular haematoma or compression between ribs and vertebrae, leading to caudate lobe bleeding. Liver trauma should always be considered with penetrating trauma to the abdomen, low thoracic wounds as well as posterior penetrating wounds below the scapula tips.

How do you grade injuries to the liver?

The AAST grading system is used. The majority of injuries are grade I and II which can be conservatively managed. They represent 80%-90% of all cases. Grade III and IV are generally considered severe enough to warrant surgery. Grade VI is incompatible with life.

What are the principles of trauma laparotomy for liver injury?

- Speak to the regional HPB centre on call surgeon and be prepared to take advice and transfer at an early stage.

- Vascular control may be established in the face of ongoing haemorrhage by performing Pringle's manoeuvre (portal triad occlusion) or supracoeliac aortic cross clamping.

- Once packing has been performed the packs should only be removed after the anaesthetist has gained control of resuscitation.

- If Pringle's manoeuvre fails to control bleeding, the source of haemorrhage may be hepatic veins or retrohepatic IVC. The management of such injuries is difficult and there is no clear consensus on how best to treat them. Packing is usually successful and sufficient. In the hands of a non HPB specialist surgeon attempts to identify the source of haemorrhage are unlikely to be successful and may make the situation worse.

- Atypical vascular anatomy may also be a possibility e.g. bleeding from a replaced left hepatic artery that arises from the left gastric artery or the commoner replaced right hepatic from SMA.

- The normal liver can tolerate up to an hour of ischaemia but the injured liver may not. Ideally the clamp should be released every 15 minutes after occlusion.

- When performing Pringle's manoeuvre care should be taken not to damage the bile duct.

- When packing a liver the packs should not be inserted in such a manner to distract the edges of parenchymal tears but to approximate them. This is followed by sequential placing of dry abdominal packs around the liver and directly onto the site of injury to provide tamponade.

- Most surgeons would close the skin only but if this compromises ventilation then a mesh can be inserted.

- As soon as such a patient is stabilized they should be transferred to the regional HPB centre.

What are the complications of perihepatic packing?

Early complications are continued haemorrhage – this is relatively uncommon as even in patients with caval or hepatic venous injury packing should control haemorrhage. Late complications include septic complications - it is recommended that packs should be removed as soon as possible. Perihepatic packing is an indication for intravenous antibiotic administration. The first relook laparotomy following packing should only be performed 48 hours later, ideally in the regional HPB centre. This would give time to correct coagulopathy, hypothermia and acidosis.

What techniques are available for surgical haemostasis?

- Argon coagulator – 'sprays' diathermy current via an argon beam producing a surface eschar without the diathermy probe becoming adherent to the liver surface

- Fibrin glue can be used as an adjunct

- Liver sutures – these are absorbable sutures on a blunt tipped needle often used in conjunction with a bolster of haemostatic material

When are anatomical resections attempted and what is their outcome?

Anatomical resection is used only when less aggressive techniques have failed. It is attempted when all other techniques have failed to gain haemostasis. Deep liver lacerations or extensive devascularisation of major hepatic venous bleeds may be appropriate indications. The mortality approaches 50%. When considered appropriate anatomical resection should only be performed by an HPB surgeon.

What is the rationale of selective hepatic artery ligation?

This is performed if the source of bleeding is not identified, if perihepatic packing fails, and when persistent bleeding occurs with unclamping. It is no longer a commonly used technique in liver trauma. The rationale is that portal blood usually provides adequate oxygenation. Acute gangrenous cholecystitis is a well recognized complication of hepatic artery ligation and cholecystectomy should be performed if the main hepatic artery or right hepatic artery is ligated.

What is total vascular exclusion?

Total vascular exclusion refers to clamping the IVC and suprahepatic cava in addition to Pringle's manoeuvre. However in a trauma situation this may not be desirable, and highly specialized interventions such as atriocaval shunting or veno-venous bypass may be required. Atriocaval shunting = tube from infrahepatic IVC to right atrium. Veno-venous bypass = common femoral vein to internal jugular or axillary vein.

Reference

Waibel BH, Rotondo MF. Damage control in trauma and abdominal sepsis. Crit Care Med. 2010 Sep;38(9 Suppl):S421-30.

Lower Gastrointestinal Bleeding

You are called to see an 88 year old man who has been admitted with dark red pr blood loss but has remained stable until now. In the last couple of hours he has suddenly passed 1.5 litres of blood pr requiring blood transfusions to maintain his systolic BP above 70mmHg. He has responded well to transfusion and resuscitation. Haemodynamic parameters are pulse 100; BP 100/50mmHg. His Hb is 72g/l and blood clotting is normal. He has a history of CVA (on aspirin 75mg od) but is otherwise mobile and independent.

What are the most likely causes of lower GI bleed in this gentleman?

The usual source of bleeding in adults is diverticular disease. Diverticulae can be located throughout the colon and may bleed from the right colon in 50% of cases. The aetiology of diverticular bleeding is not clearly understood and many theories have been proposed. Chronic injury to the vasa recta through muscular contraction is one such theory. 80% of diverticular bleeds will resolve spontaneously.

Bleeding from a neoplasia is another possibility. A personal or family history of polyps or cancer may be present. Bleeding from neoplasia is usually (not always!) slow and insidious and often presents as a chronic anaemia rather than an acute bleed.

With advancing age bleeding from arteriovenous malformations (AVMs) becomes increasingly prevalent. These lesions can be found throughout the GI tract but are usually found in the right colon. 90% of bleeding AVMs will stop spontaneously. However, re-bleeding can occur in up to 25% of patients. A history of multiple bleeds is not unusual as these lesions are difficult to detect. However, if a malformation is found it is usually amenable to endoscopic coagulation. Less common causes of massive lower GI bleeding include ischaemic colitis, post-polypectomy bleeding, haemorrhoids, nonsteroidal anti-inflammatory drug (NSAID) ulcers, radiation colitis, infectious colitis, solitary rectal ulcer, stercoral ulcers, and small bowel tumours.

How would you investigate him further?

The next best investigation would be a CT angiogram, which may demonstrate extravasation of contrast at the site of haemorrhage, and may even demonstrate the underlying pathology. If the CT angiogram localizes the bleed and there are interventional radiology facilities available, mesenteric angiograms and embolisation techniques can be employed to stem the bleed.

CT angiography (CTA) is a quick, relatively noninvasive and safe first line investigation with high sensitivity in the presence of active bleeding. A positive scan is characterized by presence and location of active extravasation of contrast-enhanced blood, characterized as an intraluminal focal collection or "jet" visible in the arterial and/or portal venous phase, but not on the unenhanced scan. CTA has a reported sensitivity of 91% to 92% when there is active bleeding but as low as 45% when the bleeding is intermittent in nature. The main limitation of CTA is the low sensitivity when the bleeding is intermittent in nature. Other limitations include the lack of a therapeutic option, exposure to the use of ionizing radiation, and risks associated with intravenous contrast media, mainly allergic reactions and renal function damage (especially in older individuals). Scintigraphy is not readily available on a 24-hour basis and therefore this test was not considered in the patient described in this scenario.

10% -15% of these patients may have an upper GI source of bleeding such as a duodenal ulcer. This needs to be considered and excluded by means of an upper GI endoscopy.

The CTA shows no contrast blush but abnormality around the sigmoid colon, the exact nature of which is uncertain. The patient is still bleeding significantly despite transfusion and now has a BP of 70mmHg systolic. You make a decision to proceed to laparotomy.

In theatre what are the key steps even before making a skin incision?

1) You may wish to perform an upper GI endoscopy to exclude a proximal cause of bleeding if that has not already been performed. However, this needs to be balanced against how unstable the patient is and should not delay the laparotomy significantly.

2) Always examine the anorectum yourself as re-bleeding from anorectal lesions such as haemorrhoids has been described following 'blind colectomy'.

3) Position the patient supine with legs-up position just in case you need to access the rectum intraoperatively.

At laparotomy you find the stomach and duodenum to be relatively collapsed but there is presence of a large volume of blood from the distal transverse colon extending distally. There is also a mass in the sigmoid colon, which feels like it may be neoplastic. What operation would you perform and why?

Having found a lesion which could account for the bleeding I would perform a segmental resection such as a Hartmann's procedure with end LIF colostomy. I would elect not to perform an anastomosis in such as patient as he is unstable. The presence of blood in the proximal colon is from reflux rather than proximal bleeding.

The most definitive operation here would be a subtotal colectomy with end ileostomy provided the patient is fit enough to tolerate this procedure. However this is a more major undertaking than a Hartmann's and an 88 year old man may struggle to tolerate an ileostomy.

What is the role of colonoscopy in Lower Gastrointestinal Bleeding (LGIB)?

Colonoscopy in an unstable patient can be attempted but it is often frustrating and technically challenging. It is best reserved for post-polypectomy bleeds, where the location of the bleed can be guesstimated and the offending bleeder can be easily stopped. In the stable patient with an LGIB that has resolved spontaneously colonoscopy has a well established role. However the timing of colonoscopy remains controversial. Some studies have examined the role of urgent colonoscopy (within 12 to 24 hours of presentation). However there is no strong evidence to suggest that this has a better yield than urgent outpatient colonoscopy, which remains the traditional practice.

What is the role of nuclear red cell scanning in LGIB?

Technetium 99m–labeled red blood cell scintigraphy (Tc-RBC) is a more sensitive test than arteriography for depicting slower rate bleeding, and is particularly useful for the patient with intermittent bleeding. This is because once the tracer has been injected it provides the ability to scan a patient multiple times within 12 to 24 hours. The rate of bleeding for the test to be positive is as low as 0.1-0.5ml/min (compared with >1ml/min for conventional CT angiography) and is especially useful in the setting of intermittent bleeding. When positive, it can help direct angiographic intervention.

What are the limitations of a nuclear red cell scan?

A lack of detail on nuclear scintigraphy scans may result in difficulty in discriminating the colon from overlying small bowel. Guiding surgical intervention based solely on the results of the Tc-RBC scan is not advised. Rather, it should be used as a screen prior to angiography or colonoscopy. Its availability may be limited in the emergency setting.

The same gentleman you took to theatre becomes unwell again. He remains in intensive care and is intubated. Although he has bled less through his colostomy there is still some dark blood coming out. He now has atrial fibrillation for which he is being rate-controlled. His blood gases show a worsening metabolic acidosis. What are your thoughts?

I am concerned that the sigmoid was not the cause of his bleed. He seems to be deteriorating and he may be developing progressive ischaemic bowel either from his splenic flexure, or worse, his entire small bowel. Further management depends on how ill he is. If he is stable I will reconsider a further CT scan to assess the extent of his ischaemia. If he is unstable, I will take him back to theatre for a relook laparotomy to assess:

a) the bowel: place warm packs, resect non-viable bowel and refrain from any anastomosis. I would consider leaving ends in the abdomen and always book for a relook in 24 hours. If there is extensive infarction, particularly that of small bowel, then it may be appropriate to consider palliation.

b) the vasculature: trace the SMA by identifying the middle colic vessel within the transverse mesocolon and going proximally. The splenic flexure will be supplied by the marginal - and hopefully the IMA will have been assessed at the time of the sigmoid resection. If the SMA is occluded and small bowel is salvageable then it may require a bypass graft with the help of vascular surgeons, as surgical embolectomy/thrombectomy rarely works. If the small bowel remains normal and I am not certain of the cause of the bleed through his stoma, I think the safest thing is to do a completion colectomy and formation of end ileostomy.

Mesenteric Ischaemia

Scenario 1

An 81 year old lady presents with sudden central abdominal pain that is constant. Past medical history includes AF and she currently has a heart rate of 140 bpm. She is hypotensive 90/50 mmHg but alert. Clinical examination reveals peritonitis and her lactate is 10mmol/l. A CT abdomen has shown extensive free fluid and poor enhancement of the terminal ileum. You decide to perform a laparotomy.

What is the most likely aetiology here?

The most likely diagnosis is acute mesenteric ischaemia from embolic occlusion of the SMA secondary to AF.

At laparotomy you find extensive small bowel infarction which if resected would leave her with approximately 2 metres of viable small bowel. There are no palpable SMA pulses and you decide to use a hand held doppler. No signals are audible with this. How would you proceed?

She certainly needs resection of the non-viable bowel and has a chance for survival based on the remaining 2 metres of viable bowel. I would also consider discussing her case over the phone with the on call vascular surgeon as this appears to be consistent with an embolic occlusion of the SMA. They may well consider performing an SMA embolectomy.

Most patients with embolic SMA occlusion will have a main stem embolus and extensive intestinal ischaemia. Open SMA embolectomy is a good treatment option. This involves laparotomy and exposure of the SMA, following which a transverse arrteriotomy is performed. A Fogarty catheter is inserted and a balloon embolectomy performed.

What postoperative medication should be considered for this patient?

During the critical postoperative period all patients undergoing revascularization of the SMA should receive treatment dose low molecular weight heparin.

Patients surviving acute mesenteric vessel occlusion need to be carefully medicated when discharged. In the case of embolic occlusion, life-long anticoagulation therapy with a vitamin K antagonist or low molecular weight heparin is indicated. Most patients with embolic SMA occlusion have synchronous embolism in other vascular territories and need to be protected from new embolic events.

Scenario 2

You see a 66 year old lady in the resus room with severe acute abdominal pain, metabolic acidosis (pH 7.1, BE-18, lactate 5.0). She has a history of advanced congestive cardiac failure (CCF) and COPD. She has a mottled abdomen and BP is 90/40mmHg. You decide to perform a laparotomy, suspecting small bowel ischaemia as the main diagnosis. She is on quadruple strength noradrenaline and dobutamine.

At laparotomy there was normal small bowel from DJ flexure for approximately 30cm. There was dusky small bowel and colon beyond this up to mid transverse colon, which was not infarcted but had no peristalsis. She has no palpable SMA pulsations.

What may be the aetiology of her small bowel ischaemia?

Although the commonest aetiology of small bowel ischaemia is embolic she has been in sinus rhythm throughout. Given her history of CCF she may well have non-occlusive mesenteric ischaemia (NOMI) due to a low flow and perfusion state.

You decide not to resect any bowel as it would leave her in a non-survivable situation. What are the options at this stage?

The patient may ultimately need to be palliated but her only real chance for survival is if mesenteric flow improves with optimisation of cardiac output and haemodynamics. Therefore I would aim to admit her onto the critical care unit admission for cardiovascular support, but not for further operative intervention should she deteriorate as this would be futile.

NOMI generally affects patients over 50 years of age suffering from myocardial infarction, congestive heart failure, aortic insufficiency, renal or hepatic disease, and patients following cardiac surgery. NOMI accounts for 20%-30% of all cases of acute mesenteric ischemia with a mortality rate of the order of 50%. It is characterized by gastrointestinal ischaemia with normal vessels. It is very common in critically ill and perioperative patients, but also occurs in pancreatitis, renal failure and sepsis. Treatment options include aggressive fluid resuscitation and careful choice of vasoactive drugs. Awareness of reperfusion-induced bowel damage is important.

Scenario 3

A 76 year old lady presents with vague central abdominal pain, at times very severe. There is abdominal distension but only mild generalised tenderness. She has a lactate of 2 on ABG. Plain abdominal film demonstrates distended small bowel with evidence of thumb printing. You request a CT scan which shows thickened small bowel with possible intramural gas and delayed filling of the portal venous system. She has previously had a right hemicolectomy for an ischaemic caecum many years ago.

At laparotomy she has 70cm of non-viable small bowel which you resect. The remaining small bowel is not frankly ischaemic but is congested, aperistaltic and has a haemorrhagic appearance. Mesenteric pulsations appear normal. She is physiologically stable and not requiring inotropes.

How would you proceed?

I would start by placing warm packs around the congested bowel to improve perfusion and speak to the anaesthetist about optimising cardiac output as well as possible. The congested appearance of the bowel and presence of arterial pulsations makes me think that she may have mesenteric venous thrombosis. I would have a low threshold to perform no more resections but to bring the patient back after 24 hours for a relook laparotomy. Therefore the resected ends of bowel can be placed back in the abdomen and mass closure performed.

An alternative approach would be to deliver the two ends as a double barrel stoma which can be reversed at a later stage.

How would you manage her post operatively?

I would reassess her regularly and ensure she is on a heparin infusion to help prevent any further clot propagation. I would book her for theatre the next day but reoperate earlier if she deteriorates.

What percentage of cases of mesenteric ischaemia are due to mesenteric venous thrombosis?

Mesenteric venous thrombosis is a rare condition and accounts for approximately 5%-15% of cases of all acute mesenteric ischaemia.

Mesenteric venous thrombosis is classified into primary (no cause found) or secondary with underlying risk factors. The non-specific and subtle presentation usually delays diagnosis, which is usually made only at the time of laparotomy or autopsy. The clinical features of this condition are usually subtle and not as dramatic as acute arterial mesenteric ischaemia. The mortality is significant at 27% and long-term anticoagulation is essential for survivors as there is a high recurrence rate for this condition.

What are the important associations of MVT?

Portal Hypertension

- Liver cirrhosis

Inflammatory

- Intra-abdominal sepsis e.g. diverticulitis
- Inflammatory bowel disease
- Acute pancreatitis

Hypercoagulable states

- Malignancy – particularly colonic / pancreatic
- Dehydration
- Thrombophilia
- Thrombocytosis e.g. post-splenectomy
- Oral contraceptive pill

Neck Trauma

You are called to see a 29 year old man who has been stabbed in the neck following a pub brawl. He is haemodynamically stable and protecting his airway. GCS15. The stab wound is 3cm anterior to the sternocleidomastoid with a haematoma. What is your approach?

This patient needs to be assessed along ATLS® guidelines and resuscitated accordingly. The priority would be to secure the patient's airway. I would call the anaesthetic team to attend straight away. Though he is maintaining his airway, the upper airway is at risk of complete obstruction and may be in danger, or may already be compromised. Therefore a low threshold for endotracheal intubation or surgical airway is indicated.

Do not wait for the airway to obstruct and what could have been a routine intubation prove to be very difficult.

What further investigations should be considered?

Once stable CT angiography (CTA) would be the most useful and practical investigation. Further investigations will depend on CTA findings, but may include bronchoscopy / endoscopy / digital subtraction angiography, depending on what structures are involved.

As a principle in trauma embedded foreign bodies must never be removed until the patient is asleep, due to the risk of precipitating bleeding from deeper structures that are being tamponaded.

What are the different zones of the neck?

Zone I: extends from the sternal notch to the cricoid cartilage. It includes the subclavian and innominate vessels, the common carotids and lower vertebral arteries and the jugular veins.

Zone II extends from the cricoid cartilage to the angle of the mandible. It includes the common carotid, carotid bifurcation, the vertebral arteries and the jugular veins.

Zone III extends from the angle of mandible to the base of the skull. It contains the branches of the external carotid artery, the internal carotid artery, vertebral artery and the internal jugular and facial veins.

Zones I and III are relatively inaccessible to physical examination and rely upon radiological imaging. **Zone II** is much more accessible and less reliant on imaging.

Penetrating injuries may extend for more than one zone and this must be kept in mind.

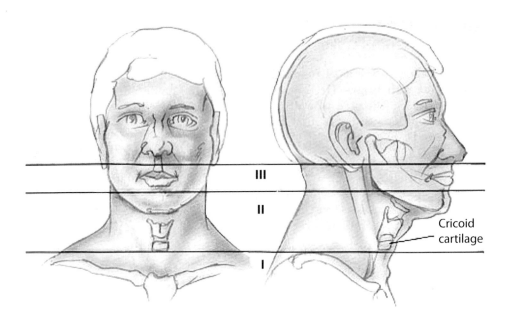

Why is the neck so prone to serious traumatic injury?

The neck is a conduit for many vital aerodigestive and vascular structures that do not have much overlying bony, muscle or soft tissue protection, thus making them vulnerable. Penetrating trauma accounts for the main mechanism for neck injuries.

What is the significance of penetrating platysma and sternocleidomastoid with a neck injury?

The extent of penetration of platysma and sternocleidomastoid are important to assess in the management of neck trauma. Injuries that do not penetrate platysma are considered to be superficial. It is therefore a vital landmark in the assessment of penetrating neck trauma. Injuries that are anterior to sternocleidomastoid have a high chance of damage to major structures whereas those that are posterior are more likely to involve the spinal cord or cervical vertebrae.

What clinical features may be evident with penetrating injuries to the neck?

Haematoma

Respiratory distress

Stridor

Odynophagia / dysphagia – suggestive of oesophageal injury

Surgical emphysema – suggestive of tracheal injury / pneumothorax / oesophageal injury

Bubbling / gurgling – suggestive of tracheal injury

Hoarseness – division or compression of the recurrent laryngeal nerves

Cranial nerve deficits

Machinery bruit – a-v fistula between IJV and carotid artery

What patterns of injury may be seen following blunt neck trauma?

Blunt neck trauma can be subtle. It most commonly affects the carotids, trachea and larynx:

- Blunt cerebrovascular injury – partial or complete occlusion, pseudoaneurysm formation or transection of carotid or vertebral arteries

- Laryngeal fractures which may present with any of the airway symptoms above – stridor etc

- Subcutaneous emphysema – tracheal injury

Describe the mechanism of blunt cerebrovascular injury.

These injuries are caused by sudden stretching or buckling of the arteries leading to intimal flaps and dissection. Initially the patient may be completely normal, only to suffer a debilitating ischaemic or embolic stroke hours to days later. Unexplained neurological findings in the face of a normal CT scan should always be viewed as suspicious.

Intra-operatively how would you deal with a penetrating injury to the carotid artery? trachea? oesophagus?

This involves employing the same principles as any vascular trauma. Direct pressure to control haemorrhage – digital pressure is preferable to large packs or swabs. Obtain proximal and distal control of the vessel. Primary repair is usually not possible. Interposition grafting is often required with PTFE, as autologous vein to carotid artery will provide a significant mismatch in size. In dire circumstances the external carotid can be ligated with minimal sequelae. However ligation of the internal carotid is a last resort due to the greater functional significance. Remember for most blunt injuries anticoagulation is the mainstay of treatment.

As a principle all tracheal lacerations should be debrided and repaired by direct suture. Oesophageal injuries should also undergo primary repair as long as the diagnosis is made early. With delayed diagnosis a drainage procedure may be wiser before delayed repair. Significant loss of oesophagus may require an oesophagostomy but usually sufficient oesophagus can be mobilized.

Necrotising Fasciitis

You are called to see a 70-year-old male diabetic patient who had a recent incision and drainage of a large right buttock abscess. You are informed that the patient is systemically unwell with a temperature of 38.5°C, P 110 and BP of 100/60mmHg. There is a worsening cellulitis around the previous incision, which is oedematous and has a foul smelling discharge. You go to review the patient and notice patchy skin necrosis surrounding the perianal region and perineum. What are your concerns?

This patient is septic and the clinical findings suggest necrotising fasciitis. This is a life-threatening surgical emergency. Senior surgical and critical care teams should be involved in his care from this point. He needs aggressive resuscitation and to be prepared for theatre for an examination under anaesthetic and appropriate debridement. Resuscitation would involve the placement of large bore venous cannulae, an arterial line, and a urinary catheter. Oxygen and crystalloid fluid should be administered. Broad-spectrum antibiotics should include cover for gram-positive, gram-negative, and anaerobic bacteria, and is best done by discussion with a senior microbiologist.

On examination on the ward you are concerned that he may require extensive debridement. Are there any other procedures you may want to consent this patient for?

This patient is unwell and needs urgent debridement. He may return to ITU ventilated, and is likely to require a second look in theatre at 24 hours. He will then require subsequent trips to theatre for further debridements, dressing changes and reconstruction. The source of the underlying infection may also be from the large bowel, and a diverting colostomy should be considered, both for the instance where the bowel is the source of infection, and to manage the faecal output while there is a significant perianal wound.

Are you aware of any scoring systems for determining the likelihood of necrotising fasciitis?

The Laboratory Risk Indicator for Necrotising fasciitis (LRINEC) may be used to determine the risk in patients presenting with what appears to be cellulitis. This involves six parameters, CRP, WCC, haemoglobin, sodium, creatinine and glucose. A score greater than six indicates a high possibility of necrotising fasciitis.

The scoring criteria are:

- CRP (mg/L) ≥150: 4 points
- WBC count
  - <15: 0 points
  - 15–25: 1 point

- >25: 2 points
- Haemoglobin (g/dL)
  - >13.5: 0 points
  - 11–13.5: 1 point
  - <11: 2 points
- Sodium (mmol/L) <135: 2 points
- Creatinine (μmol/L) >141: 2 points
- Glucose (mmol/L) >10: 1 point

Scoring systems should only be used when there is stronger clinical suspicion cellulitis. If there is a clinical suspicion of necrotising fasciitis, the patient should have exploration in theatre, and scoring systems should not be used to justify observing the patient on the ward. Cardinal features such as patchy necrotic skin, or rapidly progressing "fronts" of cellulitis, render such scoring systems redundant.

How might necrotising fasciitis be classified?

The condition is usually classified as either Type 1 (polymicrobial) or Type 2 (single organism). Type 1 comprises 85% of cases.

More recently Type 3 and Type 4 necrotising fasciitis have been described. Type 3 is mono-microbial caused by Gram negative Vibrio *spp* and has a mortality of 30%-40%. Type 4 is extremely rare and due to fungal cases of Candida necrotising fasciitis.

What are the causative organisms?

Patients with Type 1 necrotising fasciitis usually have both aerobic and anaerobic organisms present (Gram positive cocci, Gram negative rods, and anaerobes). The underlying organism for Type 2 is usually Group A Streptococci or Staphylococci. There has been an increase in the incidence of MRSA necrotising fasciitis recently.

What layers are typically affected by the necrotising infection?

Necrotising fasciitis affects the deep layer of fascia that invests the whole body. As the fascia necroses and liquefies, the infection proceeds and spreads along this layer, deep to the skin and subcutaneous fat. The extent of the process can be estimated, as reactive cellulitis of the skin progresses above the fasciitis. As the perforating blood vessels to skin, which pierce the fascia, are occluded, the skin will become ischaemic and in due course blacken and necrose also. The extent of necrotic skin is always a gross underestimation of the extent of the underlying disease.

Which patients are particularly at risk of developing necrotising fasciitis?

Type 1 is more common amongst those that are immuno-compromised. It particularly affects poorly controlled diabetics. Other risk factors include obesity, chronic renal failure, alcohol and drug abuse, leukaemia or other malignancy, old age and the use of steroids or other chemotherapy agents. It may also be associated with perforating gastrointestinal tumours.

Type 2 necrotising fasciitis may occur in otherwise fit patients with a history of recent trauma or surgery to the affected tissue.

Is there any role for imaging?

The diagnosis of necrotising fasciitis is made clinically in almost every case. Plain film, CT, MRI, or even ultrasound may be used to demonstrate soft tissue thickening and surgical emphysema. Lack of enhancement following administration of intravenous contrast may differentiate necrotising fasciitis from cellulitis. Imaging may have a role in excluding related complications such as a focal collection. Operative intervention should never be delayed to facilitate radiological investigation unless there is very significant doubt about the diagnosis and the patient is otherwise a very high risk surgical candidate.

Is there a role for histological investigation?

Where the diagnosis is equivocal, the most prescient way to proceed is often to take the patient to theatre for multiple biopsies of the underlying fascia. An on call histopathological service is able to analyse the fascia, and the presence of suppuration, extensive acute inflammation, small vessel thrombosis and overwhelming bacterial colonisation can help to make the diagnosis more certain. Gram stain and tissue microscopy can also be performed by the microbiology team. This approach has the advantage that the debridement is not unduly delayed while waiting for the investigation, and if, on opening the fascia, there is the typical "dirty dishwater" appearance of liquefying fat and fascia, then the debridement can proceed immediately.

What are the principles of operative debridement in this case ?

Debridement needs to be generous, excising all evidence of necrotic and dead tissue, which will include the deep fascia. When bleeding tissue is seen, this is a sign of having reached healthy tissue. This debridement is not for the fainthearted, and must proceed until healthy tissue is reached, regardless of the tissues involved. A diverting colostomy should be performed for cases where the process involves the anorectum and sphincter, and for patients with wounds at high risk of faecal contamination. This is best performed as an end colostomy than a loop colostomy as the former allows better defunctioning.

Second look in theatre after 24 hours should always be planned as the patient may require further debridement, and at least will require a change of dressings and wound inspection. Further trips to theatre can be titrated with reference to the clinical picture.

What do you do if the patient survives?

Early involvement of your plastic surgical colleagues is important as the patient may require a complex reconstruction. If debridement involves the perineum and involvement of the genitourinary tract is suspected then urology involvement is crucial.

What do you understand by the term Fournier's gangrene?

Fournier's gangrene is a polymicrobial necrotizing fasciitis of the perineal, perianal, or genital areas. The condition is not limited to males.

The commonest causes of Fournier's are local trauma or extension of a urinary tract or perianal infection.

Genitourinary causes include transurethral instrumentation, as well as surgery of the penis and scrotum, and transrectal prostate biopsy. Anorectal sources of infection include ischiorectal, perianal, and intersphincteric abscesses, particularly when inadequately treated.

Diverticular perforation, carcinoma of the sigmoid colon and rectum and internal haemorrhoids ligated with rubber bands are amongst other aetiologies.

Oesophageal Perforation

Scenario 1

You receive a telephone call from a peripheral hospital about a 27 year old male who was sword swallowing 5 days ago and presents with severe neck and chest pain, pyrexia and dysphagia. He is tachycardic at 110 bpm, pyrexial 38°C and BP 140/85mmHg. He feels generally unwell and examination reveals no surgical emphysema or abdominal discomfort.

How would you investigate this patient?

My main concern in this situation is that of an oesophageal perforation. It sounds like the patient is septic given his temperature, tachycardia and symptoms. In the first instance I would obtain a CT scan of his neck, chest and abdomen with some oral contrast.

The CT scan shows marked pneumomediastinum with a collection in the root of the neck as well as a small collection in the lower mediastinum. The site of perforation is not obvious and there are no pleural effusions. What further investigations may you require?

The next best investigation would be an upper GI endoscopy. This would reveal the site of perforation as well as rule out any pathology at this site.

You agree to bring the patient under your care after discussion with the consultant oesophagogastric surgeon on call. You later endoscope the patient and find a small defect just below the cricopharyngeus. Endoscopically what else would you do?

The endoscopy would also allow insertion of a draining NG tube as well as a feeding NJ tube. The NG tube would be used to empty the stomach of any contents which could potentially reflux back into the defect and would also prevent retching/vomiting.

You decide to manage the patient conservatively on HDU with iv antibiotics and antifungals. Two days into the admission the patient suddenly develops worsening pain, temperature as well as stupor. He is on maximal antibacterial treatment and not responding. His CRP is 450 and WCC 22 × 10⁹/l. How would you proceed?

His lack of progress may be due to further collections and worsening mediastinitis. I would therefore obtain a further CT scan of his neck, chest and abdomen. There is a high likelihood that he will require operative intervention and escalation to ICU.

The repeat scan shows significant deterioration since the original scan with mediastinal collections increasing in size. He continues to deteriorate clinically with worsening acidosis and gas exchange. How would you proceed?

Timely intervention and early drainage of sepsis is of paramount importance. The patient needs to have a thoracotomy and washout to clear the mediastinal sepsis. The collection in the neck may be accessible from the mediastinum. There is a good chance he will be ventilated and on inotropes, therefore cooperation with the critical care team is vital.

What are the basic principles of the operation he needs?

The patient will need to have a double lumen endotracheal tube intubation to allow single lung ventilation. The collection is best approached via a right thoracotomy. Any pleural collections are drained and appropriate cultures sent. With the lung retracted the mediastinal collection is usually noticed as a bulge, which is then opened and drained. The collection at the root of the neck may be accessible from above the azygous vein. A large Foley catheter can be inserted into the cavities and used for irrigation. Large chest drains are then left in situ along with a drain up to the neck from the mediastinum. If the neck collection has not been accessible via the chest then a right neck cervical incision may need to be performed.

Scenario 2

You are called to A & E to review a 45 year old man who is complaining of chest and abdominal pain. It is 2am and he has been out for dinner and started retching and vomiting violently. He is tachycardic at 110, pyrexial (38°C) and has a BP of 150/85mmHg and respiratory rate of 20. He feels generally unwell. He looks sweaty and clammy, and examination findings reveal reduced air entry in the left base, generalized abdominal discomfort and mild surgical emphysema in the neck.

What is your diagnosis?

Given the history of chest/abdominal pain in association with forceful retching and vomiting along with sepsis and surgical emphysema, he may have an oesophageal rupture. In the absence of any underlying oesophageal pathology this is likely to be Boerhaave's syndrome.

How would you define Boerhaave's syndrome?

Boerhaave's syndrome is a form of spontaneous perforation of the oesophagus occurring in the absence of underlying oesophageal pathology. It is characterized by a full thickness disruption of the oesophageal wall.

What is the pathophysiology of Boerhaave's syndrome?

Boerhaave's perforations are a form of barogenic injury to the oesophagus from a sudden rise of intra-abdominal pressure due to repeated vomiting and/or retching against a closed cricopharyngeus. This history is seen in almost all cases (80%-90%). The perforation is usually single and longitudinal anywhere from 1cm to 8cm long but usually approx 3cm long. Typically the mucosal injury is longer than the overlying muscular tear. They usually occur in the left lower posterolateral oesophagus above the oesophagogastric junction. The mediastinal pleura over the oesophagus is breached due to a combination of barogenic trauma as well as erosion by gastric acid. The negative intra-thoracic pressure draws food and gastric content into the mediastinal and pleural cavity, leading to a chemical pleuromediastinitis with subsequent clinical deterioration.

How is Boerhaave's different to Mallory-Weiss syndrome?

Mallory-Weiss is a mucosal tear of the oesophagus from shear stress whereas Boerhaave's is a form of barogenic trauma to the oesophagus with full thickness injury.

What is Mackler's triad?

This triad applies only to Boerhaave's syndrome and is classically a history of vomiting / retching followed by sudden onset of chest pain and development of subcutaneous emphysema. However, it is seen in only approximately 15% of cases.

What are the typical chest x ray changes that may be seen in oesophageal perforation?

- Pleural effusion (This tends to be left sided with a lower third oesophageal perforation. Higher perforations may produce a right sided effusion. Pleural effusions occur as the pleura becomes disrupted from gastric acid and content.)
- Pneumomediastinum
- Subcutaneous emphysema
- Hydropneumothorax or pneumothorax
- Collapse / consolidation

In this case how do you confirm your suspicion of an oesophageal perforation?

A CT scan with oral contrast would help define the extent of contamination and also help to exclude other diagnoses such as aortic dissection. If the patient is intubated prior to the scan, contrast media can be given via a small nasogastric tube inserted just past the cricopharyngeus. Following the CT scan I would consider seeking help from an oesophagogastric surgeon who would more than likely perform an upper GI endoscopy to confirm the presence and level of perforation, any underlying oesophageal pathology, and also allow insertion of a nasogastric tube under direct vision. The NG tube helps to prevent acid and bacteria from the stomach draining into the mediastinum.

Would you perform a contrast swallow in this patient?

At this stage a contrast swallow is not required and it will not provide the same information that a combination of CT and endoscopy would. A contrast study will be of use in subsequent follow up after definitive treatment to demonstrate healing and resolution of the leak. It would provide information on the site, extent of leakage and communication with pleural cavity. A non-ionic contrast tends to be used these days as it has a smaller risk of sequelae should the patient aspirate. Gastrografin tends not to be used due to the serious nature of gastrografin aspiration.

Your endoscopy confirms a large perforation at the lower left oesophagus with visible communication with the mediastinum. There is no underlying oesophageal lesion. The CT shows large collections in both pleurae as well as the mediastinum. How would you manage him?

In all such cases specialist help should be sought from the regional oesophago-gastric unit. Given the degree of contamination present, relatively early presentation in a young fit patient will require operative intervention. The perforation is best approached through a left thoracotomy (via 7th or 8th interspace for lower oesophageal perforations or right thoracotomy via 5th intercostal space as alternative for mid to upper perforations). The patient will require single lung ventilation, but at times the lung may have to be reinflated as he may be too sick to tolerate prolonged single lung ventilation. Thorough drainage and washout of collections in the pleural cavity along with debridement of any necrotic and devitalized tissue should be performed. A longitudinal myotomy is performed to expose the mucosal injury knowing that the mucosal injury is usually much longer than the muscular defect.

Once the perforation is located the operative options are either closure over a T tube or primary repair with or without reinforcement. In extreme cases an oesophagectomy may be required. The majority of cases are closed over a T tube. I would use a large diameter T tube (6-10 mm) placed through the defect with the limbs of the tube well beyond the perforation. The oesophagus should be loosely closed with 3.0 absorbable sutures. The T tube is then exteriorized and secured at the skin where it will form an oesophagocutaneous fistula over time.

In this particular case an argument can be made for primary closure as the patient has presented early. The leak rate is significant particularly if the repair has been delayed for more than 24 hours, as the tissues may not be healthy. The leak rate is approximately 50% for those delayed beyond 24 hours and 20% even within 24 hours, therefore primary repair has a limited role. The suture line may be reinforced with omentum, pedicled intercostal muscle flap or pericardium. However with delayed presentation it would be safer to close over a T tube. Once the thoracic phase is completed a feeding jejunostomy may be performed at the end of the procedure through a mini laparotomy incision to facilitate enteral feeding. At the end of the operation large bore chest drains are left in place, being careful to ensure that as they are placed they do not become displaced by re-inflation of the lung.

Is there a role for non-operative management of an oesophageal perforation?

Non-operative management may be pursued if the patient has no evidence of mediastinitis and there is evidence that the perforation is controlled. Such management requires very close observation on a critical care unit with a low threshold to intervene should the patient decompensate. Radiological or intercostal drains should be placed into collections as directed by imaging. The patient should be on broad spectrum antibiotics and antifungals, and an intravenous proton pump inhibitor to reduce gastric acid production. Repeat imaging should be performed to look for any further collections. Non-operative management is usually performed following iatrogenic instrumental perforation of the oesophagus where contamination may be minimal.

What is the commonest cause of oesophageal perforation?

Iatrogenic injury to the oesophagus during therapeutic upper GI endoscopy e.g. dilatation is the commonest cause of oesophageal perforation.

What iatrogenic causes of oesophageal perforation do you know?

Therapeutic upper GI endoscopy carries a risk of perforation of approximately 5%. This risk is increased in patients who have received prior chemotherapy or radiotherapy. These include dilatation for achalasia - particularly balloon pneumatic dilatation, which carries a higher risk than graded dilatation due to higher pressures and larger balloon size.

Diagnostic upper GI endoscopic procedures:

Perforation risk of a diagnostic OGD is rare at 0.03% and usually occurs at the lower oesophagus near the site of any pathology such as a tight stricture.

Trans-oesophageal echocardiography (TOE): particularly when used as prolonged placement for intra-operative monitoring during cardiac surgery. This occurs due to pressure necrosis.

Other causes include:

Anti-reflux surgery: Applies to both open and laparoscopic procedures. The risk is highest for redo surgery.

Foreign body perforation	Corrosive injury
Thoracic surgery	Spinal surgery
Surgical tracheostomy	Head and neck operations
Nasogastric tube insertion	

Further reading

Griffin SM, Lamb PJ, Shenfine J, Richardson DL, Karat D, Hayes N. Spontaneous rupture of the oesophagus. Br J Surg. 2008 Sep;95(9):1115-20.

Paediatric Trauma

What is the definition of an infant, toddler etc..?

- Infant 0-1 year
- Toddler 1-3 years
- Pre-school 3-5
- School age 6-12
- Adolescent >12
- Teens 13-19

What is the commonest mode of death in paediatric trauma?

The pattern of injuries in children differs to that seen in adults: mortality is related primarily to head injury. Head injury is the commonest cause of death in children over the age of one year. Severe cerebral oedema occurs three to four times more frequently in children than adults and often occurs in the absence of contusion, ischaemic brain damage or intracranial haematoma. Haemorrhagic shock and severe life threatening chest injuries are uncommon. Trauma is the commonest cause of death in children over the age of one year and sadly the majority of deaths occur before the child arrives at hospital.

Why are thoracic injuries less common in children compared with adults?

The child's skeleton is incompletely calcified and is therefore more compliant. Internal organ damage can occur without overlying bony fracture. A good example of this is the rarity of rib fractures in children. When they occur there is usually serious underlying lung injury and mortality increases in proportion to the number of ribs fractured.

Why are multiple injuries more common in children?

Because of the smaller body mass of children the energy imparted from trauma results in a greater force per unit body area.

How can you calculate a child's weight?

An estimate of the child's weight needs to be made as soon as possible as most drugs are given on a dose/kg basis. At birth a child weighs approximately 3 kg, this increases to about 10 kg at the age of one year. For children aged 1 to 10 years, weight can be estimated by the formula;

Weight (kg) = 2 x (age + 4)

This allows calculation and preparation of the doses of medications likely to be required.

Why is airway management particularly important in a child? How is airway management different in children?

The inability to establish or maintain an airway is the commonest cause of cardiac arrest in children. An oropharyngeal airway of the appropriate size can be inserted over the tongue under direct vision, to help maintain a patent airway. It must not be inserted "upside-down" and rotated as in an adult as this may damage the soft palate and cause bleeding. Nasopharyngeal airways are not used as they tend to damage the adenoidal tissue that is prominent in children and again this can cause significant haemorrhage. Children are at greater risk of regurgitation and aspiration because of a shorter oesophagus, a lower pressure gradient between the larynx and stomach, lower oesophageal sphincter tone and gastric distension from swallowing air. The young child's predilection to aerophagy (air swallowing) can lead to painful abdominal distension, making examination difficult and increasing the risk of regurgitation and aspiration. A naso or oro-gastric tube should be used to decompress the stomach if this is excessive, although the oral route is preferred if there is craniofacial trauma.

What are the structural differences between a child's and adult's airway?

Structural characteristics of the paediatric airway:

- Large occiput (<3years), short neck – head and neck flexes.

- Infants (<6 months) breath via the nose - complete airway obstruction may occur if blocked by blood or oedema.

- Relatively large tongue, floppy epiglottis – this obscures the view of the glottis.

- Relatively short trachea - risk of right main bronchus intubation.

- Uncuffed ETT should be used < 9 years of age. The cricoid is the narrowest part of the airway and provides a natural seal.

- The Broselow tape will provide an indication of what size airway to use. Alternatively the size of the child's little finger gives an approximation to the diameter of ETT.

Why is a surgical airway a risky procedure in children?

Most children can be oxygenated adequately using a good technique with a bag-mask and airway while expert help is obtained. If a surgical airway is required needle cricothyroidotomy is the recommended technique in children under the age of 12 years. This is a difficult, high risk procedure as paratracheal placement of the cannula and insufflation of oxygen will result in massive mediastinal emphysema that may be fatal. Furthermore, even if successful, it may cause damage to the cricoid cartilage, the only complete ring of cartilage in the airway, causing collapse of the upper airway. Healing results in tracheal stenosis and long term airway problems.

How common are C-spine injuries in children?

Even though the incidence of cervical spine injury is low in children, the child's head should be immobilised, initially by the airway person, using manual in-line stabilisation, unless the child is already immobilised.

How does haemodynamic stability differ in children compared with adults?

The absolute circulating blood volume is small (80ml/Kg in child) and the loss of relatively small absolute volumes can result in significant haemodynamic compromise. Children are extremely efficient in compensating for the loss of blood as a result of a relatively greater ability to increase systemic vascular resistance and heart rate. The signs of early haemorrhagic shock are subtle in children and the onset of decompensation is abrupt. Hypotension is therefore a late and pre-terminal sign.

The only reliable change in heart rate is an accompanying bradycardia that usually precedes cardiac arrest.

What is the best assessment of blood loss in a child?

More reliable signs are capillary refill time (CRT, normal <2 seconds), skin colour and temperature, and conscious level.

What are the most reliable sites of intravenous cannulation?

The optimal sites for peripheral venous access are the veins on the dorsum of the hand or foot and the saphenous vein anterior to the medial malleolus. The antecubital vein is often easy to cannulate but the catheter is readily kinked by flexion of the elbow. The elbow should be splinted if used. Two short, wide bore intravenous cannulae are the ideal, the size dictated by the size of the child.

Up to what age can an intraosseous needle be inserted?

In the presence of shock, if intravascular access is not achieved within 90 seconds via the percutaneous route, then the intraosseous route should be used in children up to six years of age. But some studies have indicated it is also suitable in older children and adults.

What are the sites for intraosseous cannulation?

The most common site used for intraosseous access is 2-3 cm below the tibial tuberosity on the flattened medial aspect of the tibia, or alternatively the anterolateral surface of the femur, 3 cm above the lateral condyle, and the medial malleolus. A bone injection gun may assist intraosseous entry. Entry should not be performed distal to a fracture site.

What and how much fluid should be given to the child?

Initially, a bolus of a warmed, isotonic crystalloid (10 to 20 ml/kg) is given. Any child presenting with profound haemorrhagic shock or who fails to respond to 40ml/kg of crystalloid and/or colloid should receive warmed, packed red blood cells (10ml/kg). If type specific or fully cross-matched blood is not available within 10 minutes then Group O Rh negative blood should be used.

What is an acceptable systolic blood pressure in a child?

The lower limit of systolic BP = 70 mmHg + twice the age in years. Diastolic pressure should be 2/3rds of systolic pressure. Urine output = 1.5 – 2 ml/kg/hr depending on age. The adult value of 0.5ml/kg does not apply until the child has stopped growing.

Why is temperature control particularly important in the child?

Small children have a high body surface area to weight ratio, which is at its greatest when the child is newborn. Consequently, children lose heat much more rapidly than adults do; for example, newborn children will lose 1°C every four minutes if left uncovered.

What specific abdominal injuries are more common in children?

A number of abdominal visceral injuries are more common in children than adults. Duodenal haematoma and pancreatic injury are more common due to a combination of undeveloped abdominal musculature and propensity to bicycle handlebar injury. Bladder rupture is more common in children than in adults as the bladder has a more intraperitoneal position in children. Also small bowel perforation near the ligament of Treitz may occur.

What is SCIWORA?

The high incidence of spinal cord injury without radiological abnormality (SCIWORA) in children should reinforce the importance of a detailed neurological examination as the best method of identifying cord injury.

Why is non-operative management commonly used in children?

Non-operative management is the preferred method of treatment for solid organ injury in children, as haemorrhage is generally self-limiting and responds well to fluid or blood transfusion. Figures from one paediatric trauma centre report only 4% of blunt liver injuries and 21% of blunt splenic injuries requiring operative management.

When might you suspect Non Accidental Injury (NAI)?

Children injured as a result of child abuse tend to be younger, sustain greater trauma, and are more likely to have a pre-injury medical history and retinal haemorrhages when compared to children with unintentional injuries. One recent study examining abusive head injury as a cause of death in 42 children showed 81% had retinal haemorrhages. A high index of suspicion should be maintained in all cases of paediatric injury.

Penetrating Chest Trauma

A 25 year old fit male is brought to A & E by his partner. He had an argument with his friend and was stabbed below his left nipple by a kitchen knife of unknown length. He felt short of breath initially and when you arrive to A & E, he is on 4l of O$_2$ with saturations of 93%, RR 20/min, BP 100/60 mmHg, HR 80/min. He has a 3cm wound, which is covered with sterile gauze, and during the auscultation of the chest there is decreased air entry on the left. Abdominal examination is unremarkable. Bloods have been taken, two units of blood crossmatched and the radiographer has just performed a portable CXR. The nearest cardiothoracic unit is 90 minutes drive from your hospital.

What possible organs could be injured?

The stab wound is in the region of the 'cardiac box' (border outlined by the clavicles superiorly, costal margins inferiorly and mid-clavicular lines laterally) thus cardiac and large vessel injuries should be considered.

The lung is the most commonly injured intrathoracic organ in stab wounds, and given the clinical picture of desaturation and decreased air entry, a pneumothorax or massive haemothorax could be present. The distinction could be made by percussion (hyper-resonant vs dull), auscultation (decreased air entry apically and anteriorly vs posteriorly and basally) and stability (significant desaturation vs haemorhagic shock).

The diaphragm is also at risk as this could be at the level of nipples during expiration.

Others are the intra-abdominal organs, especially stomach, colon, spleen and (less likely) the left liver lobe, left kidney and tail of pancreas.

As you are examining the patient, he starts to complain of severe shortness of breath. His RR increases to 30/min, saturation is 85%, BP 80/55 mmHg and HR 120. On examination he is cyanotic, trachea is deviated to the right, there is hyper-resonant percussion and on auscultation there is no air entry in the left chest. What would be your management of this patient?

This patient has typical signs of a tension pneumothorax and requires urgent decompression of the chest to alleviate cardiopulmonary compromise. As a temporary measure, a large bore cannula (grey) must be inserted and secured in the second intercostal space in the mid-clavicular line. Typically a hiss of air will confirm the diagnosis. The next step is insertion of an intercostal chest drain.

Be aware that tension pneumothorax is a clinical diagnosis and treatment must be immediate. One must not delay the treatment by waiting for confirmation of the diagnosis by CXR. In fact a CXR demonstrating a tension pneumothorax should not exist!

How would you insert the chest drain?

The patient should move towards the left side of the bed and sit up to 45 degrees to a convenient height and the whole chest should be exposed. Hands should be scrubbed as for any other surgical procedure and sterile gown and gloves must be used. The skin of the patient is prepped twice with betadine or chlorhexidine solution. Lignocaine 1% or 2% is used for local infiltration. The patient is draped and a 2 cm horizontal skin incision is made at the level of the fifth intercostal space anteriorly to the midaxillary line in the so-called 'safe triangle' (borders: lateral part of pectoralis major anteriorly, latissimus dorsi posteriorly, and level of the nipple distally).

A Spencer-Wells dissector is used to dissect through the subcutaneous tissue, serratus anterior, intercostal muscles and pleura. The dissector is advanced perpendicularly into the chest just above the sixth rib with good control of the depth of penetration. Once the parietal pleura is pierced the dissector is opened in the direction of the intercostal space. The index finger is introduced to the pleural cavity to confirm absence of adhesions between the lung and chest wall. A chest drain 28F is inserted apically (pneumothorax) or basally (haemothorax) and secured with a suture. A horizontal mattress suture is prepared for wound closure once the drain is removed and sterile dressing is applied. The drain is connected to an underwater seal initially without suction and swing is observed in the tubing together with drainage of air or collected blood. CXR is required to confirm the position of the drain.

After insertion of the chest drain the patient stabilises, Sat 99% on 2 l of O2, RR 10, BP 100/60 mmHg and HR 80bpm. There is a small air leak observed and 400 mls of blood is drained. There is good air entry on auscultation. CXR performed prior to your arrival is now available on a system with obvious pneumothorax and complete collapse of the left lung (Figure 1 below). Is drainage of 400 mls sufficient for surgical exploration in the stable patient?

Figure 1

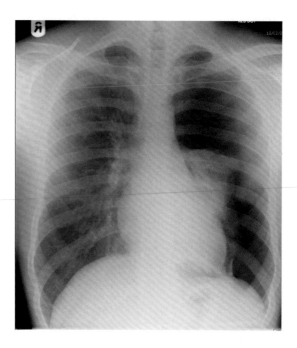

No, surgical exploration in the stable patient should be considered if there is immediate drainage of 1,500 mls or ongoing bleeding of 300 mls for three consecutive hours or 200 mls for five consecutive hours.

What would be your next step?

Early referral to the nearest cardiothoracic centre and CXR to confirm the drain position and full expansion of the lung. Pericardial effusion needs to be excluded with FAST scan or transthoracic echocardiography. If these are not available or the results are equivocal (for example poor imaging due to obesity), then a CT scan should be performed in stable patients.

The cardiothoracic unit is contacted and the cardiothoracic surgeon asks you to transfer the patient over. You are awaiting transport. Unfortunately, the patient starts to deteriorate. He becomes very anxious, his saturations are 90% on 2l of O2, BP 75/45 mmHg and HR 120bpm. There is no tracheal deviation, there is good air entry on auscultation of the lungs and the patient is peripherally cold.

He does not respond to fluid challenge. You suspect that the patient might have signs of pericardial tamponade, but echocardiography and CT are not available at the moment. What typical signs of pericardial tamponade would you look for?

Beck's triad. This consists of muffled sounds (due to blood/clot around the heart), distended jugular veins (due to impaired diastolic filling of the right atrium) and low blood pressure (due to low cardiac output).

The patient suddenly arrests, an anaesthetist is available, the crash team is on their way and CPR commenced. What would you do?

This patient is dying due to a cardiac arrest secondary to pericardial tamponade. Penetrating injury with witnessed cardiac arrest is typical and the (only) indication for emergency department anterolateral thoracotomy, and this needs to be performed without any delay. Needle pericardiocentesis is not as effective in trauma situations due to often clotted blood which cannot be removed by needle aspiration or drain insertion.

What are the chances for the patient to survive?

The success of emergency department thoracotomy is between 10% to 15% for penetrating trauma (vs 1% for blunt trauma – thus blunt trauma is currently not an indication for this procedure).

Talk me through the steps of emergency department thoracotomy?

The patient is supine with his left arm placed above the head. The skin incision starts at the edge of the sternum and runs horizontally below the nipple and then curves towards the axilla following the shape of underlying rib. The muscles are retracted between the muscle fibres or divided sharply. Intercostal muscles are divided above the rib. Care should be taken not to injure the underlying lung and mammary vessels, which are located one cm lateral from the edge of the sternum. A Finochietto retractor is used to open the intercostal space and the lung is retracted. The pericardium is opened longitudinally to preserve the phrenic nerve. The heart is frequently in ventricular fibrillation and internal paddles may be of benefit. Alternatively external defibrillator pads should be connected.

What manoeuvres can you perform to increase the chances of survival of this patient?

Pericardial opening releases tamponade and allows more effective direct cardiac massage. It also allows exposure and repair of cardiac injury (usually right ventricle) with a running Prolene 3-0 suture or pledgeted horizontal mattress suture. Clamping of the descending aorta would increase blood pressure to vital organs, increase coronary perfusion and eliminate eventual bleeding from vessels distal to the clamp. Finally clamping of the lung hilum would eliminate eventual bleeding from pulmonary vessels.

What would you do in the case of a right-sided penetrating wound and cardiac arrest due to cardiac tamponade?

The best approach would be a clamshell incision to get access to the cardiac injury (usually right atrium) and benefits of left chest access (cardiac massage, clamping of the aorta). This is achieved by continuation of an incision across the sternum and anterolateral thoracotomy on the other side. Mammary vessels should be clamped and divided. Two retractors are usually used to achieve maximum exposure to all chest organs.

Be aware that sternal or Gigli saws are not usually available, but heavy Mayo scissors are able to cut through the sternum.

Look at the CT scan from a different young healthy patient with stab wound to the left chest (Figure 2). What are the most obvious abnormalities?

Figure 2

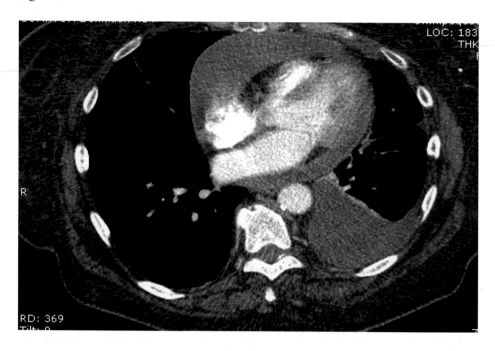

This patient has a moderate size left sided haemothorax. There is also a large pericardial effusion with typical sign of cardiac tamponade - compression of the right ventricle.

Perforated Peptic Ulcer Disease

A 71 year old man with severe COPD presents to the resus room with a 1 day history of severe central abdominal pain worse with moving and coughing. He denies any history of alcohol intake or previous ulcers. He is on prednisolone. On examination he is thin and cachectic looking. He is tachypnoeic, temp 38°C, BP:80/50 mmHg and pulse 110bpm. He is peritonitic with a rigid abdomen. Investigations reveal an elevated WCC at $18 \times 10^9/l$, CRP 320. You suspect a perforated gastroduodenal ulcer with septic shock. An erect CXR confirms pneumoperitoneum.

At laparotomy he is found to have extensive contamination within all four quadrants of the abdomen and a 2cm anterior perforated gastric ulcer sited over the distal stomach. What operation would you perform?

My operation of choice would be an omental patch repair of the ulcer, but I would always perform a biopsy of a gastric ulcer even if the ulcer looks benign. I would locate a healthy patch of omentum and use it to form a patch repair reinforced with 3.0 PDS. I do not close the ulcer itself but take good bites of the gastric wall to ensure the sutures do not cut through. I would use further 3.0 PDS sutures to reinforce the repair around the edges, particularly if the tissue was friable. The sutures are not tied too tight otherwise there is a risk of strangulating the omentum. An extensive washout (5 litres) saline is used to irrigate the peritoneal cavity.

Would you place a drain in this patient?

My practice is not to routinely place a drain but given the extent of contamination, friability of tissue and high risk nature of the patient, a drain would be wise. I would place the drain close to the site of patch repair. It is important to also ensure that a nasogastric tube is positioned into the body of the stomach prior to closure.

Towards the end of the operation the anaesthetist asks you about feeding access for this patient. They anticipate a slow recovery and for him to be intubated for at least 24 hours. Given his presentation with septic shock and poor general pre-morbid status they ask for your opinion on how to feed this patient. What are your options?

Although the patient could be given TPN through a central line, a better option would be to provide enteral nutrition. This is best provided by means of a feeding jejunostomy rather than a nasoenteric feeding tube. Although it is unconventional to place a feeding jejunostomy after this operation, it would be advisable in this scenario. Following a straightforward repair in this case it is perfectly justified given the expected slow recovery and frailty of the patient.

What are your post-operative instructions for this patient?

- Nasogastric tube to be aspirated every 2 hours for the first 24 hours. Left on free drainage in between

- Intravenous proton pump inhibitor – infusion not required

- Continue intravenous antibiotics – discuss with microbiology about which ones to use and what to change to, pending peritoneal / blood cultures. Anticipate a higher incidence of fungal positive cultures than expected requiring agents such as fluconazole

- VTE prophylaxis as per protocol

- Chest physiotherapy once awake due to the high risk of post op chest complications

- Start the jejunostomy feed at 25ml/hr on day one. Keep at this rate until bowels open and the patient is tolerating feed

- Chase up histology from biopsy. Once established on diet and fluids, eradicate for *H.pylori*

Is there any evidence for eradicating *H.pylori* following an omental patch closure of a perforated duodenal ulcer?

In a randomized trial a significant reduction in ulcer recurrence rate was shown in the group receiving *H.pylori* eradication treatment following simple omental patch repair of perforated duodenal ulcer (Ng et al).

What is the rationale for non-operative treatment of a perforated duodenal ulcer?

It has been shown that a number of these perforations seal spontaneously. In patients who are clinically stable, not peritonitic and have responded well to resuscitation, it may be possible to manage them conservatively with close monitoring and frequent reassessment. However, this is not always successful and patients can deteriorate - there should be a low threshold for operative intervention.

What is the evidence for non-operative treatment of perforated duodenal ulcers?

A randomized trial compared the outcome of non-operative treatment with that of emergency surgery in patients with a clinical diagnosis of perforated peptic ulcer. 83 patients entered in the study and it was concluded that an initial period of non-operative treatment with careful observation may be safely allowed except in patients over 70 years old, and that the use of such an observation period can obviate the need for emergency surgery in more than 70 per cent of patients. (Crofts et al)

In which patients is a higher mortality rate predicted?

There are a number of scoring systems including the Boey scoring system and the Mannheim Peritonitis Index (MPI) and more recently the Peptic Ulcer Perforation Score (PULP score). These risk stratify patients and predict outcomes of patients with perforated peptic ulcer.

The Boey score is the most commonly and easily implemented of these scoring systems, and accurately predicts perioperative morbidity and mortality.

Boey Score

Concomitant severe medical illness
Preoperative shock
Duration of perforation > 24 hours
Score: 0–3 (Each factor scores 1 point if positive)

Boey score and outcomes

Risk score	Mortality (OR)	Morbidity (OR)
1	8% (2.4)	47% (2.9)
2	33% (3.5)	75% (4.3)
3	38% (7.7)	77% (4.9)

Therefore in this patient a score of 3 would apply as he has severe COPD, shock and a >24 hour history.

Is there any evidence on relationship of the timing of emergency surgery for perforated peptic ulcer disease with outcome?

Data from the Danish Clinical Register of Emergency Surgery: A cohort study of 2,668 patients showed that every hour's delay was associated with a 2.4% decreased probability of survival compared with the previous hour (Buck et al).

What is the accepted role of laparoscopic repair of a perforated peptic ulcer?

The evidence for laparoscopic repair of perforated peptic ulcer disease remains uncertain. In a recent case control study rates of wound complications, organ space infections, prolonged ventilation, postoperative sepsis, return to the operating room, and mortality tended to be lower for the laparoscopic group, although not significantly. Length of hospital stay was, however, significantly shorter for the laparoscopic group by an average of 5.4 days. However these benefits of laparoscopic repair may be offset by the costs.

Recommendations are for laparoscopic repair for stable patients without any Boey risk factors.

What is the definition of a 'giant' peptic ulcer? What are the operative options for such ulcers?

A 'giant' peptic ulcer is defined as having a diameter greater than 2cm. Giant gastric ulcers are most commonly found on the lesser curve and often require an antrectomy with reconstruction either immediate or delayed. Giant duodenal ulcers pose a very difficult problem, particularly when close to the CBD and ampulla.

In some cases a distal gastrectomy may be required. The duodenal stump should be closed if possible. In difficult cases a Nissen closure can be carried out or alternatively a formal fistula created with tube drainage of the duodenum (using either a T-tube or foley catheter). Other described techniques include a jejunal serosal patch, tube duodenostomy, and Roux-en-Y duodenojejunostomy.

References

Mariëtta J. O. E. Bertleff, Johan F. Lange Laparoscopic correction of perforated peptic ulcer: first choice? A review of literature. Surg Endosc. 2010 June; 24(6): 1231–1239.

Buck DL, Vester-Andersen M, Møller MH; Danish Clinical Register of Emergency Surgery. Danish surgical delay is a critical determinant of survival in perforated peptic ulcer. Br J Surg. 2013 Jul;100(8):1045-9.

Lui FY, Davis KA. Gastroduodenal perforation: maximal or minimal intervention? Scand J Surg. 2010;99(2):73-7.

Crofts TJ, Park KG, Steele RJ, Chung SS, Li A. A randomized trial of non-operative treatment for perforated peptic ulcer. N Engl J Med. 1989 Apr 13;320(15):970-3.

Ng EK, Lam YH, Sung JJ, Yung MY, To KF, Chan AC, Lee DW, Law BK, Lau JY, Ling TK, Lau WY, Chung SC. Eradication of Helicobacter pylori prevents recurrence of ulcer after simple closure of duodenal ulcer perforation: randomized controlled trial. Ann Surg. 2000 Feb;231(2):153-8.

Byrge N, Barton RG, Enniss TM, Nirula R.Laparoscopic versus open repair of perforated gastroduodenal ulcer: a National Surgical Quality Improvement Program analysis. Am J Surg. 2013 Dec;206(6):957-62; discussion 962-3.

Lau H. Laparoscopic repair of perforated peptic ulcer: a meta-analysis. . Surgical Endoscopy 2004 Jul;18(7):1013-21. Epub 2004 May 12

Di Saverio, Bassi, Smerieri, Masetti, Ferrara, Fabbri, Ansaloni, Ghersi, Serenari, Coccolini, Naidoo, Sartelli, Tugnoli, Catena, Cennamo, Jovine. Diagnosis and treatment of perforated or bleeding peptic ulcers: 2013 WSES position paper. . World J Emerg Surg. 2014 Aug 3;9:45.

Perianal Sepsis

A 28 year old type 2 diabetic woman presents with a 3 day history of a painful perianal lump. She is unable to tolerate rectal examination, but there appears to be a large (7cm) perianal abscess.

What further information do you need?

I would like to know

- Is this a recurrent problem or the first presentation? *If this is recurrent it makes an underlying disease such as Crohn's more likely.*

- She is a young patient, which makes it possible that she may have underlying bowel disease such as Crohn's. Therefore questions such as weight loss, bowel habit, rectal bleeding are relevant.

- How well is her diabetes controlled? I would ask her questions pertaining to her general blood sugar control, previous diabetic problems, whether she is seeing her GP or specialist.

How would you proceed from here?

Given that it is her first episode of a perianal abscess the treatment of choice would be an incision and drainage of the abscess, which would be best performed under general anaesthetic. If this is a recurrent problem then involvement of a colorectal colleague is important as they may choose to obtain further imaging prior to proceeding. I would book and consent the patient for an EUA and incision and drainage of perianal abscess.

What preoperative tests should be performed?

This lady needs routine bloods. As she is a diabetic her blood sugar should be checked and if she has not had a recent HbA1C this should be performed. If this demonstrates poor glycaemic control then consultation with a diabetologist should be carried out to see if her blood sugar control can be optimised.

What is the pathophysiology of a perianal abscess?

This abscess originates from an infection arising in the cryptoglandular epithelium of the anal canal. Generally both internal and external sphincters act as a barrier to infections passing from the bowel lumen to surrounding tissues. However, infection can occur via the crypts of Morgagni which penetrate the sphincters and allow access to surrounding tissue.

What are the organisms commonly implicated in this type of abscess formation?

The most common causative organisms are Escherichia coli, Bacteroides species, and Enterococcus species.

Does this lady require any further imaging prior to surgery?

No, this is a first presentation of a perianal abscess, incision and drainage and an EUA are all that is required.

Are antibiotics required?

The treatment for a simple abscess is incision and drainage. However, in high-risk patients, (diabetics, immunosuppressed patients, extensive cellulitis, Crohn's disease) it is justifiable to give post-operative antibiotics. This lady has type 2 diabetes and it would be reasonable to give her antibiotics.

Describe your approach in theatre.

Firstly in these cases safe positioning of the patient is important. I would ensure the patient is put into a lithotomy position. Given the propensity for perianal procedures to induce profound vagal stimulation I would start only once my anaesthetic colleague is happy to proceed.

I would first perform a rectal examination followed by a rigid sigmoidoscopy. This is to ensure no other pathology is present such as neoplasia. It may also allow me to visualise an internal opening from a fistula.

If there are any signs to suggest HIV or Crohn's disease then appropriate histology can be taken. As a general principle as a colorectal non-specialist I would then aim to simply drain the abscess and involve a colorectal colleague should there be any more complex findings.

Your registrar completes the procedure. There is no other finding other than an abscess and she is discharged with antibiotics. The patient re-presents again three months later with a similar problem. What proportion of patients with an anorectal abscess will develop a fistula after initial incision and drainage?

This may be as high as 50% of patients.

What is the definition of a fistula?

It is an abnormal passage from one epithelialised surface to another epithelialised surface.

What is Goodsall's rule?

This states that for an anal fistula, if the fistula lies in the anterior half it will open directly into the anal canal, however if the fistula lies in the posterior half of the canal it will track towards the midline posteriorly and open at the midline posteriorly.

What is the accuracy of Goodsall's rule?

For anterior fistulae - it holds true approximately 50% of the time, and for posterior fistulae approximately 90% of the time.

What is Park's classification?

This is a classification of anal fistulae according to their relation to sphincters.

Type 1 - Intersphincteric (most common 45%)

Type 2 - Transsphincteric (30%) these enter the ischioanal space by perforating the external sphincter

Type 3 - Suprasphincteric (20%) these loop over the external sphincter and perforate the levator ani

Type 4 - Extrasphincteric (5%) these are external to the sphincter muscle, and are seen with supralevator abscesses. They may have a cryptoglandular origin but can also result from trauma, foreign body, or a pelvic abscess eg diverticular or appendiceal abscess

Repeat EUA demonstrates an anal fistula with an internal opening below the sphincters. What would you do?

This fistula can be safely laid open, which should reduce the chance of recurrence.

If a higher transsphincteric fistula had been found what would you do?

As well as draining the abscess a seton stitch can be placed to aid the drainage of sepsis. Laying open a higher fistula risks incontinence. The seton will allow drainage and a repeat EUA can be performed when infection has settled to provide definitive treatment.

What are the options for definitive treatment once the sepsis has cleared?

If there is a concern this might be a complex fistula further imaging (MRI) may be required.

For simple fistulas - (intersphincteric or low lying transsphincteric) not involving the external sphincter or puborectalis, a fistulotomy or fibrin plug/glue may be used. A fistulotomy has a recurrence rate of approximately 20% compared with 30%-60% for fibrin glue, however there is a risk to sphincter function with a fistulotomy. A further option is to carry out a fistulectomy by coring out the tract, which may then be laid open, or have a simple anatomical closure.

For complex fistulae (involvement of >30% of the external sphincter, suprasphincteric, fistulae with multiple tracts, recurrent or related to IBD, or extrasphincteric/high transsphincteric) the options include a cutting seton or a mucosal advancement flap. Cutting setons have a recurrence rate of up to 20% and incontinence rate of up to 30%, whereas an advancement flap may have a recurrence rate of up to 35% and incontinence rate of up to 13%.

Pregnant Patient with Cholecystitis

A 27 year old pregnant lady is admitted with acute cholecystitis. She is in the first trimester of her pregnancy. She has some RUQ tenderness and a low grade pyrexia. USS confirms a thick-walled gallbladder with minimal pericholecystic fluid.

The mother asks you whether cholecystectomy may lead to abortion. What would you tell her?

There is a very slight increased risk of miscarriage from surgical manipulation but in reality the risk is very small. The anaesthetic bears minimal risk of provoking spontaneous abortion. So although there is a theoretical risk of manipulation inducing miscarriage the risk is very small.

She would like to know if there would be any other risks to the baby if she had an operation.

The main risk of operating in the first trimester is the risk of teratogenesis. The majority of organogenesis is complete by the 8th week. Beyond 10 weeks the risk of teratogenic effects is negligible. Generally non-urgent surgery should be delayed until at least the second trimester and every effort should be made to treat her cholecystitis conservatively.

What are the main cardiovascular changes of pregnancy and what measure do you take to minimise their effects?

There is a 40%-50% rise in plasma volume which exceeds a red cell expansion (20%). This leads to a physiological anaemia and increased cardiac output which by term CO is approximately 140% of normal. Smooth muscle relaxation by progesterone leads to a fall in SVR hence fall in BP. Aortocaval compression by a gravid uterus can lead to decreased venous return (supine hypotension). The significance of these changes is that aortocaval compression should be avoided otherwise a further fall in BP may occur, leading to uterine hypoperfusion.

Why is pregnancy a significant risk factor for VTE?

Pregnancy not only contributes to immobility but is by itself a hypercoagulable state.

There is a rise on levels of nearly all clotting factors (except XI) along with a rise of platelet count. Fibrinolysis is inhibited by a plasminogen inhibitor derived from placenta. All of these factors contribute to an increased risk of VTE.

Having explained the specific consent for cholecystectomy she would like to know what other risks come with the operation if it were to be performed nearer term.

Gastro-oesophageal reflux is very common (70%) by the third trimester. This is due to the effects of progesterone relaxing the lower oesophageal sphincter and a pressure effect of the uterus onto the stomach. Therefore she is at higher risk of aspiration during induction of anaesthesia. She will be at increased risk of hypoxia due to a reduced FRC and a 50% increased O_2 demand.

Renal Trauma

A 57-year-old man has sustained a high-impact injury during go-karting. He presents with left loin pain and gross haematuria. He is haemodynamically stable. CT scanning reveals a grade 4 renal injury on the left side and a congenitally atrophic right kidney.

How would you manage this patient?

Haemodynamic stability is the primary criterion for the management of all renal injuries. This patient is stable and can be treated with non-operative management. This will consist of bed rest, IV fluid, IV antibiotics and regular observation of vital signs.

Extravasation of urine is not an indication for surgical intervention. Persistent extravasation or urinoma are usually managed successfully with endourological techniques. Surgical exploration is only required for an unstable patient with signs of retroperitoneal trauma or may be indicated in reno-vascular pedicle injury or pelvi-ureteric junction disruption. The majority of patients with grades 4 and 5 renal injuries present with major associated injuries, with resultant high exploration and nephrectomy rates.

What types of renal trauma do you know of?

90% of renal traumas in the UK are blunt traumas from road traffic accidents, falls and sport injuries. Gunshot and stab wounds are the most common causes of penetrating injuries. Renal traumas from penetrating injuries tend to be more severe and less predictable than those from blunt traumas.

Isolated renal trauma is uncommon, and up to 40% have associated intra-abdominal injuries. Direct blunt trauma crushes the kidney against ribs and indirect trauma can result in vascular or pelvi-ureteric disruption.

What common clinical findings may suggest renal injury?

It is very important to closely inspect the loin for bruising and swelling: gross haematuria, flank swelling with bruises or microscopic haematuria with hypotension (systolic <90mmHg). Fracture of the 12th rib may also be suggestive of an underlying renal injury. A renal pedicle injury is possible in the absence of haematuria. Pre-existing renal abnormality such as hydronephrosis due to ureteropelvic junction abnormality makes renal injury more likely following trauma.

Does the degree of haematuria correlate with the severity of renal injury?

Although haematuria is a hallmark sign of renal injury it is neither sensitive nor specific enough for differentiating minor and major injuries. Major renal injury, such as disruption of the ureteropelvic junction, renal pedicle injuries or segmental arterial thrombosis may occur without haematuria.

Which patients need to be admitted to hospital?

Patients with gross haematuria, unstable vital signs, associated other injuries and children under 16 years old.

Which patients may need radiological imaging?

The indications for radiographic evaluation are gross haematuria, microscopic haematuria and shock, or presence of major associated injuries. Since the majority of renal injuries are not significant and resolve without any intervention, not all patients need imaging.

What investigations should you arrange in a stable patient with renal injury?

A well-hydrated and stable patient should have a CT to visualize any corticomedullary laceration, extravasation of the dye, renal vessel injury, the presence of normal contralateral kidney and to exclude other associated visceral injuries. Renal USS can only accurately identify haematomas and peri-renal collections. CT has largely replaced the use of angiography for staging renal injuries. Angiography, however, is more specific for defining the exact location and degree of vascular injuries prior to possible radiological intervention.

What complications may occur following renal trauma?

Early complications may be seen within the first month and include infection, perinephric abscess, urinary fistula, hypertension, urinoma. Patients with grade III-V trauma must be followed closely and their blood pressure monitored regularly. If vascular hypertension develops, nephrectomy is indicated. Repeat imaging 2-4 days after trauma minimizes the risk of missed complications. Late complications include arteriovenous fistula, hydronephrosis or chronic pyelonephritis, and pseudoaneurysms.

Reference

European Association of Urology. Guidelines on urological trauma. EurUrol 2012 Oct; 62(4): 628-39.

Splenic Trauma

A 35 year old male suffers from blunt abdominal trauma having been knocked over by a car travelling at 40mph. He is ejected into the air and lands on the car windscreen. He has severe abdominal and shoulder tip pain. On arrival blood pressure: 140/90 mmHg pulse: 120 bpm. With intravenous fluid replacement the pulse rate is now 90 bpm and BP remains stable. Blood tests reveal a Hb: 11.1g/dl with normal biochemistry. A CT scan of his chest / abdomen and pelvis with intravenous contrast is performed and shows a grade II splenic injury with a moderate haemoperitoneum as well as fracture of lower left 7th and 8th ribs.

How would you manage this patient?

This patient's management can be divided into immediate management and specific management.

Immediate management would follow full resuscitation according to ATLS® principles ensuring Airway and C-spine control, Assessment and treatment of Breathing, Circulation, Disability.

In addition I would involve a senior member of the critical care team to help with resuscitation and further intensive care or theatre based management. The patient must be cross-matched for 6 units of type specific blood and until a decision is made regarding operative or non-operative management I would consider it sensible to inform the operating theatre co-ordinator that such a patient is in the resuscitation room.

Specific management: Given the finding of a grade II splenic injury with no involvement of the splenic hilum and a good response to fluid resuscitation, the patient can be managed non-operatively. This would involve:

1) Keeping the patient fasted in case of any surgical intervention required. Given the presence of haemoperitoneum I would be particularly aware that non-operative management may not succeed in this patient.

2) Admission to a critical care setting – HDU as a minimum with hourly monitoring of pulse, BP and urinary output. The critical care staff may choose to insert an arterial line for invasive blood pressure monitoring.

3) Strict bed rest with analgesia for 5-7 days. One needs to be aware that the patient is at risk of respiratory complications from diaphragmatic splinting. Adequate analgesia may involve the use of a patient controlled analgesia system.

4) Regular reassessment of the patient's clinical condition in case of any deterioration. A daily FBC should be performed.

5) If non-operative management proves to be successful then a follow up CT scan may be performed at ten days to look for any evidence of

splenic artery pseudo-aneurysm, which if present may require angio-embolisation. Always be aware of the risk of delayed splenic rupture which peaks between days 7 to 10.

At 6 am you receive a phone call about this patient from the high dependency unit. He has been hypotensive for the past two hours (80/50mmHg) with a pulse rate of 100 bpm. His urine output is 25ml/hr for two hours. He has failed to respond to further boluses of crystalloid. You go to see him and his abdomen is tense and more distended than earlier. How would you proceed?

Given the finding of haemodynamic instability and known splenic disruption the safest option would be to proceed to a laparotomy.

Talk me through how you would perform the trauma laparotomy.

First I would ensure I have adequate assistance as well as the necessary equipment. I would ask the theatre staff to have a full laparotomy set including vascular clamps and a sizeable retractor such as a Balfour retractor. Have two pool suckers to hand as well and ensure that a minimum of 6 units of cross-matched blood is available. Ideally I would have a cell saver set up in addition.

Prepare the patient's abdomen whilst he is fully awake and be fully scrubbed and ready even before the induction of anaesthesia. Drape the abdomen generously ensuring that xiphoid to pubis is accessible.

Once the patient is asleep I would make an incision from above the xiphoid to the pubis. I would expect a large amount of blood on entry into the abdomen and would manually remove blood and clots into a dish. The next step would be to pack all four quadrants to gain vascular control. Placing a pack beyond the spleen would help with subsequent splenic mobilisation as well as giving some control of haemorrhage.

Any adhesions and attachments lateral to the spleen need to be divided but some spleens can be highly mobile. My aim would be to try and deliver the spleen medially, which would provide better access to the hilum.

To gain access to the hilum I would divide any greater omentum overlying the gastrosplenic ligament, thereby gaining access to the short gastric vessels which may also need to be divided. Usually by this stage the hilum can be seen and a large clamp applied to the splenic artery and vein close to the spleen, ensuring that the tail of pancreas is not caught. These vessels should be ligated and divided between strong ties. The spleen is then removed from any surrounding attachments ensuring no damage is done to the fundus of the stomach in the process.

The remainder of the trauma laparotomy is completed in a systematic manner ensuring that the liver / colon / small bowel and mesentery are all carefully examined. The remaining packs are then systematically removed to ensure no further bleeding is evident. Washout is performed and a drain is placed in the left upper quadrant, a nasogastric tube would be appropriate (given the risk of gastric stasis) and the abdomen closed.

What complications may arise in the post-operative period that are specific to this operation?

Specific complications following a trauma splenectomy can be divided into immediate and late complications:

Immediate complications include bleeding which if significant may require further laparotomy. The aetiology of bleeding may be surgical but in the presence of significant blood loss then any coagulopathy, acidosis and hypothermia needs to be corrected.

Later complications include left lower lobe pneumonia due to diaphragmatic splinting, pancreatic fistula, or gastric leakage due to damage to the fundus. Overwhelming post splenectomy sepsis (OPSI) is rare and minimised by ensuring immunisation prior to hospital discharge.

What is Kehr's sign?

Kehr's sign is pain referred to the left shoulder that worsens with inspiration. This is due to irritation of the phrenic nerve from blood adjacent to the left hemidiaphragm.

What are the indications for angioembolisation in splenic trauma?

Angioembolisation (either proximal embolisation of the splenic artery or both proximal embolisation and selective distal splenic artery embolisation) may be used as an adjunct in the non-operative management of splenic trauma. Studies have confirmed higher success of non-operative management when splenic artery angioembolisation has been used in selected cases. In a ten year study by the National Trauma Registry of the American College of Surgeons the greatest benefit was seen in those patients with high grade (IV/V) splenic injuries who were haemodynamically stable but had contrast blush on CT.

How would you manage this patient prior to discharge from hospital?

Following emergency splenectomy ideally an immunisation course should be given at least two weeks following surgery. However, if the patient is discharged before two weeks, then it should be given immediately before discharge. To ensure that vaccinations against encapsulated bacteria are not forgotten following discharge it is advisable to administer them prior to the discharge. The immunisation course consists of pneumococcal vaccine (*Streptococcus Pneumoniae*) and a combined vaccine for *Haemophilus influenza B* and *Neisseria meningitidis*. In addition an annual vaccine for *influenza* needs to be given.

Antibiotics, usually penicillin V (500mg bd), may be required life-long. The duration of antibiotic prophylaxis is not well established. In the case of penicillin allergy then erythromycin / clarithromycin are the agents of choice. Antibiotics are to be started immediately post surgery for a minimum of two years but preferably lifelong.

Patients should also be warned to be more vigilant about infections and see their GP sooner rather than later.

Post splenectomy cards are usually available from pharmacy for the patient. The patient's medical records should be flagged to indicate "asplenic patient". The patient may wish to invest in a medic alert bracelet as well.

Informing the patient's GP is important, as vaccination may need to be repeated after 5 years. There is usually a Splenectomy Notification Letter to be completed and copied to the patient, GP and medical notes.

Counselling the patient is of utmost importance prior to discharge so that they remain fully compliant. They need to understand that if they develop any signs of infection e.g. sore throat, fever etc, to seek urgent medical attention. A standby course of antibiotics is advisable.

What do you understand by the term Overwhelming Post Splenectomy Infection (OPSI)?

OPSI is a major risk in patients with an absent or dysfunctional spleen (e.g. sickle cell disease) and although uncommon, is associated with a high mortality. These infections are often due to encapsulated bacteria such as *Streptococcus pneumonia, Haemophilus influenza* type b and *Neisseria meningitidis*. Other serious infections include malaria, babesiosis (caused by tick bite) and *Capnocytophaga canimorsus* (caused by dog bites) and secondary infections following influenza. OPSI can present months or years post splenectomy.

What is the incidence of OPSI?

OPSI is uncommon but serious and occurs at a rate of around 4%-5% in children and 1% of adults per year following splenectomy. It is imperative that all patients with an absent or dysfunctional spleen are appropriately immunised and receive antibiotic prophylaxis.

The patient asks you for advice regarding normal activities after discharge. What would you tell him?

Patients should be restricted from high risk activities such as skiing, contact sports, mountain biking for up to three months. The evidence base behind determining a three month wait is limited but generally accepted.

Is there a role for a follow up CT scan following non-operative management of splenic trauma?

If non-operative management has been successful then generally there is no need for a repeat CT. Delayed rupture from splenic artery pseudoaneurysm is a well-known complication after splenic injury treated with non-operative management. The timing and role of follow-up CT scanning is controversial, as the incidence of pseudoaneurysm formation is not known. Some studies suggest that a follow-up CT performed approximately one week after splenic injury may be useful to detect delayed pseudoaneurysm formation, but this is not routine practice in many centres.

Re-imaging may also be appropriate in those in whom activity restriction may need to be lifted such as professional athletes, military service personnel, and extreme sports enthusiasts.

References

Bhullar IS, Frykberg ER, Siragusa D, Chesire D, Paul J, Tepas JJ 3rd, Kerwin AJ. Selective angiographic embolization of blunt splenic traumatic injuries in adults decreases failure rate of non-operative management. J Trauma Acute Care Surg. 2012 May;72(5):1127-34.

Muroya T, Ogura H, Shimizu K, Tasaki O, Kuwagata Y, Fuse T, Nakamori Y, Ito Y, Hino H, Shimazu T. J. Delayed formation of splenic pseudoaneurysm following nonoperative management in blunt splenic injury: multi-institutional study in Osaka, Japan. Trauma Acute Care Surg. 2013 Sep;75(3):417-20.

Strangulated Femoral Hernia

A 77 year old female presents at 4am with a strangulated right femoral hernia requiring urgent surgery. She has a prosthetic mitral valve for which she takes warfarin. Past medical history includes atrial fibrillation and CVA. Her INR on admission is 5.1. You decide to operate urgently on this patient.

How would you reverse this lady's anticoagulation?

Emergency surgery can only be safely performed in this lady once the INR is below 1.5. Rapid reversal of oral anticoagulant therapy can be achieved by using fresh frozen plasma (FFP) or Prothrombin Complex Concentrates (PCCs). I would liaise with the on call haematologist to ensure rapid reversal is achieved, ideally using PCCs.

PCCs contain three or four vitamin K-dependent clotting factors and offer a number of advantages over FFP. These include a lower volume of infusion, ambient storage and reconstitution, lack of blood group specificity, a more favourable safety profile and improved efficacy. Hence many clinical practice guidelines now recommend PCC in preference or as an alternative to FFP for rapid anticoagulant reversal. In all cases these should be supplemented with oral or intravenous vitamin K. Beriplex P/N® (CSL Behring, Marburg, Germany) is one of the commonest preparations used and contains factors II, VII, IX and X, in addition to the vitamin K-dependent coagulation inhibitors protein C and protein S.

How is PCC administered?

PCC is administered intravenously (via central or peripheral venous lines) over a 10 to 20 minute period, and is given 30 minutes prior to surgery. Such cases are best discussed with the on call haematologist for guidance. A check INR is not routinely recommended prior to commencing emergency surgery, as reversal is very reliable.

What operative approach would you use to repair the femoral hernia?

I would approach the hernia through a modified McEvedy extra-peritoneal approach. This would involve a transverse incision roughly halfway between umbilicus and pubic symphysis, opening the anterior rectus sheath, retracting the rectus muscle and approaching the hernia sac in the extraperitoneal plane. The inferior epigastric vessels may have to be ligated and divided en route. The hernia sac can usually be reduced by gentle traction from inside and outside. Once the sac is opened, if the contents are non-viable small bowel then a resection can be performed if necessary. In the absence of gross contamination a prolene mesh repair in a plug manner can be performed or alternatively a suture repair done.

Other options include the classical vertical paramedian McEvedy approach or laparotomy. A low approach is not recommended as it may not be possible to safely perform a bowel resection.

As you attempt to reduce the hernia sac you have great difficulty in releasing it. How would you tackle this situation?

Anatomically it would be safe to divide any adhesions medial to the hernia sac and to divide the lacunar ligament knowing that the femoral vessels lie laterally. There is a risk of injuring an aberrant obturator vessel in doing so, and this can be a significant vessel which may need to be controlled first.

As the hernia sac is reduced there is gross spillage of enteric content as the small bowel was lacerated on delivery. There is a perforated Richter's type hernia and the bowel at the site of perforation is non viable. How would you proceed?

I would open the peritoneal lining to effectively do a laparotomy through the same incision. I would remove any contamination from the field and aim to perform a small bowel resection with a hand sewn anastomosis which is my preferred approach. Given her need for post operative anticoagulation I would take particular care with haemostasis so as to avoid any significant mesenteric haematoma. I would perform a washout before closing the wound.

How would you manage her anticoagulation post operatively?

The main concern immediately postoperatively is the risk of valve thrombosis and thromboembolism in a patient with a mechanical heart valve. In this patient postoperatively anticoagulation may be commenced with either intravenous heparin or treatment dose low molecular weight heparin once I am happy that the risk of bleeding is low. In her case she has a higher than normal risk of thromboembolism, given she has a mitral valve, previous stroke and atrial fibrillation. Each case is best discussed with the cardiology team to determine the safest anticoagulation strategy.

The risk of thromboembolism can be stratified according to the patient's age, prosthetic valve type, anatomical valve location, presence of atrial fibrillation and previous stroke or cardioembolic event. The highest thromboembolic risk is seen in patients with prosthetic mitral valve, multiple prosthetic heart valves, prosthetic heart valve and previous stroke, and atrial fibrillation.

Reference

Daniels PR, McBane RD, Litin SC, Ward SA, Hodge DO, Dowling NF, Heit JA. Peri-procedural anticoagulation management of mechanical prosthetic heart valve patients. Thrombosis Research. 2009 Jul;124(3):300-5.

Testicular Pain

You are reviewing a 16 year old boy in A & E complaining of acute onset of lower abdominal and scrotal pain for the past hour. What are the differentials?

The most likely cause is testicular torsion. Other differentials include a strangulated hernia, acute epididymo-orchitis or torsion of the hydatid of Morgagni.

What might be apparent to suggest the latter diagnosis?

A palpable blue dot discolouration on the scrotum is diagnostic of a torsion of the hydatid of Morgagni.

What is Prehn's sign?

This test is used to distinguish between epididymitis and testicular torsion. It involves gently elevating the scrotum, which alleviates the pain of epididymitis but not in a torsion.

What other clinical findings might you find?

On the affected side the testis is usually elevated and may have a horizontal lie. The cremasteric reflex will also be absent.

What is the pathogenesis of testicular torsion?

Torsion is usually divided into intravaginal and extravaginal, the latter occurring in neonates only. In the former, torsion occurs within the tunica vaginalis due to a long mesentery or because of a bell-clapper deformity which allows rotation within the tunica vaginalis.

On clinical examination of this child testicular torsion could not be excluded. How would you proceed?

Any boy with testicular pain where testicular torsion cannot be excluded requires urgent exploration. The patient needs to be consented and warned that there is a risk the testicle may be non-viable and an orchidectomy may be required.

Either a transverse incision or a median raphe incision may be performed. The latter allows access to the contralateral testicle through the same incision so that it may be fixed. This is usually carried out with three point fixation using 2-0 or 3-0 prolene.

On exploration the testicle does indeed appear to have undergone a torsion. What would you do?

The testicle should be "untorted" and wrapped in warm packs. This should be done to encourage blood flow and determine if the testicle is viable. Given the short history in this case the testicle may well be salvageable.

What is the role of doppler ultrasound preoperatively to exclude torsion?

Ultrasound cannot completely exclude the possibility of torsion, but may be used as an adjunct in patients where the clinical picture suggests the risk is low. If there is a strong concern of a testicular torsion clinically, regardless of ultrasound findings, the scrotum should be explored.

Traumatic Diaphragmatic Rupture

A 60 year old male, unrestrained, car driver travelling at 50 mph had a head on collision with a tree. He sustained blunt trauma to his upper abdomen and distal chest from the steering wheel. He complains of dyspnoea, pain in the left chest and left upper quadrant of his abdomen. On arrival his saturation is 95% on 4 l of O2, RR 22/min, pulse 85/min and BP 130/70mmHg. During the auscultation of the chest there is no air entry basally on the left. His Hb is 125 g/l with normal biochemistry. His CXR and CT scan of the chest with intravenous contrast are performed and shown below (fig 1).

What are the main CXR and CT findings?

Figure 1

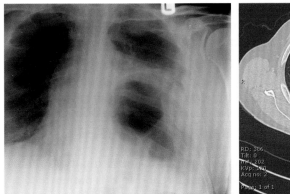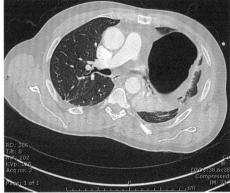

Most obvious findings on CXR are suspected herniation of abdominal contents (stomach and/or transverse colon) into the left chest and fractures of 7th-9th ribs. CT confirms these findings. Abdominal CT reveals additional small splenic subcapsular haematoma (grade I) with no signs of haemoperitoneum.

What is the typical mechanism of trauma and which part of the diaphragm has the highest propensity for rupture?

High intensity impact on the upper abdomen and distal chest is the typical mechanism leading to a sudden increase in intra-abdominal pressure pushing abdominal organs against the diaphragm and causing its rupture.

Tears in the muscular part of the left hemidiaphragm are by far the most common, usually presenting as a large longitudinal slit between the muscle fibres. Injury to the right hemidiaphragm is less common due to protection by the liver. Circumferential detachment of the diaphragm from the ribs or rupture of the central tendon (pericardial hernia) are rare.

What would be your initial management of this patient?

The immediate management should be to resuscitate the patient along ATLS principles. A NG tube should be inserted to decompress the stomach.

This patient requires an emergency repair of diaphragmatic rupture and four units of type specific blood must be crossmatched. The theatre coordinator and theatre anaesthetist need to be informed and a senior member of the critical care team should be involved in management of this patient.

You are waiting for available theatre, when the patient de-saturates to 85% on 60% FiO2, RR 35/min and BP 90/60mmHg. During the auscultation of the chest, there are no breath sounds on the left side but you can clearly hear bowel sounds. What would be your next step?

The patient needs immediate intubation and positive pressure ventilation. Negative intrathoracic and positive intra-abdominal pressure during spontaneous ventilation increases the size of intrathoracic herniation. This leads to compression of the lung, incarceration of abdominal organs and, in extreme situations, tension gastrothorax/viscerothorax with shift of the mediastinum to the opposite side. This shift causes compression of the inferior vena cava within the central tendon of the diaphragm with decreased venous return and decreased cardiac output.

The aim of the intubation is to change negative intrathoracic pressure during spontaneous ventilation to positive intrathoracic pressure during mandatory ventilation. This will aid repositioning of the viscera to the abdomen and stabilization of the patient.

The patient stabilised after intubation and a theatre slot is finally available. What would be your approach for diaphragmatic repair in this patient?

I would perform a midline laparotomy. The majority of patients with diaphragmatic rupture have concomitant splenic, liver or bowel injury. The abdominal cavity should be well explored before the diaphragmatic rupture is repaired. In this patient the splenic rupture was grade I thus not requiring any surgical attention and there was no other intra-abdominal injury.

Posterolateral thoracotomy via the 8th or 9th intercostal space would be another option. This would be considered in the case of isolated right hemidiaphragmatic rupture. The right hemidiaphragm is more accessible from this approach. Concomitant intrathoracic injury requiring surgical repair would be another indication for thoracotomy.

A third option would be combined laparotomy and thoracotomy in case of intra-abdominal and intrathoracic injury.

Laparoscopic and thoracoscopic approaches are increasingly popular.

How would you repair the diaphragm?

After reposition of the viscera to abdomen and retraction caudally, the dome of the hemi-diaphragm is exposed and the defect is closed directly from back to front with interrupted horizontal mattress non-absorbable sutures (Ethibond or Polypropylene 0 or 1). Absorbable sutures should not be used due to risk of re-herniation development. The sutures can be reinforced with the use of Teflon pledgets. Before the repair usually two chest drains (apical and basal) are placed into the chest cavity.

Do all patients present as emergency?

No, delayed presentation is common. Patients can present months or years after trauma with dyspnoea or abdominal pain with incarceration of stomach or colon. Some patients present early after injury, but diaphragmatic rupture is missed (fig 2). Repair is more challenging in these cases due to adhesions and scarring. It is usually not possible to perform direct repair and a non-absorbable mesh may be required.

Figure 2

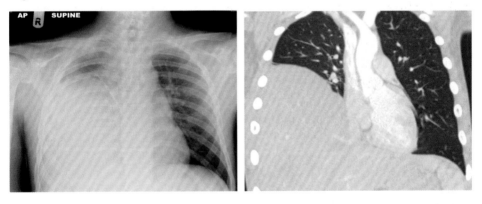

Figure 2 shows an example of a missed diaphragmatic rupture. A 17 year old male presented to hospital with dyspnoea. He underwent exploratory laparotomy due to polytrauma with liver and spleen injury two months before presentation. CXR and CT revealed herniation of the liver into the right hemithorax. The rupture was repaired from the right posterolateral thoracotomy. Figure 3 shows CXR immediately after repair.

Figure 3

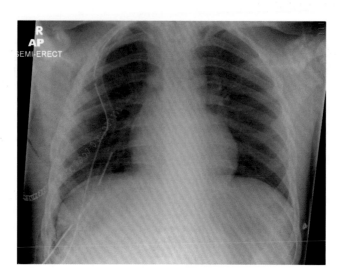

A high index of suspicion is important in patients with a typical mechanism of injury. These patients should have follow up CXR. In equivocal cases MRI or even thoracoscopy/laparoscopy are the best modalities to exclude diaphragmatic rupture.

Ulcerative Colitis

The gastroenterology team has called you to review a patient with known ulcerative colitis (UC). He has been an inpatient for four days and treated with steroids but is not improving symptomatically. What are the indications for surgery in UC patients?

There are absolute indications, and relative indications. Absolute indications include perforation and toxic dilatation. Relative indications include failure to respond to medical therapy and bleeding.

What features early in an admission for acute UC suggest surgery is likely to be necessary?

There are a number of features that are poor prognostic features for avoiding surgery - these include greater than 10 bowel movements per day all with the passage of blood, low haemoglobin and low albumin and CRP >45.

Ideally, how should such patients be managed at admission?

Patients admitted with acute flare up of UC should be under the joint care of both surgical and gastroenterology teams. This allows progress to be monitored, continual communication between the teams and swift action if required. Monitoring should involve the following parameters - stool charts, pulse, temperature, CRP and haemoglobin and plain abdominal radiographs. Further, these patients need daily physical examinations, intravenous fluids, thromboprophylaxis. Their nutrition needs to be addressed and ideally a haemoglobin of above 10 g/dl maintained. Corticosteroids (hydrocortisone 400 mg/day) should be commenced. Higher doses of steroids offer no greater benefit. Also required, withdrawal of anticholinergic, antidiarrhoeal agents, NSAID and opioid drugs and continuation of aminosalicylates.

Why might a perforation be difficult to detect?

Patients will be on high dose steroids, which may mask the clinical signs - a high index of suspicion must be maintained. Steroids may also make it difficult to distinguish from an infective colitis, hence stool cultures should be sent at the earliest possible opportunity. The treatment should not be delayed and it is appropriate to commence on both steroids and broad spectrum antibiotics, whilst waiting for the culture report.

What is rescue treatment?

If there is no improvement in acute severe colitis by day 3, colectomy may be considered or rescue therapy may be instituted. Rescue therapy is either with IV cyclosporine 2mg/kg/day or Infliximab 5mg /kg (0,2 and 6 weeks). Infliximab is used if cyclosporine is contraindicated or some times as first line rescue therapy in acute severe UC.

What is infliximab, what is it licenced for?

Infliximab is a monoclonal antibody that binds to free and membrane-bound tumour necrosis factor-α (TNFα). It is licenced for inducing and maintaining remission in active severe Crohn's disease patients whose disease has not responded to conventional therapy, and fistulating Crohn's disease. It is also used in acute severe colitis.

What are the complications of infliximab?

Possible complications include risk of infection especially resurgence of TB, infusion reactions, malignancy including T-cell lymphoma, demyelination and drug induced lupus.

Are you aware of any criteria for assessing disease activity?

The Truelove and Witts criteria.

Criteria of Truelove and Witts for Assessing Disease Activity in Ulcerative Colitis		
	Mild Activity	Severe Activity
Daily bowel movements (no.)	< or = to 5	> 5
Hematochezia	Small amounts	Large amounts
Temperature	< 37.5°C	> or = to 37.5°C
Pulse	< 90/min	> or = 90/min
Erythrocyte sedimentation rate	< 30 mm/h	> or = to 30 mm/h
Hemoglobin	> 10 g/dl	< or = to 10 g/dl
Patients with fewer than all 6 of the above criteria for severe activity have moderately active disease		

What are the Travis criteria?

The Travis criteria predict the likely need for surgery after three days of intensive treatment. A stool frequency of >8/day or 3-8 bowel movements per day and a CRP >45 mg/l at day three appears to predict the need for surgery in 85% of cases.

How would you counsel this patient if they require surgery due to failure of medical therapy?

This patient should be informed that he will need an operation to remove most of the large bowel. Importantly he will have a stoma and this would be a good opportunity to ask a specialist colorectal nurse/stoma nurse to speak with the patient about stomas. The patient will obviously have a number of concerns regarding this, but should be informed that theoretically the stoma may be reversed in the future once he has recovered.

What operation would you carry out in this situation?

This patient should have a subtotal colectomy and end ileostomy.

What mortality would you quote in this patient?

Emergency surgery for UC carries with it a significant mortality risk. This is up to 8% in non-perforated cases, rising to 40% in those who have a perforation.

What are the principles in carrying out an emergency sub-total colectomy?

This procedure may be carried out laparoscopically but is more commonly performed as an open laparotomy. The patient should be positioned in a Lloyd-Davies, and ideally the potential stoma site should have been marked pre-operatively. The distal division of the colon should be at the sigmoid colon with sufficient length to be able to bring the end to the abdominal wall to form a mucus fistula. Alternatively some surgeons prefer to place the end subcutaneously, and not form a formal mucus fistula, in the knowledge that should the end "blow" it will create a fistula due to its placement.

An end ileostomy should be formed at the proximal division. A Foley catheter may be placed in the rectum to remain post-operatively and encourage drainage, or daily proctoscopy carried out.

GENERAL SURGERY

**Mohamed Ahmed Waleed Al-Singary Brice Antao
Bhaskar Kumar Liam Masterson Ramez Nassif
Brendan O'Connor Alexander Phillips
Eunice Tan Robert Winterton**

Contents

Classification of Complications

You are asked by your consultant colleagues to start a prospective database of elective work done by your department. What information do you think should be recorded as part of this database?

Such a database would require the recording of baseline demographics of the patient (age, gender), as well as the procedures undertaken, and other factors such as co-morbidities and ASA. Other factors that one might wish to include are BMI, whether or not they smoke, and alcohol intake. For those patients undergoing oncological resections, disease stage and use of neoadjuvant treatments may be beneficial, and perhaps CPEX testing if appropriate. Post operatively, morbidity and mortality would need to be recorded as well as factors such as length of stay, or critical care bed days.

The actual information recorded would be dependent on the nature of the department's work load, which may mean some information is more valuable than others.

With respect to complications - what systems for classifying them are you aware of?

There are a number of mechanisms used for recording and classifying post-operative complications. Perhaps the two most commonly employed are the Clavien-Dindo classification and the Accordion Score.

Can you tell me anything more about these scoring systems?

The Clavien-Dindo classification defines a complication as a deviation from the ideal post-operative course. It is graded 1 to 5, with grade 5 equating to death. The Accordion Score grades complications as mild, moderate and severe with a final classification of death.

Score	Clavien-Dindo	Accordion
1	Any deviation from the normal postoperative course without need for significant intervention (eg surgery/ radiology/ pharmacological). Allowed are fluids, analgesics, antiemetics.	Mild complications- requiring only bedside interventions- catheter, NG tube, fluids, analgesics, antiemetics.
2	Complications requiring pharmacological treatment (other than those in Grade 1). Also includes transfusions and TPN	Moderate complications requiring medications (other than those in grade 1). Includes transfusions and TPN
3	Complications requiring surgical intervention. (3a not under GA, 3b requiring GA).	Severe complications requiring surgery, endoscopic or radiological intervention. Also includes complications leading to organ failure.
4	Life threatening complications requiring intensive care. (4a is single organ dysfunction, 4b multiorgan dysfunction)	Death.
5	Death	

What are the advantages and disadvantages of such systems?

Both of these scoring systems are simple to use and have been widely employed within medical literature as a means of standardising complications. They allow comparison of outcomes and can be used to help evaluate the safety of procedures.

Their disadvantages include observer variability and also differing management plans for the same complications. Whilst one surgeon may take a conservative approach for a complication that might involve only fluid resuscitation and antibiotics, another surgeon may feel that the same complication in addition merits surgical, radiological or endoscopic intervention, which would change the grading of the complication.

Using the above information can you classify the below complications according to the Clavien-Dindo score?

A 65 year old man is admitted with generalised peritonitis. CT scan suggests a perforated DU and the patient is listed for a laparotomy. During intubation the patient aspirates. The laparotomy is performed and an omental patch is used to repair the perforation. Post operatively the patient develops pneumonia and has acute renal failure. He requires vasopressor support. The patient spends seven days in ITU and a further fortnight recovering on the ward.

This patient had developed multi-organ dysfunction and thus the complications should be graded as IVb.

A 25 year old man is brought into A & E having been shot in the abdomen. He was intubated at the scene and is haemodynamically unstable. A decision is made to proceed directly to laparotomy, where multiple bowel and mesenteric injuries are found, and a large laceration to the liver. A damage control laparotomy is carried out achieving haemostasis and stapling of injured bowel. The patient requires 18 units of packed red blood cells as well as platelets and FFP. Post operatively the patient went to ITU and remained intubated and ventilated. He is returned to theatre at 36 hours, bowel continuity is restored and the abdomen closed. He remains in ITU intubated for five days and then spends two weeks on the ward recovering.

This patient has not had any actual complication and thus should not be classified using the system.

Complications of Pneumoperitoneum

You are carrying out a laparoscopic cholecystectomy in an otherwise fit and well 45 year old lady.

What techniques are you aware of for establishing a pneumoperitoneum?

There are a number of different techniques for establishing a pneumoperitoneum and choice lies with the surgeon. Variation may be made according to the clinical picture and operation being performed.

The most frequent method, and advocated by the Royal College of Surgeons, is an open Hasson cut down.

Other methods include the use of a Veress needle, and also an optical trocar.

What are the risks of a pneumoperitoneum?

Pneumoperitoneum is associated with a number of risks, including acidosis, dysrhythmia, pneumothorax and gas embolism. It can cause extraperitoneal dissection (which may be intentional in TEP hernia repairs).

You are establishing pneumoperitoneum and the anaesthetist tells you he has a problem. There has been a sudden drop in end tidal CO2 and blood pressure. What are your concerns?

This clinical picture suggests the possibility of a gas embolism - a very rare occurrence.

How would you manage the situation?

Insufflation should be stopped, gas allowed to escape and the patient ventilated with 100% oxygen. Further, the patient should be placed in a steep head down left lateral decubitus position (Durant's position) in order to allow gas bubbles to rise to the apex of the right atrium and prevent entry into the pulmonary artery. Theoretically insertion of a central line may allow gas aspiration and improve haemodynamic status.

What techniques can be used to minimise the risk of a gas embolus?

The incidence of gas embolus is unknown but it is regarded as very rare, but may be fatal if it occurs. The most frequent cause recorded is accidental puncture of a vessel with a Veress needle at induction. Use of the Hasson (open) method should minimise this risk. Other techniques that should be employed are the use of low intra-abdominal pressure and low insufflation rates.

Why is the term "pneumoperitoneum" misleading?

This implies the use of air for insufflation, when in fact carbon dioxide is used and should thus be referred to as a capnoperitoneum.

What are the advantages and disadvantages of using carbon dioxide for laparoscopy?

Carbon dioxide has a number of benefits- it is a chemically inert colourless gas. Further, it is inexpensive, easily accessible and not combustible. It is also rapidly absorbed in the blood stream. However, it can cause hypercapnia, and metabolic acidosis. Experimental models have even suggested that it can have an adverse effect on intraperitoneal immune function, possibly increasing the risk of port-site metastases in oncological cases.

What insufflation pressure would you normally use?

Generally the lowest adequate intra-abdominal pressure should be used. A pressure of 14mmHg or less is regarded as being safe in healthy patients.

Day Case Unit

You are tasked by the clinical director to start a day case service for treating patients requiring laparoscopic cholecystectomy. How would you go about this task?

There are a number of factors that need to be considered. It would be helpful to carry out an audit of the current practices which would demonstrate the demographics of the patients that are currently being referred, how long they are typically staying in hospital and what pre-operative assessment is currently in place. This may allow reasonable service planning and help provide an estimate of the resources that are likely to be required.

Those involved in providing the service:- surgeons, anaesthetists, nursing staff, should be involved in drawing up specific protocols for the service. These protocols should help assess a number of factors including:

1) Patients' social circumstances and whether day surgery would be suitable

2) Co-morbidities and likelihood of complications

3) Appropriate anaesthetic assessment

4) Post-operative management and pain control

Discharge is often nurse-led. Specific criteria need to be established to ensure that patients are not inappropriately discharged with an unrecognised complication, and other nursing staff need to be aware of who to contact when problems do arise.

Dissemination of the protocol that is finally agreed on needs to occur so that patients can be appropriately referred into the system in order for it to realise its full potential.

What are the advantages and disadvantages of a day service?

Patients may prefer to spend a minimum time in hospital. A day service also frees up inpatient beds for other patients and can reduce the risk of hospital acquired infections. Ultimately day case surgery may lead to improved cost effectiveness.

To contrast this, patients may feel that they are part of a "conveyor belt", and that the swift discharge means they are not being looked after properly. There is also a burden on family/ friends to help with convalescence.

How could some of these disadvantages be alleviated?

Surgeons should review patients prior to discharge. Clear written post-operative guidance should be supplied with specific instructions of who to contact if problems arise in the early post-operative period.

Diathermy and Pacemaker

You are reviewing a 70 year old lady in clinic who has been having problems with biliary colic and has had several admissions in the last six months due to symptoms. You have listed her for a laparoscopic cholecystectomy. She has a pacemaker in situ. What are your concerns about this patient?

This patient has a pacemaker in situ which may lead to problems with the use of diathermy. In patients with pacemakers and implantable cardioverter defibrillators (ICDs) diathermy can cause electrical interference which may place the patient at risk. Potentially energy can be transferred through leads and cause tissue heating at the tips with high frequency current.

Is there any risk in patients if bipolar diathermy is used instead of monopolar?

A risk still exists, however the possibility of electrical inference is greatly diminished with bipolar diathermy.

What is the difference between a pacemaker and an ICD?

Pacemakers are generally small devices that maintain heart rate and may be used particularly in patients susceptible to bradycardia. It functions only when required. An ICD is a larger device that serves to prevent cardiac arrest by providing a shock. It is placed in patients with potentially life threatening rhythm disturbances.

What information should be acquired about the pacemaker preoperatively?

Patients with both pacemakers and ICDs usually carry a "passport" with specific information including manufacturer details, model and serial number, where and when the device was fitted and the reason for the placement. Further, the last time the device was checked should be established.

Prior to surgery discussion with the team involved in looking after the device (usually a cardiac physiologist) should be carried out. A check should have occurred within the last three months particularly with regard to battery life. Device functionality should also be checked after surgery. (ICDs may need to be placed in a monitor mode to prevent accidental shock delivery due to electrical interference).

What considerations should be made during surgery?

Diathermy should be avoided if possible, however if it is required it should be employed in short bursts and the plate kept away from the implant.

The ECG should be carefully monitored and the potential need for external pacing should be kept in mind. The anaesthetist should be vigilant and if there is any detectable pacemaker inhibition the surgeon should be informed to allow diathermy to be discontinued.

What role do magnets place in managing pacemakers during surgery?

Magnets secured over the pacemaker site may place it into an asynchronous mode (non-sensing). However, this is not true of all pacemakers and this should be checked with the manufacturer/ cardiac physiologist to determine the settings, as with some pacemakers a magnet may result in the initiation of a period of device diagnostics. (In ICDs a magnet may inhibit shock delivery, but again this is dependent on the device setup.)

How does diathermy work?

Diathermy works by passing high frequency alternating current through the body to produce heat. The electrical frequency involved may range between 300 kHz and 10MHz.

What are the different modes of diathermy?

These are cutting, coagulation and blend. Cutting involves a continuous low frequency current in a sinus wave which produces a very high temperature of up to 1000°C. Coagulation, contrastingly, involves high frequency current in a square form at brief intervals. Blend involves the cutting continuous low frequency current with episodes of high frequency superimposed.

What is the difference between monopolar and bipolar diathermy?

Monopolar diathermy involves the passage of current from an instrument held by the surgeon to a plate/pad placed on the patient to allow return to the generator. In bipolar diathermy no plate is required and the current passes between the two forceps ends. A plate of at least 70cm^2 should be used in monopolar diathermy away from bony prominences and metallic implants to prevent burns.

Are there any alternatives that may be employed instead of diathermy in this case?

It may be possible to carry out the operation using an harmonic scalpel. This may make operating more challenging using a different instrument, but it is a viable instrument not associated with causing any pacemaker interference.

Elective Inguinal Hernia

Your registrar is reviewing a normally fit and well 75 year old man in clinic who has been referred with bilateral inguinal herniae. Both are reducible, the right side has been causing increasing discomfort whereas the left is asymptomatic. What are the treatment options.

The treatment options include open or laparoscopic repair. Since he has bilateral inguinal herniae laparoscopic repair would be particularly beneficial. As he is fit and well he should be able to tolerate a general anaesthetic.

What are the pros and cons of laparoscopic compared to open inguinal hernia repair?

Laparoscopic repair has

- Less post operative discomfort
- Earlier return to normal activities (3 days in 7 RCTs)
- Lower incidence of chronic pain / numbness (2%)
- Fewer wound complications. When complications did occur they were generally more severe with laparoscopic approach (vascular injury or bowel injury)
- Having said that rates of complications should be low if done by a surgeon appropriately trained in laparoscopic repairs
- However, recurrence is 2% compared to 1% with an open repair

What are the NICE guidelines regarding the use of laparoscopic inguinal hernia repair?

Laparoscopic repair of inguinal hernia was likely to result in considerably less postoperative pain and numbness than open repair. There was uncertainty over the rates of recurrence and of serious complications associated with laparoscopic surgery for primary repairs.

The preferred technique for the repair of recurrent and bilateral hernias should be laparoscopic. Consideration should be made for primary repair of unilateral hernias because of the reduced incidence of long-term pain and numbness and the potential for earlier return to normal activities.

The gentleman is listed for a laparoscopic repair. You receive a letter from the cardiologists 8 weeks later which informs you that he has just been discharged after a five day stay for a myocardial infarction. What would you do?

Recent MI is a considerable risk factor for non-cardiac surgery. Ideally surgery should be postponed for six months in this patient. Risk of post-operative MI decreases as the time since the original MI increases. Within 30 days the risk may be as high as 33%, decreasing to 19% between 31 and 60 days, 8.4% at 61-90 days and 5.9% for 90-180 days.

However, if a hernia is particularly bothersome, repair under local anaesthetic could be contemplated.

How do you consent this patient?

There are both general risks and risks specific to this procedure. General risks include bleeding (usually a self limiting haematoma), infection (of wound or mesh), thromboembolism.

Specific risks include recurrence, seroma, chronic pain and numbness. It should be noted that the incidence of chronic pain may approach 20% and is often under quoted. Risk of recurrence is 1- 2%.

What is the mid-point of the inguinal canal, and what is the midinguinal point? What is the clinical significance of each of these?

The mid-point of the inguinal canal is the point half way between the anterior superior iliac spine and the pubic tubercle. The deep ring lies about 2.5cm above this point.

The mid-inguinal point is the point half way between the anterior superior iliac spine and the pubic symphysis, and marks the point of the femoral artery.

What local anaesthetic would you use for this patient and what doses would be permissible?

A combination of lignocaine with adrenaline and chirocaine would be reasonable (half and half)

Doses for these are: Lignocaine with adrenaline (1:200,000) 7mg/kg

Lignocaine 3mg/kg

Chirocaine with adrenaline (1:200,000) 2.5mg/kg

Chirocaine 2mg/kg.

What does 1% lignocaine mean?

This means there is 10mg of lignocaine in each millilitre of solution.

What are the arguments for and against repair of an asymptomatic inguinal hernia?

Argument *for* repair

- 9/10 will eventually cause pain

- Risk of complications is small but not insignificant. 5% will require an emergency repair and 30-day mortality in the acute scenario is 3%

- Watch and wait policy never cures, but delays the inevitable that most do develop symptoms or serious complications

Argument *against* repair

- Cost of repairing all hernias under the NHS when only 5% will eventually require repair for a serious complication of it

- Mortality for elective repair is 0.15%, and for emergencies 3%. However the patients who have emergency repair are arguably more likely to have never been candidates for elective repair

- Chronic pain post operatively is 30% overall. In 11% it will interfere with daily living

Further reading:

Livhits M, Ko CY, Leonardi MJ, Zingmond DS, Gibbons MM, de Virgilio C. Risk of surgery following recent myocardial infarction. Ann Surg. 2011 May;253(5):857-64.

NICE guidelines on laparoscopic hernia repair http;//www.nice.org.uk/guidance/TA83/chapter/1-guidance

Enhanced Recovery Pathway

What do you understand by the term enhanced recovery pathway?

Enhanced recovery programmes/pathways are a multidisciplinary strategy designed to improve patient outcomes. Originally conceived by a Danish surgeon, Henrik Kehlet, his objectives were to provide a pain and risk free procedure for patients.

What components are involved?

These pathways are multi-factorial comprising pre-admission, admission, intraoperative and post-operative components.

Preadmission: In general this involves patient optimisation. Co-morbidities should be addressed, significant anaemia corrected and patient education initiated. This not only involves explaining to patients what to expect and how their lifestyle may need to be adapted postoperatively, but also teaching about items like stomas so they can become more proficient at managing them at an earlier stage. The consent process should start at this early point.

Admission: Most patients on enhanced recovery pathways are admitted on the day of surgery. Fluid balance should be optimised and carbohydrate loading is often used. In bowel surgery bowel preparation has been discarded.

Intraoperatively: A minimally invasive approach is usually employed where appropriate. Goal directed fluid management, and individualised pain management often with the use of epidurals or PCAs. Where possible the use of drains is discouraged and nasogastric tubes removed.

Postoperatively: Early mobilisation and early use of enteral nutrition are key components. Discharge planning should be commenced at an early opportunity and most pathways include daily goals for the patients to achieve.

Which specialties have implemented these principles?

Originally this was conceived for patients undergoing colorectal resections. The principles have subsequently been adopted by a variety of general surgical procedures - including oesophagectomy, hepatobiliary surgery, gynaecology and orthopaedics. In all of these groups it has been found to be effective and safe, usually significantly reducing the length of stay with no increase in morbidity.

When are patients able to go home?

Fearon stipulated four criteria that should be met to determine if patients are fit for discharge. These are that the patients:

1) Have good pain control with oral analgesics

2) Are eating and drinking and not requiring iv fluids

3) Are independently mobile or have reached their preoperative level

4) Have met all of the above criteria and are willing to go home

How have enhanced recovery pathways affected outcomes?

These pathways have led to decreased lengths of stay, a reduction in complication rates, and also a reduction in costs.

The reporting on re-admission rates has been variable, however pathways have not been associated with increased re-admission rates and in many cases there has been a fall.

There is also a reported increase in patient satisfaction. In addition pathways have not been found to compromise patient care.

Lastly, a number of studies have suggested that these pathways shorten stay and consequently this leads to a considerable cost saving for each patient, although some argue that the cost saving is due to a reduction in complications rather than reduced hospital stay.

Further reading:

Fearon, KCH Ljungqvist O, Von Meyenfeldt M, Revhaug A, Dejong CHC, Lassen K, Nygren J, Hausel J, Soop M, Andersen J, Kehlet H. Enhanced recovery after surgery: a consensus review of clinical care for patients undergoing colonic resection. *Clinical Nutrition.* 2005; **24**: 466–477.

Groin Lump

You have been referred from the GP a 70 year old lady who has noticed a painless left groin lump. The GP is concerned that this may be an incarcerated femoral hernia. What are the differential diagnoses for a groin lump in this patient?

There are a number of possibilities and the history and examination may make one more likely. However, without further information the possibilities include (i) a groin hernia - either femoral or inguinal, lymphadenopathy raising the possibility of a tumour which drains to that region or (ii) lymphoma or even (iii) an aneurysm/ pseudoaneurysm.

How would you distinguish between a femoral hernia and an inguinal hernia clinically?

Classically an inguinal hernia is described as lying above and medial to the pubic tubercle, whereas a femoral hernia lies laterally and below the tubercle. However, this is not always true as a small direct inguinal hernia may lie lateral to the pubic tubercle as the internal ring lies lateral to the femoral canal (thus lying lateral and above the tubercle!)

What other examination would you carry out other than the groin?

As well as examining the contralateral side, a full abdominal examination should be performed. If the diagnosis is not clear and there is a concern that this is lymphadenopathy, neck, axillae and perineum will all require examination, and the lower limb to exclude the possibility of a malignant melanoma or squamous cell skin cancer.

What structures drain into the superficial groin lymph nodes?

These lymph nodes receive drainage from the skin and subcutaneous tissue of the abdominal wall below the level of the umbilicus, perineum, buttocks, external genitalia and lower limbs.

Clinically this appears as a lymph node rather than a groin hernia. There are no other abnormalities that you can find. How would you investigate this further?

As well as routine blood tests (especially a full blood count) a lymph node biopsy should be carried out. An initial FNA may be performed, and if this suggests the possibility of lymphoma then a formal excision/ partial excision biopsy will be required. This may be carried out under local or general anaesthetic.

What is the Ann Arbor Staging system?

This is the system used to stage both Hodgkin's and non-Hodgkin's lymphomas. It involves four stages (I-IV) dependent on degree of spread and location. It is localised to a single region; II involves two regions on the same side of the diaphragm; III both sides of the diaphragm and IV disseminated disease. The stages may also be modified with A or B indicating absence (A) or presence (B) of constitutional symptoms such as sweats, fevers or weight loss.

Gynaecomastia

A 52 year old man presents to the breast clinic with bilateral enlargement of breasts over the last few years. You suspect he has gynaecomastia.

What is gynaecomastia and what are the common causes?

Gynaecomastia is benign proliferation of glandular male breast tissue. Pseudogynaecomastia can have a similar appearance but is due to excess adipose tissue and not breast tissue. True gynaecomastia is caused by an imbalance between androgens and oestrogens, thus can result from either reduced androgen or increased oestrogen production.

- Physiological gynaecomastia is the commonest cause (~30%). This has a trimodal distribution in neonatal, puberty and old age.

- Drug induced causes (~20%) commonly arise from prostatic cancer drugs, cardiac and retroviral medication. Common drugs include spironolactone, H2 antagonists and anabolic steroids. Cannabis can also cause symptoms by inhibition of testosterone action.

- Pathological cases (~25%) can include hyperthyroidism, excess alcohol intake, liver disease, cirrhosis and renal failure. Testicular or bronchogenic malignancies that secrete βHCG can result in increased oestrogen secretion, usually resulting in more rapid progression of symptoms.

- Idiopathic (~25%).

Should all gynaecomastia be investigated?

As gynaecomastia in senescence is a common finding due to the peripheral aromatization of testosterone (>60% of men over 65) only selected cases require further investigation. Similarly pubertal gynaecomastia does not routinely require assessment and in the majority of cases can be reassured and managed in primary care. Cases requiring further investigation include:

- Unilateral symptoms.

- Suspicious mass, nipple discharge or nipple changes.

- Known Klinefelter's syndrome, as such cases can have a breast cancer risk similar to the female population.

What are the principles of assessment of gynaecomastia?

Triple assessment is required as per any breast lump to exclude a male breast cancer. Either mammogram or ultrasound scanning can be used pending local expertise. Mammogram can be both sensitive and specific though it is unusual for male breast cancer to have small/subtle lesions. Core biopsy is usually performed for any suspicious lesions as fine needle aspiration cytology is likely to be indeterminate

(C3) due to the presence of hyperplasia, which would then require a subsequent core biopsy.

If no cause is found on local assessment then a systemic cause would be considered. This can be investigated by checking renal, liver, thyroid function and imaging to assess for a bronchogenic lesion (initially chest x-ray).

What endocrine tests would you perform?

βHCG, LH, testosterone, oestrogen, prolactin and AFP levels would be checked if renal, liver and thyroid function were normal. If all of these are normal, it is unlikely a serious cause will be missed. If βHCG is also normal this excludes a βHCG secreting testicular tumour. Testicular examination is thus not always required. If any abnormalities in biochemical assessment are discovered and no malignant source is identified then such cases are best referred to an endocrinologist.

What treatment options are there?

Reassurance is often all that physiological gynaecomastia requires. In drug related causes, medication can be reviewed and amended if appropriate.

There is limited evidence on the use of medication for gynaecomastia from small non-randomized trials. Danazol is licensed in the UK for treatment with a recommended short course. Tamoxifen at a lower dose (10mg) can also be effective, particularly with florid proliferative gynaecomastia. Although regression may occur, less is known about the long term outcomes.

Surgical correction can be performed with liposuction and/or excision of residual nodular areas. Liposuction is often used in younger patients with softer gynaecomastia. This allows feathering of edges and subsequent skin contraction. For more extensive areas subcutaneous mastectomy (Webster's procedure) can be considered. These can often be difficult to correct and achieve a good cosmetic outcome, particularly if there is marked breast development and redundant skin. This is best undertaken by a specialist plastic surgeon.

What are the complications of surgery for gynaecomastia?

Poor cosmetic outcome following gynaecomastia surgery is a common reason for litigation. Patients should be warned about infection, bleeding, scarring, nipple necrosis, alteration in nipple sensation, persistent pain, unsatisfactory cosmetic outcome (saucer deformity), tethering of nipple to pectoral muscle (nipple animation) and recurrence.

Hidradenitis Suppurativa

You are reviewing a 23 year old lady who has been having recurrent axillary abscesses and has been diagnosed with hidradentitis suppurativa. She presents again with two large painful axillary nodules. What other sites are typically affected by hidradenitis suppurativa?

Other sites include groin, perineum, infra-mammary folds, perianal region and buttocks.

What risk factors are there for this condition?

Hidradenitis suppurativa is more common amongst females and those overweight. Smoking is also a risk factor, as is uncontrolled type 2 diabetes.

What is the aetiology of the disease?

This remains unknown although a number of theories exist. Arguably the most likely cause is due to follicular occlusion with involvement of the sweat glands.

What are the three classical stages of the disease?

Hurley (1989) described three clinical stages of the disease. These are:

Stage 1: Single or multiple abscesses. No evidence of sinus tracts or cicatrisation.

Stage 2: Recurrent abscesses, with tract formation and cicatrisation. These may be single lesions or multiple.

Stage 3: Multiple tracts and abscesses involving a whole area.

How would you manage this lady?

This patient needs incision and drainage of the abscesses that are present and laying open of any tracts. Cultures should be taken from the area and a culture of any pus from the abscess.

She may also benefit from antibiotics - usually metronidazole, clindamycin or tetracycline. If she has had previous cultures taken then antibiotic therapy can be tailored to this and discussed with microbiology. Long term combination treatment of clindamycin with rifampacin for 12 weeks may be used.

Lifestyle factors should be addressed as appropriate: weight loss, smoking cessation and control of blood sugar if a diabetic. Deodorants should also be avoided as they can exacerbate the condition.

If control of the condition cannot be achieved with the above interventions, input from the plastic surgeons may be needed and a wide excision with skin flap.

What other treatments are used to manage the disease?

As well as antibiotics, antiseptic wash such as chlorhexidine may be used to try and reduce colonisation.

In women flares may also be associated with menses, and anti-androgens may be used as part of the OCP. In severe cases immunosuppressants such as steroids, ciclosporin, and methotrexate may all be used. However, these may have side effects that cannot be tolerated and can result in a flare in disease when stopped. More recently, biological TNF alpha blockers have been used.

Cryotherapy and laser ablative therapy have also been tried for more severe cases, with minimal proven benefit.

Hydrocoele

You are reviewing a 24 year old man in clinic with a large left sided testicular swelling. He reports that it fluctuates in size depending on activity. Examination reveals a soft scrotal swelling with a bluish tinge and fluid shift. What is the likely diagnosis and what test can you do to help confirm this?

This is likely to be a hydrocoele, and transillumination could be carried out to demonstrate that the nature of the swelling is a fluid collection.

What is a hydrocoele?

This is an accumulation of fluid around the testis in the tunica vaginalis. They are usually congenital and present before a child reaches two years of age. Most congenital hydrocoeles will resolve spontaneously, however surgical correction may be required if they persist.

How can hydrocoeles be classified?

Broadly they can be classified as communicating and non-communicating. The former indicates the presence of a small inguinal hernia which allows fluid to pass. The history of this patient suggests a communicating hydrocoele, as he reports that it changes in size.

A non-communicating hydrocoele indicates closure of the processus which leaves a loculated collection of the cord.

What is the aetiology of hydrocoeles?

These may be congenital, but frequently in adults the cause is unclear.

There may be an association with an underlying condition such as infection, tumours and can even be associated with torsion.

This patient is concerned that the hydrocoele will affect fertility. What will you tell him?

Hydrocoeles in themselves are not associated with fertility issues. However, there may be an associated condition that may affect fertility.

Do all hydrocoeles require treatment?

No, small and non symptomatic hydrocoeles do not require any intervention. While aspiration can be performed in larger hydrocoeles fluid will reaccumulate and surgical intervention is required.

Are there any other investigations that need to be performed?

The diagnosis should be possible to make clinically. However, larger hydrocoeles may mask an underlying tumour. An ultrasound scan is advisable.

What surgical techniques are available to treat a hydrocoele?

It may be approached as either an inguinal operation or scrotal.

The inguinal approach allows high ligation of the patent processus vaginalis and is frequently carried out in infants.

A scrotal approach may be carried out and several different techniques have been described:-the Andrews procedure involves an incision at the superior part of the hydrocoele and tacking the cut edges to the cord or leaving the everted sac open.

The Jaboulay procedure involves resecting the majority of the sac leaving a small cuff by the testicle which is everted and sutured along the cord.

The Lord's procedure described in 1964 involves a small incision which allows the testicle to be delivered. The sac is opened circumferentially and the edges plicated which when tied form an accordion-plicated ring around the testis and epididymis.

Laparoscopic Cholecystectomy

You have been referred a 24 year old lady with sickle cell anaemia (SCA) who has been having problems with cholelithiasis. What are the concerns for this patient?

Patients with SCA may experience vaso-occlusive crisis (VOC) due to blockage of small vessels. This may be precipitated by infection, acidosis, dehydration cold, hypoxia and surgical trauma. Thus there is a high risk of this occurring during a general anaesthetic. These patients need to be treated carefully. Baseline haemoglobin should be checked and transfusion may be required to ensure an Hb>10g/dl.

Care needs to be taken to avoid the above precipitants of a VOC, so patients should be adequately filled, adequately warmed, hypoxia needs to be avoided and pain controlled.

What proportion of patients with SCA may develop problems due to gallstones?

Cholelithiasis is extremely common in patients with sickle cell anaemia with approximately 70 % of these patients having gallstones by the age of 30. Thus cholecystectomy is the most common elective operation required in these patients.

What affect does laparoscopic surgery have on post-operative complication rate?

This appears to lower the rate of complications and thus should be advocated if possible.

What other arrangements should be considered for this patient?

Pre-operative assessment by an anaesthetist should be carried out. It may also be worth considering a post-operative stay on HDU to ensure careful monitoring.

How do vaso-occlusive crises tend to manifest clinically?

These usually present as venous thrombosis, organ infarction and severe pain. The latter is normally present in bones and joints due to bone marrow ischaemia and sickling in bone marrow sinusoids.

What is acute chest syndrome (ACS) and how is it managed?

This is a VOC affecting pulmonary vasculature. It tends to present 2-3 days post surgery and risk correlates with drops in haemoglobin. It manifests as fever, cough or chest pain and there may be evidence of pulmonary infiltrates on the chest x-ray. It can also be triggered by pneumonia and thus broad spectrum antibiotics may be required. Good pain control must be maintained and exchange transfusion may need to be considered.

Malignant Melanoma

You are reviewing a 45 year old man who has been referred with a skin lesion by the GP. This is on his neck, is approximately 2cm in diameter and irregularly shaped. It is a heterogeneous black/ brown colour and has bled once on scratching and has changed in appearance recently according to the patient's partner. How should this be managed?

This history is highly suspicious of a malignant melanoma. A full thickness biopsy should be carried out for staging. Complete excision with a narrow margin (1mm) of normal skin should be included.

Are you aware of any scoring systems to determine if a suspicious lesion should have further investigation?

Ultimately any lesion which raises concern should be further investigated. MacKie produced a seven point checklist which suggested whether a lesion needs further evaluation. A score of 3 or more indicates a lesion does require investigation.

Major features: each scores 2 points

    1) *Change in size*

    2) *Irregular pigmentation*

    3) *An irregular shape*

    4) *Diameter 6mm or greater*

Minor features: each scores 1 point

    1) *Inflammation of the lesion*

    2) *Bleeding/ weeping*

    3) *Itchiness or change in sensation.*

What are Clark's level and Breslow's thickness?

Clark's level is a staging system used to describe the degree of melanoma invasion. However, it has been shown to have a poorer predictive value than Breslow's depth and is used in lesions of less than 1mm depth. There are five levels:

    1) Melanoma in situ = confined to the epidermis

    2) Invasion into papillary dermis

    3) Invasion to the junction of papillary and reticular dermis

    4) Invasion into the reticular dermis

    5) Invasion into subcutaneous fat

Breslow's thickness is a prognostic classification based on actual depth of invasion. It is a better guide than Clarke's level for prognosis.

	5 Year Survival
Stage 1- up to 0.75mm depth.	90%
Stage 2- 0.75 to 1.5mm depth	80%
Stage 3- 1.50 to 2.25 mm depth	65%
Stage 4- 2.25 to 4.0mm depth	50%
Stage 5- Greater than 4.0mm depth.	35%

Stage 3 lesions and above are associated with a higher incidence of nodal metastases.

The excision biopsy confirms a superficial spreading melanoma with a Breslow's thickness of 2.6mm. What further investigations should be carried out?

This patient needs to be fully staged with a head, chest, abdomen and pelvis CT. Discussion at a skin cancer MDT should also be organised on an urgent basis.

A wide local excision with a margin of at least 2cm should be carried out.

A sentinel lymph node biopsy should be carried out - this involves using isosulfan blue or technetium-99 to identify the node. If this proves negative, no further surgery is required, however a positive finding will indicate the need for regional lymph node clearance.

What is the role of adjuvant therapy if there is a finding of lymph node involvement?

There is no definitive evidence for the use of adjuvant therapy in managing malignant melanoma.

Interferon has been used in patients from low to high risk and clinical trials are still ongoing.

One meta-analysis concluded that it was associated with relapse-free survival, but a very small effect on overall survival with a five year benefit of only 3%.

The impact of adjuvant radiotherapy is also unclear. The Tasmanian Radiation Oncology group showed a 15% improvement in local control in high risk patients. However the risk-benefit of this treatment is not quantified.

Reference

MacKie RM. Clinical recognition of early invasive melanoma. BMJ. 1990;301:1005–6

Meckel's Diverticulum

You are carrying out a laparoscopy in a 21 year old male for suspected appendicitis. The appendix appears normal. There is some free fluid. How would you proceed?

The use of laparoscopy allows good visualisation of the internal viscera. With a normal looking appendix the next step would be to walk the small bowel to ensure there is not an inflamed Meckel's diverticulum.

What is a Meckel's diverticulum?

Meckel's diverticulum is a remnant of the vitellointestinal duct due to incomplete closure of the duct. It is a true diverticulum as it contains all the layers of the gastrointestinal tract.

What proportion of the population have a Meckel's diverticulum?

It is the commonest congenital anomaly of the gastrointestinal tract and is found in approximately 2% of the population – it may remain completely asymptomatic throughout life, particularly if it has a broad base and does not contain ectopic gastric mucosa.

Anatomically where is a Meckel's diverticulum usually located ?

Usually they are found on the antimesenteric border of the distal ileum approximately 2 feet (45-60 cm) proximal from the ileocaecal valve. However, its site may be more proximal.

What type of mucosa does it contain ?

A Meckel's diverticulum is a true diverticulum and contains all layers of the bowel wall. It frequently contains ectopic tissue – ectopic gastric mucosa being the commonest. It may also contain ectopic liver, pancreatic tissue, jejunal mucosa, combined gastric and pancreatic tissue as well as duodenal mucosa.

What is the "rule of two's" with respect to a Meckel's diverticulum ?

- 2% of the population have a Meckel's diverticulum.
- Male to female ratio = 2:1.
- 2 feet from the ileocaecal valve.
- 2 inches in length.
- Often contains 2 types of mucosa.

How else may a Meckel's diverticulum present?

The majority of Meckel's diverticula are asymptomatic and are only discovered during autopsy, laparotomy or barium studies. Presentation occurs usually following a complication of the condition:

- Intestinal obstruction:
  - commonest presentation
  - A fibrous band may exist between the Meckel's and umbilicus
  - Intussusception of the diverticulum into the ileum may occur if the diverticulum invaginates and then is pushed forwards by peristalsis
  - Volvulus
  - Incarceration of the diverticulum into a hernia (Littre's hernia)
  - Tumours originating in the diverticulum
- Meckel's diverticulitis:
  - the next most common presentation
  - often indistinguishable from acute appendicitis
- Gastrointestinal bleeding:
  - Usually affects children and adolescents
  - Usually from a bleeding peptic ulcer on the wall opposite the Meckel's
  - Bleeding may be massive, especially in children – usually bright red blood per rectum or anaemia secondary to chronic bleeding
- Neoplasms in a Meckel's are rare but have been reported to present with symptoms such as anaemia

What does a Meckel's scan show?

99mTc-pertechnetate is preferentially taken up by ectopic gastric mucosa in the diverticulum. Radionucleotide scans may provide evidence of a Meckel's diverticulum when uptake of ectopic gastric mucosa occurs.

How would you manage the findings in this patient?

Traditionally an open wedge resection of the diverticulum can be made. In this case a laparoscopic wedge resection should be carried out.

Would you resect an incidental finding of Meckel's diverticulum if this did not appear to be the source of the problem?

This is controversial, wide based diverticula are unlikely to cause problems in the long term, and some surgeons advocate resection in narrow based diverticula.

Neck Lumps

A 39-year-old woman presents to the ENT outpatient department with recurrent swelling of the left submandibular gland that has lasted six months. It occurs a few times a week, usually after a meal. The swelling is associated with a dull ache and usually subsides after one to two hours. On examination of the submandibular area she has no obvious swelling or skin involvement. Intra-oral palpation reveals a well-defined hard mass in the right floor of mouth region. A plain x-ray of the oral cavity is obtained (Figure 1).

Figure 1: Oral cavity x-ray demonstrating an intra-oral lesion (arrowed)

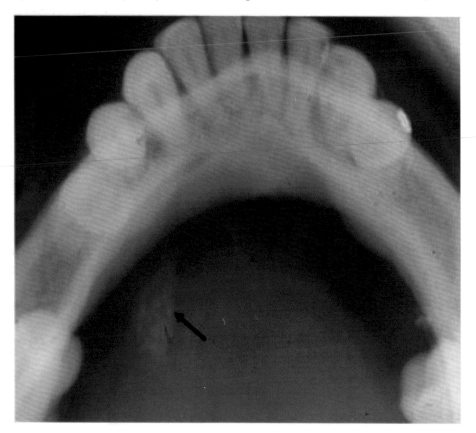

What is your differential diagnosis? What is the pathogenesis of this condition?

The history and examination suggest a submandibular duct calculus. Sialolithiasis is the formation of a stone within the salivary gland duct or parenchyma. The pathognomic feature in this scenario involves the description of localised pain after meals. Approximately 85%-90% of the cases of sialolithiasis occur in the submandibular gland because of a more viscid and alkaline saliva in comparison to the other salivary glands. Other factors that predispose to stasis in the submandibular duct (Wharton's duct) may play a role e.g. wider lumen, tighter orifice, dependent gland requiring an upward course. The parotid gland will account for about 10%-15% of sialolithiasis cases. Stones are generally not found in sublingual or minor salivary glands.

What are the anatomical features of the submandibular gland?

The submandibular glands are located deep under the mandible and superior to the digastric muscles. They weigh about 15 grams and produce around 60%–70% of the total volume of mucinous saliva (more viscid compared to parotid gland serous saliva). They are divided into superficial and deep lobes by the mylohyoid muscle. The marginal mandibular branch of the facial nerve lies superficial to the gland in the platysmal layer of the neck. The hypoglossal and lingual nerves run deep to the gland. Secretions are delivered into the submandibular duct (Wharton's duct) on the deep portion, after which they hook around the posterior edge of the mylohyoid muscle. The excretory ducts are crossed by the lingual nerve and ultimately drain into the sublingual aspect of the tongue (Figure 2).

What other investigations can be utilised to provide a diagnosis?

Plain x-ray of the affected region can be helpful in the diagnosis. The floor of mouth x-ray is simple and available in most departments. In this particular situation no further imaging may be necessary. Other investigations include ultrasound, non-contrast enhanced computed tomography and magnetic resonance imaging. Sialography is mainly reserved for the evaluation of chronic sialadenitis.

What are the management options?

The treatment for small stones is designed to preserve the passage of the stone and restoration of salivary flow. This may include sialogogues (e.g. sugar-free citric boiled sweets), increased fluid intake and massage. Non-steroidal anti-inflammatory drugs (or other simple analgesia) can be used for pain control if no contraindication exists. Intra-oral resection can be performed for isolated stones in the distal duct i.e. close to the ampulla. For proximal stones located in the proximal duct (lateral to the mylohyoid muscle), the surgeon may decide to treat the patient with resection of the gland. This is also the preferred treatment for patients with recurrent bouts of sialolithiasis.

Why are these patients predisposed to poor dental hygiene?

Submandibular gland stones may be associated with poor dentition or recurrent pharyngitis that is resistant to antibiotic therapy. Streptococcus *viridans* is a common bacterial infection associated with prolonged obstruction / stasis of saliva.

Figure 2: Surgical anatomy of the submandibular gland

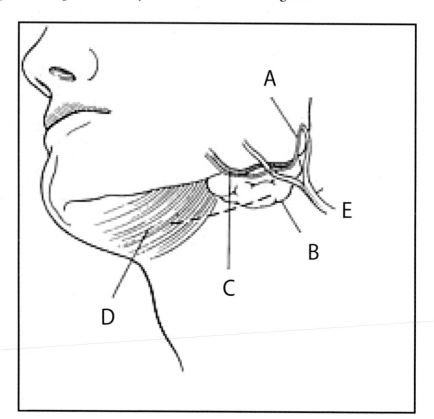

A, Marginal mandibular nerve; B, Submandibular gland; C, Facial artery;

D, Mylohyoid muscle; E, Common facial vein

What are the steps of submandibular gland excision?

- Endotracheal intubation with neck extended and head tilted away from side of lesion, shoulder bolster and head ring. Check patient is not paralysed. Draping is done in such a way that the lower lip, lower margin of the mandible, and upper neck are exposed.

- Local anaesthetic infiltration e.g. 2.2ml of 2% lidocaine with 1:80,000 adrenaline. Linear skin crease incision approximately two fingerbreadths below the angle of mandible extending from the sternocleidomastoid muscle.

- Dissect carefully through skin, subcutaneous fat and platysmal layer to expose the capsule of the submandibular gland (SMG), common facial vein and external jugular vein posteriorly.

- A subcapsular dissection with exposure of the SMG is performed. Contraction of the angle of the mouth will alert the surgeon to the proximity of the marginal mandibular nerve.

- At the superior margin of the SMG, dissect with a haemostat in the fatty tissue above the gland to ligate and divide the facial artery and vein (keeping immediately above the SMG so as to avoid injury to the marginal mandibular nerve).

- The surgeon next frees the anterior margin of the SMG from the anterior belly of digastric muscle, and proceeds in a posterior direction, elevating the SMG from the lateral surface of the mylohyoid muscle.

- By retracting the mylohyoid anteriorly and by using careful finger dissection, the lingual nerve, submandibular ganglion, and submandibular duct are exposed.

- The SMG can then be reflected inferiorly, and the facial artery is identified, ligated and divided where it exits from behind the posterior belly of digastric muscle.

- Once the hypoglossal nerve has been identified, one may safely clamp, divide and ligate the submandibular duct and the lingual nerve, taking care not to place the tie across the main nerve.

- The SMG is then finally freed from the tendon and posterior belly of the digastric and removed. The final view of the resection demonstrates the hypoglossal nerve, lingual nerve, and transected duct on the lateral aspect of the hyoglossus muscle.

- Haemostasis, drain and close in layers.

- Complications include haemorrhage; marginal mandibular / lingual / hypoglossal nerve injury and dry mouth due to reduced saliva production.

Thyroglossal cyst

A 59-year-old male noted a midline neck lump that has become more prominent recently, having had the lump for over 30 years. It has lately become inflamed on an intermittent basis with associated discharge of a yellow liquid. Examination in the clinic reveals a 1cm x 1cm mobile neck lump at the level of the hyoid bone. An ultrasound scan and FNAC suggested a cystic lesion with no malignant features on cytology. Due to the recurrent nature of the swelling and the cosmetic appearance, the patient was keen on surgical excision.

What is the embryological background of a thyroglossal cyst?

In the 4th week of life, the embryo develops a thickening at the tongue base called the foramen caecum. This will eventually form the thyroid gland, which migrates downward to the level of the fifth cervical vertebra between the first and second branchial arches. Along this tract, midline neck lumps can present as either thyroglossal cysts or residual thyroid tissue that has failed to migrate fully. The common location is at or below the level of the hyoid bone. Cysts can present either in early childhood or in the 3rd or 4th decade of life, when they could present with recurrent infection as an abscess.

What examination technique can distinguish between a thyroglossal cyst and thyroid gland swelling?

Thyroglossal duct cysts most often present with a midline neck lump, which may or may not be asymptomatic. Common symptoms include throat pain or dysphagia. A thyroglossal cyst will move with swallowing or on protrusion of the tongue due to its attachment to the tongue base via the tract of thyroid descent. This is in contrast to thyroid gland masses, which move with swallowing (deglutition) only.

What is the operation of choice to remove the cyst?

The operation of choice involves removal of the hyoid bone along with remnants of the thyroglossal tract (Sistrunk's procedure). The Sistrunk operation requires excision of the central portion of the hyoid bone to ensure complete removal of the tract. This will reduce the likelihood of recurrence and subsequent infection. At times antibiotics can be indicated if there is sign of infection. In the past thyroid uptake scans were ordered preoperatively, however, most units have now stopped this practice due to the very low incidence of thyroid tissue failing to migrate fully.

Parotid gland

A 53-year-old woman was referred to the outpatient department after noticing a right neck lump. It had gradually increased in size and was not painful. Examination of the ear, nose and throat was unremarkable and in particular the facial nerve was fully functional. Palpation of the neck confirmed a firm 2cm mass under her right ear lobule. She went on to have an ultrasound scan which confirmed 20 x 15 x 12 mm mass in the superficial right parotid extending to the tail. An FNAC showed evidence of a pleomorphic adenoma. Due to the possibility of malignant change it was recommended to remove the lump, and a pre-operative MRI neck was organised (Figure 3).

Figure 3: Cross-sectional MRI neck revealing homogenous right parotid mass

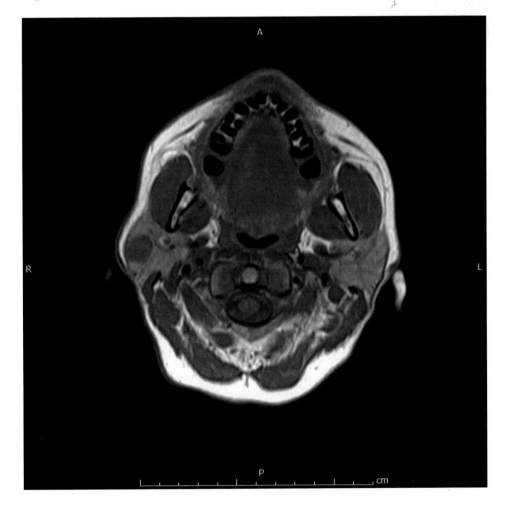

What are the important anatomical features of the parotid gland?

The gland is located at the angle of mandible and produces serous saliva. It is divided into a superficial and deep lobe by the facial nerve that has motor branches supplying the muscles of facial expression (temporal, zygomatic, buccal, marginal mandibular, cervical). The most important nerves to preserve supply the eyelid and angle of mouth. For most lesions of the parotid gland it is necessary to formally identify the facial nerve main trunk and follow the peripheral nerve fibres distal to the lesion.

What diagnostic imaging techniques can be obtained?

In small, mobile tumours of the parotid, US scan may suffice to assess the parotid mass and its location in the superficial lobe. However, clinical features which suggest a carcinoma (i.e. facial nerve weakness, other cervical lymph node enlargement, pain, tethering to deep structures) should mandate imaging ideally in the form of an MRI neck. Imaging may provide useful important information regarding the relationship between the tumour and facial nerve i.e. superficial or deep to the retromandibular vein, or invasion of local structures.

Is it advisable to obtain a pre-operative biopsy?

In most cases pre-operative diagnosis can aid patient counselling and informed consent regarding the exact procedure required (e.g. total or superficial parotidectomy, neck dissection, adjuvant therapies). Needle biopsy (FNAC) can be utilised to diagnose tumours pre-operatively with a high level of specificity and sensitivity.

What are the steps of a parotid gland excision?

- Endotracheal intubation with neck extended and head tilted away from the side of lesion, shoulder bolster and head ring. Check patient is not paralysed. Draping is done in such a way that the eye, angle of mouth and upper neck are exposed.

- The facial nerve monitor is optional in this procedure but usually recommended.

- Local anaesthetic infiltration e.g. 2.2ml of 2% lidocaine with 1:80,000 adrenaline.

- Skin crease incision (Modified Blair) extending from pre-auricular skin crease and extending posteriorly to the level of the sternocleidomastoid muscle.

- Dissect carefully through skin, subcutaneous fat and platysmal layer to raise a flap by using the natural plane on the surface of the parotid gland (SMAS layer). This incision is carried beyond the extent of the tumour to expose parotid fascia anterior to the lesion.

- A posterior flap is then raised to allow division of the anterior branch of the greater auricular nerve branches.

- The facial nerve trunk can be identified after identification of the posterior belly of digastric muscle, the styloid process, tympanomastoid suture line and the tragal pointer (a triangular extension of cartilage inferiorly off the tragus which suggests the location of the facial nerve in the direction of its inferoanterior point).

- Once the main trunk has been seen, it is followed to the pes anserinus, the structure marking the separation of the temporofacial (upper) and cervicofacial (lower) divisions.

- Smaller branches are then followed carefully with the aim of mapping their relation to the tumour.

- A common technique for nerve dissection is to use a small, fine haemostat to gently elevate the parotid tissue in the natural plane just superficial to each nerve. The tissue lateral to and between the tines of the instrument is sealed with a bipolar cautery and divided, and the process is continued.

- Once the tumour has been resected, the facial nerve can be tested with a handheld stimulator to confirm that it is unharmed.

- Haemostasis, drain and close in layers.

- Complications include infection, haematoma, facial nerve paralysis (temporary versus permanent), Frey's syndrome or salivary duct fistula.

Solitary lumps in the neck can present to any medical practitioner. The aetiology will change with the age of the patient, location of the mass, mode of presentation and associated symptoms (i.e. pain, fever, etc...). It is therefore important to conduct a comprehensive head and neck examination.

History

Note the duration of the lump, size, site of origin and duration of onset. The presence of red-flag symptoms (e.g. voice change; dysphagia; weight loss; haemoptysis; persistent sore throat;) may suggest a malignant process, while the presence of B-symptoms (e.g. night sweats / bone pains) could indicate a haematological malignancy such as lymphoma (Table 1) to follow.

In most adult patients, a history of upper respiratory tract infection suggests an infective or inflammatory aetiology, while high alcohol or smoking consumption may be associated with malignant lumps. Congenital neck masses present mainly in children and often enlarge over a longer time period, although this will not always be the case.

The patient should be screened for foreign travel and local inflammation within the head and neck region. Evidence of immunosuppression such as intravenous drug abuse, diabetes, HIV/AIDS, tuberculosis, or autoimmune diseases are important to note as these may indicate an inflammatory cause.

Examination

The neck is divided into two triangles (anterior and posterior), by the sternocleidomastoid muscle (Figure 4). Midline neck lumps may arise from the thyroid isthmus, or can represent a thyroglossal or dermoid cyst or plunging ranula. Lumps in the anterior triangle have a large differential, whereas posterior triangle lesions mainly result from localised inflammation (with the notable exception of lymphoma, nasopharyngeal carcinoma or infectious mononucleosis). Lumps in the supraclavicular region may represent a metastasis from lung, breast or abdominal cancer.

Figure 4: Common pathologies located in the neck

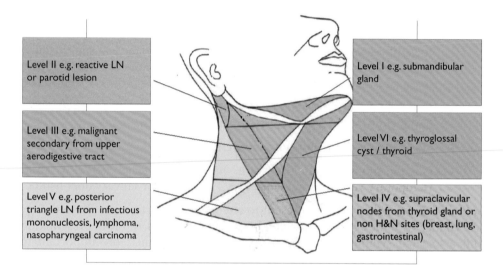

Examination should focus on finding out the site and anatomical structure from which the lump may arise i.e. skin, lymph node, parotid / submandibular / thyroid gland or other connective tissue (e.g. neurovascular). Palpation includes assessing the size, attachment to deeper structures, temperature, pain and consistency. The oral cavity, oropharynx and larynx should be part of the specialist examination trying to exclude any primary lesion if there is high suspicion of malignancy of the neck mass. Lastly, a general examination should include looking for hepatosplenomegaly, chest signs, or axillary / groin lymphadenopathy.

Investigation

Further investigation is based on the clinical impression obtained from the history and examination. Urgent referral to ENT should be considered at first consultation if any red flag symptoms are present (Table 1) e.g. >1cm size, oral cavity lesion (as above), hard / rubbery consistency.

Investigations that may be appropriate include needle biopsy (e.g. fine needle or core biopsy), blood tests (e.g. CRP, FBC, Infectious mononucleosis screen, ACE, toxoplasma), CT or MRI neck (+/- angiography if a vascular lump), ultrasound if a thyroid lump, chest x-ray (to look for pulmonary metastases or TB), panendoscopy or surgical biopsy (incisional / excisional).

Table 1: Differential diagnoses for neck lump*

Inflammatory	Infective	**Bacterial** Staphylococcus, streptococcus (tonsillitis / pharyngitis), mycobacterium tuberculosis, mycobacterium avium (Atypical TB), bartonella (cat scratch disease), brucellosis
		Viral Epstein Barr Virus (Infectious mononucleosis); HIV; rhinovirus, adenovirus, cytomegalovirus
		Fungal Histoplasmosis, coccidiomycosis, blastomycosis
		Protozoa Toxoplasmosis, leishmaniasis
	Autoimmune related	Lupus, sarcoidosis, rheumatoid arthritis, Sjogren's syndrome
Neoplastic	Malignant	• Metastatic head-neck squamous cell cancer (if patient younger age / male consider human papillomavirus aetiology) • Metastatic carcinoma from lungs, breast, upper GI (lower neck or supraclavicular region) • Lymphoma, leukaemia (especially posterior triangle) • Primary cancer from salivary gland, tail of parotid, lung apex (may be associated with Horner's syndrome) • Sarcoma • Thyroid cancer
	Benign	Pleomorphic adenoma, neurogenic (schwannoma, neurofibroma, paraganglioma), vascular (e.g. carotid body tumour, aneurysm, aberrant subclavian / brachiocephalic artery)
Congenital		Thyroglossal cyst, cystic hygroma, dermoid cyst, branchial cyst, vascular lesions (haemangioma, lymphangioma)
Miscellaneous		Sebaceous cyst, lipoma, laryngocoele, prominent cervical rib (thin neck), sialectasia / sialolithiasis

***Red flag symptoms (local)** = dysphagia / odynophagia; voice change; persistent sore throat; unilateral nasal obstruction / epistaxis / otalgia / glue ear.

Red flag symptoms (systemic) = Unintentional weight loss; malaise / loss of appetite; haemoptysis; shortness of breath; abdominal pain; bruising or bleeding; generalised itch.

B-symptoms (Fever / Night sweats / Bone pains).

Paediatric Inguinal Hernia and Hydrocoele

You are called to the accident and emergency department to review a 7 week old male infant with sudden onset of unilateral scrotal swelling. The parents noticed the swelling for the first time today and the baby remains well. On examination, his abdomen is soft. You note an irreducible, non-tender right inguino-scrotal swelling, the upper margin of which you can get above (Figure 1). What is the most likely diagnosis?

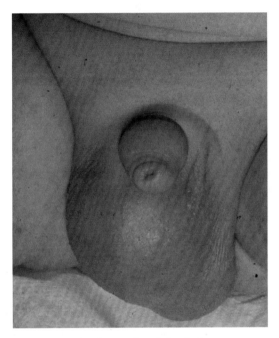

This infant is likely to have a hydrocoele of the left testis, given that you can get above the swelling. Transillumination is not reliable in differentiating between hydrocoeles and inguinal hernias as the bowel can transilluminate just as brightly as fluid in young infants.

What other conditions present with scrotal swelling in this age group?

Possible differential diagnoses in this scenario include inguinal hernia, testicular torsion, epididymitis or epididymo-orchitis, trauma and testicular tumours.

What is the pathophysiology of hydrocoele in children?

Paediatric hydrocoele is due to incomplete obliteration of the processus vaginalis, allowing peritoneal fluid to accumulate around the cord structures or testis. The processus vaginalis remains patent throughout life in approximately 20% of normal adults. The processus vaginalis is a peritoneal diverticulum that extends through the internal ring at approximately 3 months gestation. As the testis migrates downwards from the posterior abdominal wall towards the scrotum between 7 and 9 months gestation, it pulls with it an extension of this lower abdominal peritoneal surface. After completion of testicular descent, the portion of the processus vaginalis surrounding the testis becomes the tunica vaginalis.

The derivation of the processus vaginalis in females is less clear. Cord hydrocoele may occur with complete sealing of the processus vaginalis proximally and distally, leaving a patent, fluid-containing midportion. This may present as a groin mass and be confused with an incarcerated inguinal hernia. In females, the equivalent is known as a hydrocele of the canal of Nuck. A communicating hydrocoele is similar to a fluid containing inguinal hernia, in that the fluid is in continuity with the peritoneal cavity via a narrow but patent processus vaginalis (PPV) and can potentially be reduced, or reduce spontaneously when recumbent. Hydrocoeles secondary to testicular or epididymal pathology are much less common in children.

How is a hydrocoele treated in children?

Hydrocoeles are common in the first months of life, with the majority resolving spontaneously by one year of age. Surgery is generally only required if the hydrocoele persists beyond the age of 2 years, or is very large and compressing the testis or cord structures. The PPV is transfixed and divided at the level of the internal inguinal ring. The fluid should be expressed from the distal sac but the whole sac need not be removed. Using diathermy to divide the sac aids haemostasis and reduces the risk of post-operative scrotal haematoma.

You have been asked to review a 1 week old female neonate in the Neonatal Unit with a right-sided inguinal swelling that has been coming and going since birth. She was born at 34 weeks gestation. The child became unwell and the swelling has increased in size. It is no longer reducing spontaneously. How are you going to assess this patient further?

The patient must be reviewed urgently as the history is suggestive of an incarcerated inguinal hernia. A general assessment of the neonate must be made, including abdominal and inguinal examination. The swelling must be assessed for site, size, contents and reducibility. The patient must be resuscitated and given adequate analgesia.

The swelling is not easily reducible. What is your working diagnosis and management plan?

This presentation is consistent with an incarcerated inguinal hernia. In a female infant, the hernia sac may contain omentum, small bowel, fallopian tube, ovary or rarely, the uterus or appendix. In girls with bilateral inguinal hernias, consideration must be given to the possibility of bilateral inguinal testes in association with a disorder of sexual differentiation.

Non-operative reduction of an inguinal hernia is the treatment of choice in a stable patient. There is a very low likelihood of reducing strangulated bowel in young children and the complication rates are much higher with emergency operations for irreducible hernias. Initially, the infant should be placed in the Trendelenburg position to provide mild traction on the hernia contents and relieve oedema. Adequate sedation should be given to relax the abdominal musculature. If the hernia does not reduce, an attempt at manual reduction is performed by applying constant gentle pressure on the fundus of the hernia sac (in the direction of the cord). The vast majority of incarcerated hernias can be reduced using these conservative techniques. An elective herniotomy can then be planned in 24-48 hours once oedema and swelling of the sac and investing tissue have subsided.

Failure to reduce the hernia in this setting is a neonatal surgical emergency. The friable sac is difficult to handle and the child will require specialist perioperative care. Urgent transfer to the nearest tertiary referral paediatric surgical centre should be arranged.

How would your management plan differ if the hernia had remained easily reducible?

Surgery is necessary in all cases of paediatric inguinal hernia because of the danger of strangulation, which is highest in the first 6 months of life, when the risk of incarceration exceeds 60%. Up to 30% of infants with an inguinal hernia initially present with a strangulated hernia. In premature infants, inguinal hernias should be repaired prior to discharge from the neonatal unit. In term infants, elective herniotomy should be scheduled on the next available elective list, within 1 month of making the diagnosis. If the patient is being discharged home in the meantime, it is crucial to inform the parents to seek medical attention if the child becomes unwell or the swelling becomes persistent at any time.

What are the complications of inguinal hernia repair in children?

The overall complication rate after elective herniotomy is approximately 2%, increasing to 8%-33% in the case of emergency repair of incarcerated hernias. Complications include bleeding and haematoma formation, infection (<1%), injury to cord structures (<2%), recurrence (0.5-1%), increasing up to 8% for herniotomy performed in the neonatal period and iatrogenic cryptorchidism (1%). Intestinal resection is necessary in 3%-7% of patients, in whom the hernia is not reduced, leading to potential added morbidity.

What is the epidemiology of paediatric inguinal hernia?

The incidence of indirect inguinal hernia in full term neonates is between 1%-5%. Incidence in preterm infants is much higher at 9%-11%. The incidence approaches 60% in babies with a birth weight between 500g – 750g. There is a male preponderance with a ratio of males to females of 5-10:1. Of all inguinal hernias, 60% occur on the right side, 25%-30% on the left and 10%-15% are bilateral.

Bilateral hernias are more common in premature patients, occurring in 44%-55%. The risk of metachronous contralateral hernia is 7%-31%.

Should contralateral inguinal exploration be performed in children with unilateral inguinal hernia?

This has long been a subject of debate. In studies where contralateral exploration was performed at the time of herniotomy, infants 2 months or younger had a 63% rate of contralateral PPV, decreasing to 40% of children over the age of 2. Given the rate of metachronous contralateral hernia of 7%-31%, one can surmise that a contralateral PPV will only become clinically significant in 25%-50% of cases. Considering the increased risk of complications with bilateral repair, it is likely not routinely indicated. However, it may be considered in premature infants with a higher likelihood of contralateral hernia, or in children with significant co-morbidities in whom anaesthetic risk is increased.

References

Lau, ST, Lee, YH, Caty, MG. Current management of hernias and hydroceles. *Semin Pediatr Surg.* 2007 16(1):50-7.

Hutson, JM, O'Brien, M, Woodward, AA and Beasley SW. (Eds.) (2008) *Jones Clinical Paediatric Surgery*, 6th Edition. Australia: Blackwell Publishing.

Paediatric Intussusception

A 6 month old boy is brought to the A & E department with a 48 hour history of being unwell. He appears to have intermittent, colicky abdominal pain for periods lasting a few minutes, associated with screaming and drawing his knees up. He has been vomiting, and is pale, clammy and lethargic between episodes. On examination, you feel an abdominal mass in the right hypochondrium. In the emergency department he passes a bloody stool mixed with mucous. What is the likely diagnosis?

This boy likely has intussusception, which is the invagination of a proximal segment of bowel (the "intussusceptum") into the distal contiguous intestine (the "intussuscipiens"). 80%-90% of intussusception occurs in children between 3 months and 3 years of age, with a peak incidence between 5-7 months. Pain is the presenting symptom in 85% of patients, typically consisting of colicky pain lasting for 2-3 minutes at intervals of 15-20 minutes. After 12 hours the pain tends to be more continuous. Vomiting almost always occurs, a couple of times in the first few hours, then again once intestinal obstruction is established. Infants tend to become intermittently pale and clammy, and progressively more exhausted and lethargic between spasms. Normal or loose stools are often passed at or soon after the onset of symptoms. The "red currant jelly" stools seen in about half of patients are formed by the diapedesis of red cells through the congested mucosa of the intussusceptum. Intussusception results in intestinal oedema, lymphatic obstruction, local venous hypertension, vascular stasis and subsequent mucosal sloughing. The combination of intraluminal fluid, blood and mucosal tissue fragments results in the typical red currant jelly appearance. The classical triad of abdominal pain, vomiting and bloody stools is present in less than half of patients. 5% of patients are in hypovolaemic shock at presentation. The majority of patients have ileocolic (85%) or ileoileocolic (10%) intussusception. Ileoileal or colocolic intussusceptions are rare and associated more often with a pathological lead point. In 90% of such cases, intussusception is fixed and does not reduce spontaneously.

Outline your initial management and investigation of this boy.

Once I have made my initial diagnosis and assessed the patient's general condition and degree of dehydration, I would establish dependable intravenous access, commence rehydration with a fluid bolus, replace deficits, maintenance fluids and ongoing losses and insert a nasogastric tube for intestinal decompression. Abdominal examination is relatively non-specific, but may reveal a sausage-shaped abdominal mass anywhere between the line of the colon and umbilicus, abdominal tenderness or distension. Digital rectal examination may reveal blood, or the apex of the intussusceptum may be palpable within the rectum. I would contact the radiologist to arrange an abdominal ultrasound and prepare for pneumatic or hydrostatic pressure reduction if an intussusception is confirmed. Plain abdominal x-rays have a low accuracy for diagnosing intussusception and may be normal or show non-specific abnormalities such as partial or complete small bowel obstruction. The apex of the intussusceptum may rarely be seen as a radio-opacity. Free intraperitoneal air is indicative of a perforation.

Ultrasound imaging is the method of choice, with an accuracy approaching 100% in the diagnosis of intussusception. The typical findings are the "target", "doughnut" or "pseudo-kidney" signs (Figure 1). Ultrasound is non-invasive and does not expose the patient to ionising radiation, may detect pathological lead points (Figure 2) and is useful for identifying differential diagnoses. Ultrasound may also be used to monitor pneumatic reduction attempts.

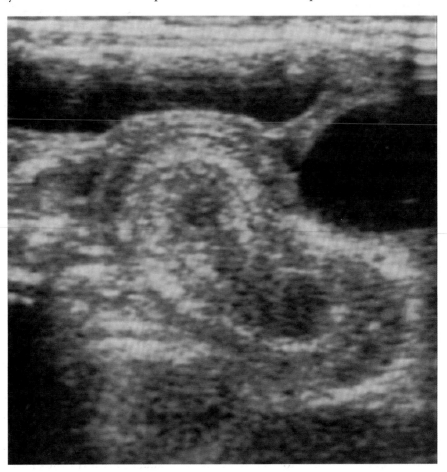

Figure 1: Ultrasound scan showing the doughnut appearance (target lesion) of an intussusception

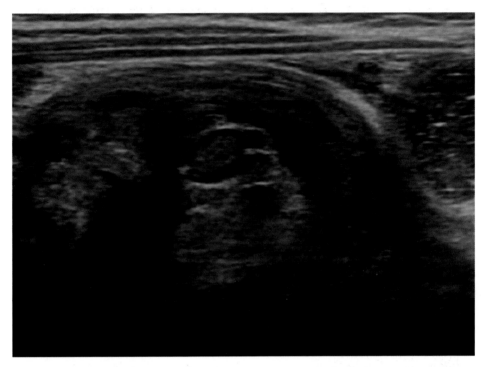

Figure 2: Intussusception with lead point on ultrasound scan.

What are the definitive treatment options?

Non-operative reduction is the treatment of choice for uncomplicated intussusception in a haemodynamically stable patient. This may be performed by pneumatic or hydrostatic pressure enemas with fluoroscopy or ultrasound monitoring. Pneumatic reduction with ultrasound monitoring is now widely accepted and increasingly used, with success rates of 85%-90%. Pneumatic reduction results in less contamination of the peritoneal cavity compared to hydrostatic reduction if a perforation occurs, but there is a risk of creating a tension pneumoperitoneum in this event. Perforation is a complication of enema reduction in approximately 0.8% of cases. Hydrostatic reduction by contrast enema reduction is also a safe and effective method. Complete reduction is confirmed when air or contrast is seen to flow freely into proximal bowel with reflux into the terminal ileum.

If a first attempt at non-operative reduction is unsuccessful, but the patient remains haemodynamically stable and at least partial reduction was achieved, it is acceptable to perform a delayed repeat enema 30 minutes to 2 hours later. Enema reduction is less successful when symptoms are present for greater than 24 hours, in children younger than 3 months or older than 2 years of age, or when there is established small bowel obstruction. Providing there is no evidence of peritonitis, enema reduction should still be attempted in these children.

Indications for operative reduction include irreducibility by enema, peritonism, perforation, haemodynamic instability and strong evidence of a pathological lead point. Laparoscopic reduction is often successful and probably associated with a shorter time to full feeds and hospital stay, but has a high rate of conversion. Laparotomy is performed via a transverse right supra-umbilical incision and gentle manipulation is used to push the intussusceptum out of the intussuscipiens, rather than by pulling with traction. If attempts at reduction cause undue injury to bowel wall, if bowel necrosis or perforation is present or if a pathological lead point is identified or suspected, then segmental resection and primary anastomosis is indicated.

Is the problem likely to recur after successful treatment?

Successful reduction does not always prevent subsequent recurrences, which are seen in 5%-11% of children. Recurrence is more likely after enema reduction than after surgery, but operative reduction still maintains a 1%-4% risk of recurrence, even if resection is performed. Recurrence usually occurs within 2-3 days of the initial reduction. Some children experience multiple recurrences, and any recurrence should raise suspicion of a pathological lead point.

What is the aetiology of intussusception?

90% of cases are idiopathic, or associated with a viral infection. Idiopathic intussusception usually occurs in the first 2 years of life and may be due to enlarged submucosal lymphoid tissue in the distal ileum (Peyer's patches) that undergoes reactive hyperplasia and becomes an apex or lead-point for the intussusception. This apex is propelled forward by peristalsis, causing telescoping of proximal bowel into distal bowel and subsequent intestinal obstruction. Pathological lead points are more commonly, although not exclusively, seen in older children. These refer to an intraperitoneal abnormality that tethers or obstructs the bowel, initiating the process of intussusception. Potential causes include Meckel's diverticulum, intestinal duplication cysts, haemangiomata, adhesions, cystic fibrosis, worm infection, intramural haematoma, malignancies such as lymphoma, intestinal polyps, Henoch-Schonlein Purpura, indwelling enteral feeding tubes and ventriculoperitoneal shunts.

Paediatric Umbilical Hernia

A well 3 year old infant is referred to your clinic for an opinion on a persistent umbilical swelling (Figure 1). The umbilical cord detached normally 5 days after birth and the infant's mother noticed an intermittent swelling at the umbilicus a few weeks later. It is covered with skin and becomes quite pronounced when the child cries, leading to a lot of parental concern. On examination, the lump is easily reducible and gurgles on compression, but does not seem to cause any discomfort. A 1cm defect is palpable in the linea alba deep to the umbilicus. The parents want this lump removed. What is the likely diagnosis in this case?

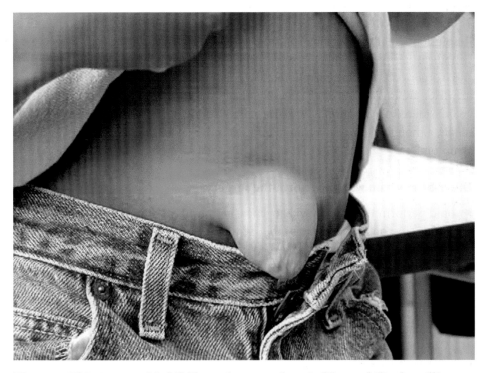

Figure 1: This 3-year-old child has a large proboscis-like umbilical swelling

This child has an umbilical hernia, which is one of the commonest paediatric surgical disorders, seen in 20% of the general population. Patients of African descent have a 10-fold increased incidence of umbilical hernia and they are seen in 75% of very low birth weight infants. Umbilical hernias are also common in children with conditions associated with increased abdominal pressure such as trisomy 21, trisomy 13, congenital hypothyroidism, ascites and mucopolysaccharidoses.

How does the umbilicus form?

The umbilicus is the region of closure of the anterior abdominal wall in the developing embryo around the structure formed by fusion of the vitelline duct (the attenuated connection between the extra coelomic yolk-sac and midgut) with the body stalk containing the umbilical vessels and allantois (the developing bladder). Closure of the body wall at this point is usually complete by birth. Delayed contraction of this fibromuscular ring can allow the peritoneum and abdominal contents to bulge through the defect, resulting in an umbilical hernia.

When should umbilical hernia repair be performed?

The majority of umbilical hernias close spontaneously without intervention. Resolution usually occurs by 12 months of age, but can take up to three years. Umbilical hernias which persist beyond 3 years of age are unlikely to resolve, and surgery should be considered. Hernias with a defect greater than 1.5cm diameter are unlikely to close spontaneously at any stage. Very large hernias may be considered for closure at an earlier age to allow an easier and more cosmetic repair, although the risk of strangulation is minimal and the hernias are felt to be symptomless.

Describe how you would perform the surgery.

I would perform the surgery via an infra-umbilical incision. I would identify the sac, reduce its contents and excise the sac to the level of strong fascia. I would close the defect transversely with absorbable suture and maintain normal umbilical inversion in my skin closure.

What alternative diagnoses might you consider if there was discharge from the umbilicus?

The nature of the discharge must be ascertained. A bloody or mucous discharge may be due to an umbilical granuloma, or ectopic bowel mucosa. Both may be treated by silver nitrate cautery, although surgical excision of ectopic mucosa may very rarely be required. A small opening on the surface of ectopic bowel mucosa may make you suspicious of a persistent vitellointestinal duct. Persistent vitellointestinal duct may also present with bilious, faeculent or persistent purulent discharge. Drainage of urine from the umbilicus is due to a patent urachus. The suspicion of either of these conditions warrants referral to a paediatric surgeon for further evaluation and investigation with contrast studies and an ultrasound scan of the umbilical region. Operative intervention to remove these remnants will be required if identified.

Patients on Anticoagulants

For patients on warfarin what threshold would you tolerate for proceeding with a surgical procedure?

In patients undergoing elective surgery this would be dependent on the procedure. For minor procedures e.g small skin lesions, an INR <2 would be permissible, for major surgical procedures INR should be lowered to an INR < 1.5. The need for continuing anticoagulation depends on their risk of thromboembolism.

What conditions would indicate a patient is high risk for thromboembolism?

- Older mechanical valve model (single-disk or ball-in-cage) in mitral position
- Recently placed mechanical valve (< 3 months)
- Atrial fibrillation plus mechanical heart valve in any position
- Atrial fibrillation with history of cardioembolism
- Recurrent (two or more) arterial or idiopathic venous thromboembolic events
- Venous or arterial thromboembolism within the preceding 1–3 months
- Known hypercoagulable state, such as ......
  - Protein C deficiency
  - Protein S deficiency
  - Antithrombin III deficiency
  - Homozygous factor V Leiden mutation
  - Antiphospholipid-antibody syndrome (primary antiphospholipid and secondary)

Intermediate risk for thromboembolism: bridging anticoagulation therapy may be required in the following scenarios

- Newer mechanical valve model (eg, St. Jude) in mitral position
- Older mechanical valve model in aortic position
- Cerebrovascular disease with multiple (two or more) strokes or transient ischemic attacks without risk factors for cardiac embolism
- Atrial fibrillation without a history of cardiac embolism but with multiple risks for cardiac embolism (eg, ejection fraction < 40%, diabetes, hypertension, nonrheumatic valvular heart disease, transmural myocardial infarction within preceding month)
- Venous thromboembolism > 3–6 months ago

Low risk for thromboembolism: bridging anticoagulation therapy not advised

- Atrial fibrillation without multiple risks for cardiac embolism
- One remote venous thromboembolism (> 6 months ago)
- Intrinsic cerebrovascular disease (such as carotid atherosclerosis) without recurrent strokes or transient ischemic attacks
- Newer-model prosthetic valve in aortic position

How may bridging anti-coagulation therapy be given?

This may be done by heparin or using low molecular weight heparin. Use of warfarin should be discontinued 4-5 days prior to surgery. Once the INR is less than 2.5 heparin should be commenced in high risk patients (and less than 2 in intermediate risk patients). The APTT should be checked and rate of infusion of heparin adjusted according to protocol.

When should the heparin be stopped, and when should it be restarted?

Heparin should be continued until six hours before surgery and resumed 6–12 hours after surgery, when surgically feasible. Oral anticoagulation can be resumed 1–2 days after surgery and once the INR is > 2, heparin can be discontinued.

How would you use LMWH to bridge stopping wafarin?

Again warfarin should be stopped 4-5 days before surgery. A therapeutic dose of LMWH should be commenced using the same parameter as for heparin. It should be continued until 24 hours before the procedure, and restarted 12-24 hours after the procedure when haemostasis is established. Warfarin may be recommenced on either the evening after the procedure or the following day.

You are reviewing a patient who needs an emergency laparotomy and is on warfarin for a mechanical heart valve. His INR is 3.5 on admission. How can this be corrected?

Immediate reversal can be achieved by FFP transfusion. However for semi-urgent procedure (that can wait >12hrs) IV Vitamin K can be tried in the first instance.

Fresh-frozen plasma (FFP) if given at the dose of 15 mls/kg body weight can reverse anticoagulation immediately without causing any resistance to warfarin. However, it is associated with the risks of transfusion, and its effects are short-lived.

After transfusion ensure that INR < 1.5 before starting surgery. If necessary more FFP will be required.

Vitamin K: smaller doses of IV vitamin K (1.25 – 2.5 mg) should be used to avoid postoperative resistance to warfarin. One study found that the median time to reversal of anticoagulation after a 1-mg IV vitamin K was approximately 27 hours. (range 0.7–147 hours).

What is Beriplex®? Beriplex® is a prothrombin concentrate complex (PCC), able to provide a more rapid and complete reversal of warfarin than FFP.

How is Beriplex® administered? Most hospitals have their own protocol for the use of beriplex® which involves consultation with a haematologist. It is usually given at 30 units/ kg, and vitamin K is usually given at the same time. The INR should be checked 10-15 minutes after administration to check reversal, and if this has not worked then further discussion with a haematologist is recommended.

Pyloric Stenosis

You are asked to review a 4 week old boy who was well until 3 days ago, when he began vomiting all feeds. His mother describes projectile, non-bilious vomits. The boy is otherwise well, and is always hungry despite the vomiting. Mum is concerned that he is losing weight and has much fewer wet nappies than normal. What diagnosis do you suspect and how will you confirm it?

I suspect that this boy has hypertrophic pyloric stenosis (HPS). It is possible to diagnose HPS based on clinical features in 80%-90% of cases. The usual presentation is with severe, projectile, non-bilious vomiting, between 3 and 6 weeks of age in an otherwise well baby. The vomitus contains milk, with some gastric mucous, and is practically never bile-stained. In approximately 18% of babies there may be some coffee-ground flecks of altered blood; this is due to oesophagitis or irritative gastritis secondary to gastric outlet obstruction. A key feature is the child's readiness and ability to feed again immediately after vomiting. Dehydration and weight loss become apparent early in the course of the disease due to inadequate fluid and caloric intake. Jaundice occurs in 2% of babies due to a decrease in glucuronyl transferase activity which occurs in starvation.

The important examination features of HPS are the observation of visible gastric peristalsis and a palpable pyloric tumour. Peristaltic waves of gastric contraction indicate hypertrophy of gastric muscle secondary to slowly progressive obstruction, and whilst non-specific, their observation makes HPS likely. Palpation of the pyloric "tumour", or "olive", is diagnostic of HPS, with a 99% positive predictive value. This is best performed when the baby is relaxed and not crying, with an empty stomach. A nasogastric tube can be passed to facilitate this if initial palpation is inconclusive. Palpation is best performed with the hips flexed, in the angle between the liver and the lateral border of the right rectus, or in the gap between the recti, midway between the umbilicus and the xiphisternum. It may help to allow the infant to feed or suck a dummy. Palpation should be performed at the start of a test feed and repeated a few hours later if initially unsuccessful.

There is a trend towards increased reliance on imaging to diagnose HPS. Ultrasonography is the investigation of choice in pyloric stenosis with sensitivity of 99.5% and specificity of 100%. A transverse thickness of greater than 3mm of a single wall of the pylorus, or a pyloric length greater than 15mm is felt to be abnormal (Figure 1). Another important real-time observation on ultrasound is the failure of relaxation of the pyloric canal. Upper gastrointestinal contrast meal has 95% sensitivity for the diagnosis of HPS and usually confirms the diagnosis in patients in whom clinical and ultrasound examination is not definitive (Figure 2). It may also reveal other pathologies such as gastro-oesophageal reflux or intestinal malrotation. The characteristic radiological feature of HPS is the "string" sign, caused by compressed, invaginated folds of mucosa within the pyloric canal. Contrast studies however give only indirect information about the pyloric canal, and pylorospasm can give similar radiological findings. The emptying speed of contrast to the distal bowel is important in distinguishing between these conditions.

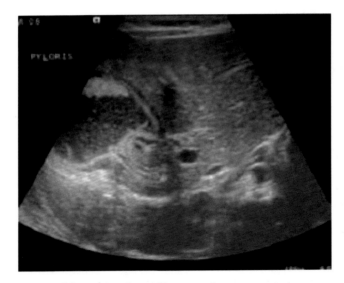

Figure 1: Ultrasound features of pyrolic stenosis

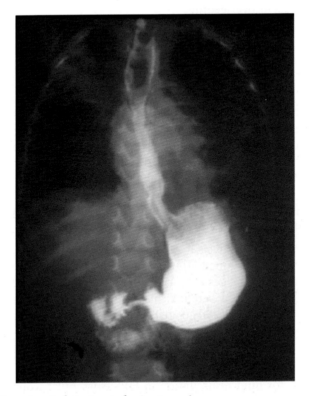

Figure 2: UGI contrast showing pyloric stenosis

Tell me about the epidemiology and aetiology of HPS.

HPS is the most common surgical condition producing emesis in infancy, with an incidence of 2-4 per 1,000 in Western populations. Boys are affected 4 times more commonly than girls, and there is some recent evidence that the incidence is increasing in parts of Britain, with a drastic increase in incidence in males but not in females, so that the sex-specific rates are 6.2 and 0.9 per 1,000 infants per year respectively. HPS seems to be more common in bottle-fed babies, in rural populations and in the summer months, for unknown reasons. The aetiology of HPS is still unknown, but may be partly genetic, with over 20% of babies affected having a positive family history. It is almost unknown in stillbirths, associated anomalies are uncommon, and HPS is exceptionally rare in infants younger than 10 days, which leads to the suggestion that it is an acquired condition. Various environmental, mechanical, genetic, hormonal, neural and physiological factors have been shown to play a role in the pathogenesis of HPS.

What other causes of vomiting might present at 1 month of age?

Other potential causes of vomiting in this baby could be grouped into infectious causes; such as meningitis, urinary tract infection or septicaemia, mechanical causes; such as gastro-oesophageal reflux, strangulated inguinal hernia, or malrotation with volvulus, or other causes; such as metabolic disorders, congenital adrenal hyperplasia or overfeeding.

What are the typical signs of dehydration in an infant?

Dehydration severity is estimated from the history and findings on clinical examination. Infants with mild dehydration (1%-5% of total body fluid volume) typically have a history of less than a day of diarrhoea and vomiting with minimal examination findings. Moderate dehydration (6%-10%) is identified by a history of abnormal fluid loss, with the findings of loss of skin turgor, weight loss, sunken eyes and fontanel, slight lethargy and dry mucous membranes. In severe dehydration (11%-15%), infants develop skin mottling, cardiovascular instability, and neurologic involvement such as irritability and coma.

What is the typical electrolyte and acid base balance seen in pyloric stenosis and explain the physiology behind its development?

Infants with HPS typically have a hypokalaemic, hypochloraemic, hyponatraemic metabolic alkalosis. This is due to the loss of fluid and large volumes of hydrogen and chloride ions from the gastric secretions in the vomitus. Infants with severe dehydration often develop a paradoxical aciduria, as the renal mechanisms for resorption of hydrogen are lost in an attempt to retain potassium and sodium ions, further compounding the metabolic alkalosis.

Describe how you would fluid resuscitate this child.

Several protocols for fluid resuscitation in HPS exist, but I would use a solution containing 0.45% saline and 5% dextrose at 1.5 times normal maintenance rate.

Infants with severe dehydration should initially receive boluses with isotonic saline solution. When urine output has been demonstrated, 10mmol potassium per 500ml of resuscitation fluid can be added. Further measurements of serum electrolytes and acid-base parameters must be undertaken to ensure complete correction of the electrolyte disturbances before surgery is undertaken. Serum bicarbonate of less than 28mEq/L and serum chloride greater than 100mEq/L is required for safe anaesthesia.

Describe the surgical treatment and post-operative management of a child with pyloric stenosis.

Ramstedt's pyloromyotomy is the operation of choice for HPS and can be performed by a supraumbilical or right transverse incision, or laparoscopically. After delivery of the pylorus through the incision, or with the duodenum grasped just distal to the pylorus in laparoscopy, an incision is made on the anterosuperior part of the pylorus, beginning at the pyloroduodenal junction, 2mm proximal to pyloric vein and extending onto the gastric antrum. The pyloric muscle is then split widely down to the mucosa and spread apart until the mucosa is bulging. Mucosal integrity is confirmed by insufflating air down the nasogastric tube and witnessing its passage onto the duodenum without bubbling out through a mucosal defect. If a mucosal defect is identified, it can be repaired with a few interrupted sutures, with or without the addition of an omental patch. Alternatively, the myotomy can be closed, the pylorus rotated 180 degrees and a second myotomy performed on the posterior surface of the pylorus.

The supraumbilical approach provides better cosmesis compared to the right transverse approach, but it can be difficult to deliver the pyloric tumour through a small incision, increasing the risk of serosal trauma to the stomach or duodenum.

Some studies have observed an increased rate of infection with the supraumbilical approach. Laparoscopy does provide improved cosmesis, but may have a slightly increased risk of mucosal perforation and incomplete pyloromyotomy. Some studies have shown a shorter time to full feeds and hospital stay, as well as less post-operative emesis and analgesic requirements with the laparoscopic approach.

Surgeons differ in their approach to the recommencement of feeding post pyloromyotomy. Some advocate a 24 hour period of fasting with nasogastric drainage, followed by slow re-introduction of feeds over 3 to 4 days, in the hope of minimising post-operative emesis. It has recently been shown however that there is no increased morbidity and a shorter hospital stay with early reintroduction of feeds on demand post-operatively. The exact regimen used is a matter of surgeon preference.

References

Van Heurn, LWE, Pakarinen, MP, Wester, T. Contemporary management of abdominal surgical emergencies in infants and children. *BJS*. 2014; 101: e24-e33.

Aspelund, G, Langer, JC. Current management of hypertrophic pyloric stenosis. *Semin Pediatr Surg.* 2007 16: 27-33

Splenectomy

You are referred a patient by the haematologists for consideration of splenectomy. What are the indications for elective splenectomy?

Most elective splenectomies are for haematological problems. The most common of these is idiopathic thrombocytopenic purpura (ITP). Other conditions include hereditary spherocytosis (IgG variety, which should be delayed until the patient is older than 6 years), autoimmune haemolytic anaemia, and in staging of haematological malignancies such as Hodgkin's disease, although this is rarely required.

It may also be required as part of a radical gastrectomy or distal pancreatectomy

Rarer causes include splenic tumours, which are usually haemangiomas, splenic abscesses and the treatment of splenic artery aneurysms.

Why is splenectomy effective for ITP?

Splenic B cells are the site of antiplatelet antibody production and subsequent antibody sensitized destruction occurs in the spleen.

How is a diagnosis of ITP made?

It is a diagnosis of exclusion once other causes of thrombocytopenia have been excluded and a normal bone marrow is present. The spleen size tends to be normal **to small** in these patients. A palpable spleen should draw doubt on whether the diagnosis is a correct one.

What is the response rate following splenectomy for ITP?

Approximately 85% of patients respond to splenectomy and maintain a normal platelet count.

What are the haematological changes that can be screened for indicating asplenia?

Blood film may show an absence of nuclear inclusions such as Howell-Jolly bodies, target cells, acanthocytes, siderotic granules and Pappenheimer bodies.

Treatment failure is usually due to splenic remnants or splenosis. This may be detected by a special nuclear scan known as a liver-spleen scan or CT / MRI.

How do you prepare a patient for an elective splenectomy?

Much of this will depend on the indication for splenectomy. For example ITP patients may be on steroids and therefore this will need to be taken into account.

Patients with myelofibrosis may have a massive splenomegaly and associated cardiac dysfunction, pulmonary hypertension which may need to be optimised.

Patients with thalassemia may have lowered white cell counts and a higher risk of infection therefore may require antibiotics.

One would have to work closely with anaesthetic colleagues to ensure a safe pre-operative preparation and anticipate and plan for any post-operative problems.

What are the complications of splenectomy ?

General complications that apply to an operation e.g. infection, DVT, PE, anaesthetic complications

Immediate

- Haemorrhage

Early

- Left basal pneumonia
- Gastric stasis
- Acute gastric dilatation
- Thrombocytosis
- Pancreatic leak from damage to tail
- Pancreatic fistula
- Gastric necrosis
- Pancreatic pseudocyst
- SMV thrombosis
- Abscess

Late

- OPSI is uncommon but is important as it has a mortality of 80%.
- Splenosis
- A-V fistula (if splenic artery and vein are clamped together)

After carrying out a laparoscopic splenectomy you find there is a high output from the drain left. What tests might you do to identify the nature of the fluid and what would this suggest?

The fluid should be sent for an amylase test. Gross elevation >10,000 would indicate a pancreatic injury.

What are the treatment measures for this?

Pancreatic injury is usually due to damage to the pancreatic duct at the tail. Treatment is usually supportive in the first instance with octreotide, and NJ feeding and it usually resolves.

What haematological changes may be observed in the post operative period?

Rise in WCC – common and may reach above $>50 \times 10^9/l$ This may be confused with sepsis

Thrombocytosis – may require antiplatelet agents if $>1,000$

What are the indications/contraindications to laparoscopic splenectomy ?

Indications are the same as for an open splenectomy

Portal hypertension and liver cirrhosis are major contraindications

Severe cardiopulmonary disease

Splenomegaly is a relative contraindication for laparascopic splenectomy, with a spleen size of $> 1,000$g representing an approximate guide.

How is laparoscopic splenectomy performed ?

This is performed under general anaesthesia with the patient in a right lateral position. A 30° laparoscope is usually used and ultrasonic dissector. The vessels are taken with a vascular stapler. The spleen once mobilized is placed in a bag and "morcellated" to allow retrieval through one of the ports (which may require extending).

What are the specific complications of laparoscopic splenectomy ?

1) Concern exists that laparoscopy may result in missing accessory splenic tissue due to a less thorough abdominal exploration.

2) There is some evidence that pancreatic injury is more common in laparoscopic splenectomy.

Where can accessory splenic tissue be found ?

Splenic hilum, greater omentum, close to the greater curvature of the stomach, gastrocolic, gastrosplenic and splenocolic liagaments.

What organisms may lead to OPSI ?

Most commonly implicated are the encapsulated bacteria:

Streptococcus pneumoniae - accounting for 90% of OPSI cases

Haemophilus influenzae

Neisseria meningitides

Other causative bacteria include

E coli

Pseudomonas aeuroginosa

Capnocytophagia canimorsus - usually from a dog bite

Group B streptococci

Enterococcus

Protozoa such as *plasmodium* species which can lead to malaria

How does OPSI usually present ?

Classically OPSI presents with a prodromal illness that rapidly escalates into a fulminant infection. This occurs most frequently within the first two years of splenectomy but may occur at any time and has been described up to ten years later. The overall lifetime risk of OPSI is 5% with an annual risk is 0.18% per year.

What prophylaxis should be provided post splenectomy ?

All patients following splenectomy need prophylactic immunization against

Haemophulus influenzae B – most UK children would already have had this

Neisseria meningitides – conjugate vaccine

Streptococcus pneumoniae – this needs to be boosted every 5 years

In the elective setting these vaccines should be given two weeks prior to surgery to allow for the greatest antibody titre rise.

What other risk factors are there for OPSI ?

The main risk factors are:

Age at splenectomy – the greatest risk exists in children.

Indication – there is a greater risk in elective patients compared to emergency splenectomy patients. (With an incidence of 14% in those undergoing splenectomy for haematological indications, compared with 1% of trauma patients)

As stated above the highest risk exists in the first 2 years.

The mortality from OPSI is between 50-90%

How should patients be counseled following splenectomy ?

- Patients should be advised to seek medical attention in the event of a febrile illness
- Patients should be told to take treatment dose of antibiotics in the event of a febrile illness
- The risk of OPSI should be explained and information leaflets provided
- A MEDIC alert bracelet should be worn
- Travel advice should be given to avoid areas endemic for malaria and animal bites

Thromboprophylaxis

What is the incidence of thromboembolic events in general surgical operations?

DVTs may occur in over 20% of patients undergoing major procedures. The risk of pulmonary embolism may be up to 5% in high risk patients undergoing major procedures.

What patient risk factors for DVT are you aware of?

There are a large number of factors that may increase the risk of DVT. Amongst these are:

Patient-related risk factors for VTE

- Obesity (body mass index $\geq$ 30 kg/m2)
- Personal or family history of VTE
- Active heart or respiratory failure
- Immobility (for example, paralysis or limb in plaster)
- Continuous travel of more than 3 hours approximately 4 weeks before or after surgery
- Inherited thrombophilias, for example:
  - High levels of coagulation factors (for example, Factor VIII)
  - Hyperhomocysteinaemia
  - Low activated protein C resistance (for example, Factor V Leiden)
  - Protein C, S and antithrombin III deficiencies
  - Prothrombin 2021A gene mutation.
- Acute medical illness
- Inflammatory bowel disease (for example, Crohn's disease or ulcerative colitis)
- Age over 60 years
- Active cancer or cancer treatment
- Antiphospholipid syndrome
- Behcet's disease
- Central venous catheter in situ
- Myeloproliferative diseases
- Nephrotic syndrome

- Paraproteinaemia

- Paroxysmal nocturnal haemoglobinuria

- Pregnancy or puerperium

- Recent myocardial infarction or stroke

- Severe infection

- Use of oral contraceptives or hormonal replacement therapy

- Varicose veins with associated phlebitis

By how much does the oral contraceptive pill increase the risk of DVT?

The OCP approximately doubles the risk of DVT.

What methods can be employed to reduce the risk of thromboembolism?

All patients admitted for both elective and emergency reasons should be assessed for thromboembolic risk.

NICE guidelines stipulate that surgical patients should be regarded at increased risk if they are undergoing a procedure that lasts greater than 90 minutes or greater than 60 minutes if the surgery is pelvic or lower limb. Acute admissions with inflammatory or intra-abdominal conditions, if they have reduced mobility or one of the above factors mentioned above, should be regarded as at increased risk.

Patients should be encouraged to mobilise as swiftly as possible and dehydration should be avoided.

Mechanical prophlyaxis involves the use of thromboembolic deterrant stockings (TEDS) and also intermittent pneumatic compression devices.

Pharmacological prophylaxis should also be employed in those regarded at risk. This involves the use of low molecular weight heparin, or unfractionated heparin in those with renal failure.

What is the impact of mechanical prophylaxis in reducing DVT risk?

- TEDS reduce DVT by 51% (No difference between knee and thigh length)

- Intermittent Pneumatic Compression reduces DVT by 56% (PE no difference) Cf. NICE CG92. Venous Thromboembolism. Reducing the risk of venous thromboembolism (deep vein thrombosis and pulmonary embolism) in inpatients undergoing surgery

What other factor should patients be assessed for before implementing pharmacological prophylaxis?

The risk of bleeding should be determined. Patients with the following conditions should be considered at risk from bleeding:-

Active bleeding

Acquired bleeding disorders

Concurrent use of other anticoagulants

Lumbar punctures/ spinal/ epidural anaesthesia in the last 4 hours or expected in the next 12.

Acute stroke

Thrombocytopenia (Platelets $<75 \times 10^9$ /l)

Uncontrolled systolic hypertension (>230mmHg)

Untreated bleeding disorders (eg von Willebrand, haemophilia)

In which patients should TEDS not be used?

A number of conditions contraindicate the use of TEDS. These include known peripheral artery disease, peripheral artery bypass grafting, severe leg oedema due to congestive cardiac failure, dermatitis, gangrene. Caution should also be used with venous ulcers.

What is the Wells score?

NICE guidelines recommend the use of the two-level Wells score for estimating the probability of DVT and PE. The original Wells score involved nine components to predict the presence of a DVT. Patients are classified as high, intermediate or low risk. Alternatively known as the Hamilton score.

This was revised in 2003, to include previously documented DVT as a component. The post-operative risk was also increased from 4 weeks to 12 weeks. The two-level refers to the risk categories as being likely or unlikely. Scores are from -2 to 9, with likely risk being deemed a score of 2 or more.

Wells score or criteria: (Possible score -2 to 9)

1) Active cancer (treatment within last 6 months or palliative) -- 1 point
2) Calf swelling >3cm compared to other calf (measured 10cm below tibial tuberosity) -- 1 point
3) Collateral superficial veins (non-varicose) -- 1 point
4) Pitting oedema (confined to symptomatic leg) -- 1 point
5) Swelling of entire leg - 1 point

6) Localized pain along distribution of deep venous system -- 1 point

7) Paralysis, paresis, or recent cast immobilization of lower extremities -- 1 point

8) Recently bedridden > 3 days, or major surgery requiring regional or general anaesthetic in past 12 weeks -- 1 point

9) Previously documented DVT -- 1 point

10) One alternative diagnosis at least as likely -- Subtract 2 points

Interpretation:

Score of 2 or higher - deep vein thrombosis is likely. Consider imaging the leg veins – duplex ultrasound.

Score of less than 2 - deep vein thrombosis is unlikely. Consider a blood test such as the D-dimer test to further rule out deep vein thrombosis.

Further reading:

http://www.nice.org.uk/nicemedia/live/13767/59714/59714.pdf

http://www.nice.org.uk/guidance/cg92/chapter/1-recommendations

Thyroid Nodule

You are reviewing a 30 year old woman in clinic with a neck lump. How do you proceed?

A full history and examination need to be carried out. In particular, features of the history to help determine the thyroid status of the patient should be sought. Further examination should be carried out if this appears to be a thyroid nodule, looking for any thyroid eye signs, and features of the lump.

The patient has noticed the neck swelling being present for just over one year. She feels it has gradually increased in size so that it is now noticeable on inspection. There are no skin changes, no history of shortness of breath, and a vague history of 3kgs weight loss in the last six months. The rest of her history suggests she is clinically euthyroid.

Clinical examination is unremarkable, no evidence of eye signs, P84 and regular, respiratory rate 16 and BP 140/80mmHg. Neck examination reveals a 3 x3 cm irregular swelling with a firm consistency on the right side. It moves with deglutition. There is no evidence of lymphadenopathy.

What further investigations would you order?

This patient needs routine blood tests (FBC, U&Es, LFTs) and thyroid function testing. Imaging should be carried out - initially an ultrasound of the neck. However a CT is likely to be required. FNA (fine needle aspiration biopsy) is compulsory in all patients with palpable thyroid nodules – the slides have to be reviewed by a pathologist with experience in thyroid cytology.

Blood tests including thyroid function tests are all within normal range. The biopsy suggests papillary thyroid cancer, THY 4. What does this mean?

The THY classification is used to grade thyroid cytology specimens and ranges from THY 1 to THY 5.

THY1: is non diagnostic and a repeat specimen is required.

THY2: benign / Non-neoplastic. However up to 10% may be 'upgraded' after a repeat biopsy, hence all such patients should have a repeat test in 6-12 weeks.

THY3: follicular neoplasm. Such samples have a 1 in 4 risk of being malignant (3/4 patients have follicular adenomas). The difference between benign versus malignant is based on histological assessment of invasion through the capsule, hence all these nodules are removed (diagnostic lobectomy).

THY4: Highly suspicious of cancer.

THY5: Diagnostic of thyroid cancer (e.g. papillary thyroid cancer, medullary thyroid cancer, anaplastic).

What is the problem with cytology results in suspected follicular cancer?

These are often classified as THY3 and this is due to uncertainty of the diagnosis which requires histology rather than cytology. Thus these patients will often require a lobectomy in order to make the diagnosis.

What proportion of nodules are cancerous?

This is estimated <1%. Remember that 50% of adults might have thyroid nodules seen on thyroid ultrasound while thyroid cancer remains a very rare diagnosis, with approx. 2,200 cases diagnosed yearly in the UK.

Nodules in men are more likely to be cancer (although cancer is more common in women).

Staging suggests no evidence of disease spread. How should this patient be managed?

This lady requires a total thyroidectomy and central compartment lymph node removal. Papillary cancer is a multifocal disease so lobectomy leaves the risk of residual disease. Radioiodine therapy is then used six weeks post-operatively to destroy any remnant thyroid tissue and demonstrate whether there is evidence of metastatic disease. In the long-term, patients remain on life-long levothyroxine replacement and have measurements of thyroglobulin at 6-12 months intervals (Thyroglobulin is only produced by thyroid cells so it is likely to become unmeasurable after radical surgery and radioactive iodine ablation. Therefore any rise in the concentration of TG can raise suspicion of cancer recurrence).

Umbilical Hernia in Liver Failure

You are reviewing a 55 year old former alcoholic with known alcoholic liver disease and ascites who has an umbilical hernia. He has a defect of approximately 5cm which is easily reducible but has been causing him increasing bother.

What are the effects of giving a general anaesthetic on the liver?

This can lead to hepatic ischaemia. In patients with cirrhosis there is a hyperdynamic circulation with decreased blood flow to the liver. These patients are more susceptible to hypoxaemia and hypotension.

A number of surgical factors can also contribute to liver ischaemia- these include use of a pneumoperitoneum, positive pressure ventilation, and bleeding.

Further, the anaesthetic gas used is of importance, with halothane causing hepatotoxicity.

What problems can arise post-operatively in patients with liver failure?

There is an increased risk of coagulopathy in these patients due to decreased production of clotting factors and depletion of vitamin K stores. Further there is increased fibrinolytic activity and thrombocytopenia.

Patients with cirrhosis have higher rates of ICU admission as well as aspiration pneumonia, pulmonary complications, metabolic problems and myocardial infarction.

What is hepatic encephalopathy?

This is a disorder of the central nervous system and can manifest as problems with consciousness, behaviour and personality. In the late stages it may lead to confusion, stupor and ultimately coma.

There are a number of factors that can precipitate these problems post-operatively, including infection, bleeding, and hypokalaemia.

How can risk be stratified in these patients?

Patients can be scored using the Child-Turcotte-Pugh scoring system. This allows peri-operative morbidity and mortality to be assessed in cirrhotic patients. Patients are classed A-C, which correlates with risk of morbidity and mortality.

Clinical and Lab Criteria	Points*		
	1	2	3
Encephalopathy	None	Mild to moderate (grade 1 or 2)	Severe (grade 3 or 4)
Ascites	None	Mild to moderate (diuretic responsive)	Severe (diuretic refractory)
Bilirubin micromol/1	< 34	34-50	> 50
Albumin (g/dL)	> 3.5	2.8-3.5	<2.8
Prothrombin time			
Seconds prolonged	<4	4-6	>6
International normalized ratio	<1.7	1.7-2.3	>2.3
Child-Turcotte-Pugh Class obtained by adding score for each parameter (total points) Class A = 5 to 6 points (least severe liver disease) Class B = 7 to 9 points (moderately severe liver disease) Class C = 10 to 15 points (most severe liver disease)			

From http;//depts.washington.edu/hepstudy

- Operative Mortality
    - Class A: 10%
    - Class B: 30%
    - Class C: 76-82%

Further, emergency surgery is associated with a higher mortality than elective surgery. Generally those classified as Class A should tolerate surgery well, those that are Class B surgery may be viable but may require optimization, and surgery is contraindicated in Class C.

Are there any other scoring systems for liver disease that you are aware of?

The MELD scoring system (Model for End-Stage Liver Disease) is a system for determining the severity of chronic liver disease. The MELD score uses a formula including several parameters – bilirubin, INR and Creatinine. Mortality risk is as follows:

- Mortality rates
    - MELD <7: 5.7%
    - MELD 8-11: 10.3%

- MELD 12-15: 25.4%

What are the outcomes of surgical repair of these umbilical herniae?

A number of studies have been carried out in cirrhotic patients with ascites. A review by McKay over 20 years suggested a mortality rate of approximately 2.7%, but patients were not stratified according to risk. A prospective trial by Marsman compared operative over conservative management. This suggested a complication rate of 18% in those receiving surgery and 77% in the conservatively managed group. They concluded that patients with an umbilical hernia and ascites should have prompt repair, due to the risk of incarceration.

Further reading:

McKay A, Dixon E, Bathe O, et al. Umbilical hernia repair in the presence of cirrhosis and ascites: results of a survey and review of the literature. *Hernia* 2009; 13:461-468.

Marsman HA, Heisterkamp J, Halm JA, et al. Management in patients with liver cirrhosis and an umbilical hernia. *Surgery* 2007; 142:372-375.

Undescended Testis

A 6 month old boy is referred to your outpatient clinic by his GP as she has had difficulty palpating his right testis. His parents are unsure if they have seen both testes. Examination reveals an underdeveloped right scrotum, with the left testis palpable in a normal scrotal position. There is no palpable testis on the right side. What is your diagnosis and how are you going to proceed?

This boy has an impalpable right testis, which is most likely undescended. Congenital undescended testis (UDT), or cryptorchidism, is the most common disorder of the male genitalia, which affects 2%-5% of male infants and is seen more commonly in premature infants. A UDT is one that has failed to descend to its normal intrascrotal position by 3 months of age. Postnatal testicular descent may continue for up to 3 months, at which time the incidence of cryptorchidism falls to 1%-2%. Further descent after this time is unlikely. The problem is unilateral in 90% of cases, and 70% of these occur on the right hand side. UDT is idiopathic in the majority of patients, but may be due to any abnormality in the anatomical structures involved in testicular descent, or their hormonal regulation. About 25% of UDT are impalpable. Of these, 40% are "vanished" testes, having undergone prenatal or perinatal atrophy, 30% are in the inguinal canal, 20% are intra-abdominal and thus truly cryptorchid, and the remaining 10% are ectopic. Ectopic testes descended normally through the external ring but are then diverted to abnormal locations, such as a perineal testis, which may be due to aberrant location of the genitofemoral nerve (Figure 1). The exact optimal timing of orchidopexy to preserve fertility and reduce malignant potential is as yet unknown, but current best evidence dictates that this boy should have surgery performed before 12 months of age.

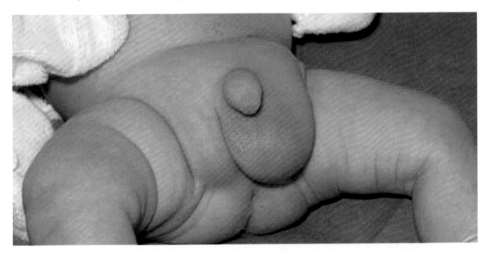

Figure 1: Right ectopic testis. Empty right hemiscrotum, and a visible swelling (ectopic testis) in the perineum to the scrotum

Why operate prior to 12 months of age?

The aim of surgical treatment for these patients is to relocate the testis to a normal position before secondary dysfunction and degeneration occur, in the hope of preserving fertility, facilitating testicular self-examination and affording cosmetic and psychological benefits in the future. Animal studies suggest that postnatal maturation of gonocytes to type-A spermatogonia occurs in the first 6-12 months after birth and that this transformation does not effectively occur in cryptorchid testes. Prospective trials have shown that orchidopexy prior to 12 months of age leads to better testicular growth as measured by ultrasound compared to when surgery is delayed until 3 years of age.

What procedure will you plan for this boy, assuming that you have the appropriate paediatric surgical experience?

I must initially confirm that the testis is truly impalpable, so I will perform an examination under anaesthesia to assess if the testis is palpable within the inguinal canal or in an ectopic position when the child is asleep and relaxed. I will consent the parents for orchidopexy +/- diagnostic laparoscopy +/- first stage Fowler Stephen's orchidopexy.

If the testis is palpable within the inguinal canal, I will perform a groin crease incision, identify the testis and dissect it from surrounding tissue to gain as much length on the spermatic cord as possible. The testis is then brought down to the scrotum and fixed in a sub-dartos pouch via a second scrotal incision. An associated inguinal hernia is seen in many cases, and concurrent herniotomy should be performed.

In the event that the testis is impalpable, I will proceed to diagnostic laparoscopy. If an intra-abdominal testis is identified, this can be brought to the scrotum by a one or two-stage procedure. If an intra-abdominal testicular nubbin is present and there is a normal scrotal testis on the opposite side, I would consider excising the nubbin to avoid the risk of malignant potential. A closed internal inguinal ring, with vas and vessels passing into the canal, may signify a small or atrophied inguinal testis, which will necessitate groin exploration and either orchidopexy, if the testis is likely to have some function, or orchidectomy. In this scenario, consideration must be given to fixation of the contralateral, healthy testis, to avoid its loss also by subsequent torsion. The parents must be made aware that surgery could lead to damage to the only remaining testis, and the pros and cons must be considered on a case by case basis, taking into account the parents' wishes.

What are the sequelae of testicular non-descent?

The main concerns are infertility and increased risk of malignancy. The fertility potential of the testis correlates with the length of time it remains outside the scrotum, due to a deficient pool of stem cells for postpubertal spermatogenesis as mentioned previously. Impaired fertility occurs in up to 33% of men with a history of unilateral UDT and 50%-66% of bilateral cases. Undescended testes which are left untreated carry an increased risk (up to 5-10 fold) of developing tumours, approximately 60% of which are seminomas arising from malignant germ cells. These tumours tend to arise between 20 and 40 years of age. Orchidopexy does not necessarily decrease the risk of malignancy developing, but facilitates earlier identification of tumours by testicular examination.

What is a retractile testis?

A retractile testis may be in the groin or upper scrotum on initial examination, but can be manipulated to a normal position at the bottom of the scrotum and will remain there for a time. It is of a normal size and present in the scrotum at least some of the time, such as during a warm bath. Retractile testes are due to a hyperactive cremasteric response, which is maximal in normal circumstances between 2 and 8 years of age. The testes should descend spontaneously to a normal scrotal position by early adolescence, without any negative consequence. There is a small potential risk of acquired UDT in this setting, so the boy and parents should observe the testicular position and return for review if there are concerns.

References

Hutson, JM, Balic, A, Nation T and Southwell, B. Cryptorchidism. *Semin Pediatr Surg.* 2010 19, 215-224.

Besner, GE. (2001) "Testicular Problems and Varicocoeles". In: Glick, PL, Pearl, RH, Irish, MS and Caty, MG. (Eds.) *Pediatric Surgery Secrets*. Philadelphia: Hanley & Belfus

Hutson, JM. (2011) "Male Genital Anomalies". In: Puri, P (Ed.) *Newborn Surgery*. London: Hodder Arnold.

BREAST SURGERY

Sunil Amonkar Adam Critchley Alice Townend

Contents

Adjuvant Chemotherapy

You are in a breast results clinic with a 52 year old lady who has recently undergone Breast Conserving Surgery (BCS) and Sentinel Lymph Node Biopsy (SLNB) for a 27mm Grade III invasive ductal carcinoma (ER 8/8, HER 2 +ve) with 1/3 SNBs containing a 1.5mm metastasis. Surgical margins are adequate. She is otherwise fit and well. Would you offer completion axillary clearance and would this influence subsequent adjuvant therapy decisions?

No, because this is a micrometastasis. The presence of a micrometastasis does not warrant specific axillary treatment as the rate of axillary recurrence is proven to be very low. All patients undergoing SNB should undergo pre-operative axillary ultrasound. Therefore by definition this lady had a clinically and sonographically normal axilla pre-operatively and in this context less than 30% of completion axillary clearance will yield further nodal metastasis.

The decision regarding adjuvant chemotherapy is increasingly driven by tumour biology and not final nodal yield. However, local staging is still important. In a sonographically normal axilla it is very unlikely that completion axillary clearance will yield a total of 4 involved nodes triggering the need for CT staging and regional nodal irradiation.

How would you define the role of adjuvant chemotherapy (ACTx)? Would you recommend this lady to undergo ACTx and do you know of any decision making tools which may support this?

ACTx is a systemic treatment given in order to reduce the future risk of disease recurrence and improve disease free and overall survival. Breast cancer is often regarded as a systemic disease from the outset. However, the estimated benefits of adjuvant treatment must outweigh the risks. I would recommend this patient to have ACTx on the basis of tumour grade, size, HER2 positivity, nodal involvement and her relatively young age. The crux of the decision is based on the tumour biology rather than the presence of a micrometastasis. The St Gallen guidelines recommend all patients under 70 with nodal involvement or ER negative disease should be referred for an oncological opinion.

Adjuvant Online (AO) provides breast cancer outcome estimates for patients who have undergone definitive surgery for unilateral, unicentric, invasive breast adenocarcinoma with no known metastasis. It provides estimated percentage improvements in disease recurrence and mortality with the use of ACTx, Adjuvant endocrine treatment and a combination of the two. AO does not take into account the HER2 status and the data is based on US breast cancer patient outcomes which are not directly analogous to UK patients. A similar online model, Predict, is based on UK breast cancer population data and does include HER2 status.

Adjuvant treatment decisions are becoming increasingly individualised. Do you know of any decision making tools based on the analysis of that patient's own cancer tissue?

Oncotype DX is a 21 gene assay (16 known breast cancer genes + 5 control genes) that produces a Recurrence Score (RS(0-100)) specific to that individual patient. This RS predicts the 10 year risk of recurrence and the likely benefit of adjuvant systemic treatment. Oncotype DX is validated for use in ER+ve, Her 2 –ve women that are node negative or in post-menopausal women with low burden node positivity (1-3+ve LN). Despite NICE recommending its use in September 2013, uptake remains relatively constrained due to the high cost (~£2000/pt). Although the tissue is still assessed centrally by Genomic Health in the US results are still available within 2 weeks. Mammaprint is an alternative gene assay that assesses 70 genes to provide a recurrence risk score.

What level of risk reduction does ACTx offer and what regimes are currently used in the UK?

The Absolute Risk Reduction (ARR) is determined by the absolute risk of that individual patient. In terms of Relative Risk Reduction (RRR), anthracycline containing polychemotherapy (e.g. FEC) reduces the annual mortality by 38% in the under 50s and by 20% for those aged 50-69.

Node negative – Anthracycline containing regimens e.g. FEC x 6

Node positive – Anthracycline/Taxane containing regimen e.g. FEC-T.

Increased cardiac risk/Previous anthracycline use – Taxane based regimens e.g. TC – Docetaxel/Cyclophosphamide.

Ideally ACTx should commence within 31 days of completion of surgery. Delays beyond 6-8 weeks are proven to be detrimental. Similarly, reductions in dose intensity and/or number of cycles have been shown to reduce the benefit of ACTx.

What are the most significant complications of Taxane and Anthracycline based chemotherapy and how can they be prevented?

Neutropenic sepsis can affect up to 20% of patients during treatment with Taxane containing chemotherapy. G-CSF reduces this risk significantly and is often given prophylactically as standard. Long term effects of taxanes include peripheral neuropathy.

Cardiac toxicity is the most significant long-term complication of anthracyclines and certain patients (>65, hypertensive, previous heart failure or myocardial infarction) should undergo monitoring with an ECHO or MUGA scan.

Alopecia can be minimised with cold cap treatment. Treatment begins around 1 hour prior to infusion lasting 3-4 hours in total.

How is HER2 status assessed and why does HER2 positivity influence the likelihood of being offered ACTx and Herceptin?

HER2 positivity is a poor prognostic factor and it increases the likelihood of disease recurrence and therefore reduced survival. It is determined by immunohistochemical grading (1=negative, 2=borderline, 3= positive). Borderline cases are submitted for in-situ hybridisation testing in the form of FISH, CISH or SISH to produce a definitive result.

Around 20% of invasive breast cancers over-express HER2. In these cases the absolute benefit of receiving ACTx and Herceptin is increased.

What is the evidence to support the use of Herceptin?

Several large RCTs (NSABP B-31/ N-9831/ HERA) demonstrated significant improvements in disease recurrence and overall survival, with relative risk reductions approaching 50% and 40% respectively.

The UK HERA trial demonstrated no benefit of Herceptin treatment given for 2 years over 1 year, which is why treatment is currently for 12 months in the UK. The FinHER study demonstrated significant benefits with just 9 weeks of treatment although these results have not been replicated elsewhere. There is ongoing research comparing 6 month and 12 month regimens (PERSEPHONE trial).

What are the side effects of Herceptin?

A large meta-analysis demonstrated a 7.2% increased risk of a significant drop in cardiac function and a 1.6% increased risk of inducing significant cardiac failure (NYHA III/IV) during a 12 month course. However these changes are reversible. Anyone demonstrating a significant decline in cardiac function should stop Herceptin and commence an Angiotensin Converting Enzyme Inhibitor. Once cardiac function returns to pre-morbid levels Herceptin can be re-started according to clinical judgment.

Adjuvant Endocrine Treatment

Your 52 year old premenopausal patient is returning to the clinic following breast conserving surgery and SLNB for a 10mm, grade 2, lymph node negative, ER positive, invasive ductal carcinoma. Along with breast radiotherapy, what other adjuvant treatment would you recommend and what is the evidence for this?

I would recommend adjuvant endocrine therapy in the form of Tamoxifen because she is ER positive.

The NATO RCT, published in 1983, was the first trial to demonstrate significant benefit for patients on adjuvant Tamoxifen compared with controls. Following this, NSABP B14, a multicentre RCT of 3,000 ER positive patients comparing 5 years of Tamoxifen with placebo, demonstrated a significant improvement with Tamoxifen in disease free survival, overall survival and contralateral breast cancer at 15years.

The 2005 Early Breast Cancer Trialists' Collaborative Group (EBCTCG) meta-analysis including approximately 15,000 patients, demonstrated a reduction in the annual breast cancer death rate of 31% in patients taking Tamoxifen for 5 years compared with controls. The cumulative mortality reduction persisted to 15 years.

Could she be offered an aromatase inhibitor (AI) instead of Tamoxifen?

Not routinely. AIs work by blocking the aromatase enzyme, responsible for the conversion of androgens to oestrogen, the principal mechanism of oestrogen production in postmenopausal women. By contrast, premenopausal women synthesise most oestrogen in their ovaries, independently of aromatase, and therefore unaffected by AIs. Hence they are ineffective in these women.

For AIs to be effective in a premenopausal woman, she must undergo ovarian ablation (oophrectomy or ovarian irradiation) or suppression (LHRH agonists). Recent evidence from the combined SOFT (Suppression of Ovarian Function Trial) and TEXT (Tamoxifen and Exemestane Trial) multicentre RCTs of approximately 4,700 ER positive, premenopausal, early breast cancer patients, suggests that patients treated with adjuvant Exemestane and ovarian function suppression (OFS) have a relative reduction of 34% in the risk of breast cancer recurrence at 5 years compared with Tamoxifen and OFS. These results compare favourably with the results of RCTs comparing AIs with Tamoxifen in postmenopausal women, and may pave the way for a change in adjuvant endocrine therapy recommendations for premenopausal women in the future.

Can adjuvant Tamoxifen be used in patients with ER negative breast cancer?

The NATO trial reported in 1983 that Tamoxifen was equally beneficial in ER positive and ER negative patients, and Tamoxifen was initially recommended as adjuvant treatment to all breast cancer patients. However subsequent studies, including the quinennial EBCTCG meta-analyses, have demonstrated no benefit in ER negative patients. The NATO (Nolvadex Adjuvant Trial Organisation) trial findings in ER negative patients are likely due to it being underpowered for subgroup analysis, and the relatively inaccurate ER measurement technique used. The lack of evidence of benefit in ER negative patients, in conjunction with the risk of endometrial cancer and thomboembolism, means that it is not recommended in these patients.

What is the mechanism of action of Tamoxifen?

In ER positive breast cancers, oestrogen binds to and activates the oestrogen receptor, driving cancer cell growth. Tamoxifen acts as a competitive antagonist to the oestrogen receptor, with its metabolites binding without activation, blocking oestrogen and thereby oestrogen mediated cancer cell growth.

Discuss the changes in recommendations you would you make if your patient was postmenopausal? Discuss the available evidence behind your recommendation.

In line with the 2009 NICE guidelines I would recommend adjuvant treatment with Anastrozole / Letrozole. I would request a baseline DEXA scan to assess her bone density.

Two large RCTs have demonstrated the beneficial effects on recurrence of adjuvant AIs against Tamoxifen in postmenopausal patients. There is no evidence for improved overall survival, possibly due to proportional increase in non-breast cancer deaths in older postmenopausal patients. The incidence of serious side effects was less in patients taking AIs during the 5 years of therapy, but similar following completion of treatment.

The ATAC (Arimidex or Tamoxifen Alone or in Combination) trial randomised approximately 9,300 postmenopausal patients to the 3 groups described. There was no benefit to taking both and the combination arm was closed early. In the remaining ER positive patients (5,200) there was significantly improved disease free survival (HR 0.86) and time to local (HR 0.79) or distant recurrence (HR 0.85) in patients on Arimidex compared with Tamoxifen at 10 years.

Part of the BIG 1-98 (Breast International Group) trial compared Letrozole and Tamoxifen in 4,800 postmenopausal ER and PR positive patients. Those taking Letrozole showed significant improvements in disease free survival (HR 0.81), particularly distant disease free survival (HR 0.73), with these benefits persisting up to 8 years.

What is the evidence for extended adjuvant endocrine treatment?

Two large multicentre RCTs, ATLAS (Adjuvant Tamoxifen, Longer Against Shorter) and aTTom, (adjuvant Tamoxifen To offer more) (approximately 7,000 and 3,000 ER positive women respectively), demonstrated that 10 years of adjuvant Tamoxifen reduced the risks of recurrence and breast cancer specific mortality as compared with the standard 5 years, contrasting with the NSABP B-14 (National Surgical Adjuvant Breast and Bowel Project) which found no benefit. Given that the benefits of 5 years Tamoxifen extend well beyond the 5 years of treatment, it is not surprising that the maximal benefits of extended adjuvant Tamoxifen are seen after 10 years. In the aTTom trial women continuing Tamoxifen for 10 years had a 25% lower recurrence rate and 23% lower breast cancer mortality rate in the second decade after diagnosis compared with women who underwent 5 years of treatment. Moreover, despite an associated increased incidence of thromboembolic disease and endometrial cancer there was no significant difference in overall mortality.

The MA.17 RCT randomised 5,200 ER positive women to 5 years of Letrozole versus placebo following 5 years of Tamoxifen. Patients in the Letrozole arm demonstrated significantly reduced recurrence and contralateral breast cancer, with improved disease-free survival in node positive patients at 2.5 years, and latterly in node negative patients. The effects were enhanced in pre or perimenopausal patients who became postmenopausal during Tamoxifen treatment. However, later analysis is unreliable since following the first interim analysis demonstrating clear benefits in favour of Letrozole, the trial was unblinded and patients in the placebo group offered selective crossover to the Letrozole arm.

NSABP B42 has randomised 4,000 patients completing 5 years of adjuvant endocrine therapy, including at least 2 years with an AI, to either 5 years Letrozole or placebo. The results are awaited.

There is no evidence to date on the efficacy or safety of 10 years adjuvant AI treatment.

What would you recommend for adjuvant endocrine treatment for a 57 year old woman who has completed 5 years adjuvant Tamoxifen and is now postmenopausal?

In line with the current NICE guidelines (2009) I would recommend extended adjuvant treatment with Letrozole for 2-3 years.

The current 2014 ASCO guidelines recommend postmenopausal patients who have completed 5 years Tamoxifen should be offered the choice to continue Tamoxifen or switch to an AI for a total of 10 years endocrine therapy. In light of the existing evidence in favour of 10 years total endocrine treatment, and a scheduled update to the NICE guidelines in 2015, I would advise her that the recommended treatment duration may change.

What is meant by endocrine switching and would you recommend this as a treatment strategy?

Endocrine switching is the term used to describe an adjuvant endocrine treatment regime of 2-3 years on either Tamoxifen or an AI followed by a switch to the other treatment for 2-3 years, completing 5 years total endocrine treatment. Two large RCTs have failed to demonstrate a benefit to a switch strategy compared with standard adjuvant Letrozole (BIG 1-98) or Exemestane (Tamoxifen Exemestane

Adjuvant Multinational (TEAM)) in 6,000 and 9,800 postmenopausal ER positive women respectively.

However, more early relapses (before 2 years) were seen in patients taking Tamoxifen followed by Letrozole (BIG 1-98). Moreover, the Intergroup Exemestane Study (IES) which randomised 4,700 postmenopausal patients disease-free on 2-3 years of Tamoxifen to either continue Tamoxifen or switch to Exemestane, demonstrated significantly improved disease-free survival at 56 months in patients who switched to Exemestane, compared with those who continued on Tamoxifen.

While there is no evidence of a benefit to endocrine switching, and it is not recommended in the current NICE guidelines, the evidence suggests that it is a safe strategy should it become necessary, for example in the case of significant side effects or the development of contraindications to treatment.

References

Nolvadex Adjuvant Trial Organisation. Controlled trial of tamoxifen as adjuvant agent in management of early breast cancer. Interim analysis at four years. Lancet 1983;1(8319):257-61.

Fisher B, Jeong JH, Bryant J. et al. National Surgical Adjuvant Breast and Bowel Project randomised clinical trials. Treatment of lymph-node-negative, oestrogen-receptor-positive breast cancer: long-term findings from National Surgical Adjuvant Breast and Bowel Project randomised clinical trials. Lancet 2004;364(9437):858-68.

Early Breast Cancer Trialists' Collaborative Group (EBCTCG). Effects of chemotherapy and hormonal therapy for early breast cancer on recurrence and 15-year survival: an overview of the randomised trials. Lancet 2005;365(9472):1687-1717.

Pagani O, Regan MM, Walley BA, et al., for the TEXT and SOFT Investigators and the International Breast Cancer Study Group. Adjuvant Exemestane with ovarian suppression in premenopausal breast cancer. NEJM 2014;371:107-118.

National Institute for Health and Clinical Excellence. Early and locally advanced breast cancer: diagnosis and treatment. 2009 NICE clinical guideline 80 guidance. nice.org.uk/cg80

Cuzick J, Sestak I, Baum M, Buzdar et al, ATAC/LATTE investigators. Effect of Anastrozole and Tamoxifen as adjuvant treatment for early-stage breast cancer: 10-year analysis of the ATAC trial. Lancet Oncology 2010;11(12):1135-1141

Regan MM, Neven P, Giobbie-Hurder A, et al, BIG 1-98 Collaborative Group, International Breast Cancer Study Group (IBCSG). Assessment of Letrozole and Tamoxifen alone and in sequence for postmenopausal women with steroid hormone receptor-positive breast cancer: The BIG 1-98 randomised clinical trial at 8.1 years median follow-up. Lancet Oncology 2011;12(12):1101-1108.

Davies C, Pan H, Godwin J, et al. on behalf of the Adjuvant Tamoxifen: Longer Against Shorter (atlas) collaborative group. Long-term effects of continuing adjuvant tamoxifen to 10 years versus stopping at 5 years after diagnosis of oestrogen receptor–positive breast cancer: atlas, a randomised trial. Lancet 2013;381:805–16.

Gray RG, Rea D, Handley K, et al, on behalf of the aTTom Collaborative Group. aTTom: long-term effects of continuing adjuvant tamoxifen to 10 years versus stopping at 5 years in 6,953 women with early breast cancer. J Clin Oncol 2013:31(suppl; abstr 5).

Goss PE, Ingle JN, Martino S, et al. Impact of premenopausal status at breast cancer diagnosis in women entered on the placebo-controlled NCIC CTG MA17 trial of extended adjuvant letrozole. Ann Oncol 2013;24(2):355-61.

Fisher B, Dignam J, Bryant J, Wolmark N. Five versus more than five years of Tamoxifen for lymph node-negative breast cancer: updated findings from the National Surgical Adjuvant Breast and Bowel Project B-14 randomized trial. J Natl Cancer Inst 2001;93:684–90.

Mamounas EP, Lembersky J, Jeong J-H, et al . NSABP B-42: a clinical trial to determine the efficacy of five years of Letrozole compared with placebo in patients completing five years of hormonal therapy consisting of an aromatase inhibitor (AI) or Tamoxifen followed by an AI in prolonging disease-free survival in postmenopausal women with hormone receptor-positive breast cancer. Clin Breast Cancer 2006;7(5):416-21.

Burstein HJ, Temin S, Anderson H, et al. Adjuvant endocrine therapy for women with hormone receptor-positive breast cancer: American Society of Clinical Oncology clinical practice guideline focused update. J Clin Oncol 2014;32:2255–69.

The BIG 1-98 Collaborative Group. Letrozole Therapy Alone or in Sequence with Tamoxifen in Women with Breast Cancer. N Engl J Med 2009;361:766-76.

van de Velde CJ, Rea D, Seynaeve C, et al. Adjuvant Tamoxifen and Exemestane in early breast cancer (TEAM): a randomised phase 3 trial. Lancet 2011;377(9762):321-31.

Bliss JM, Kilburn LS, Coleman RE, et al. Disease-related outcomes with long-term follow-up: an updated analysis of the intergroup Exemestane study. J Clin Oncol 2012;30(7):709-17.

Adjuvant Radiotherapy

How would you define adjuvant treatment?

Treatment given in addition to surgery in the absence of demonstrable disease in order to improve long term survival and reduce disease recurrence. Adjuvant treatments can be local or systemic.

What is breast radiotherapy and who should receive this?

High energy x-rays generated by a linear accelerator to target the site of excision, thereby reducing local recurrence and improving survival.

Most patients with invasive breast cancer will receive Whole Breast Irradiation (WBI) following Breast Conserving Surgery (BCS). Certain subgroups of patients following mastectomy will be recommended chest wall radiotherapy. This includes

High risk:

- All T3/T4 tumours
- ≥4 metastatic axillary lymph nodes (axillary and/or supraclavicular fossa radiotherapy may also be indicated)
- Posterior margin less than 1 mm to invasive cancer

Intermediate risk (2 or more factors including)

- age <40
- Grade 3
- 1-3 lymph node positive (SUPREMO trial)
- Lymphovascular invasion (LVI)

What is the evidence for radiotherapy following breast conserving surgery?

The Oxford (EBCCTG) overview demonstrated:

1) 75% of local recurrences occur within five years
2) Radiotherapy reduces local recurrence following breast conserving surgery by two thirds in both node positive (45% to 15%) and node negative groups (30% to 10% at fifteen years)
3) 5% survival benefit in node negative and 7% survival benefit in node positive patients at 15 years

What is the evidence for post mastectomy radiotherapy?

The Oxford overview again demonstrated:

1) Radiotherapy reduced local recurrence by two thirds in node negative (8% to 3%) and node positive (30% to 8%) at 15 years.

2) 5% survival benefit in node positive patients only

When could radiotherapy be omitted following breast conserving surgery?

- Low/intermediate DCIS with adequate surgical margins

- Patients > 65 with Grade I/II < 3 cm, ER positive, node negative cancers can be considered for entry into the PRIME II trial which is assessing radiotherapy versus observation in this group

- The CALGB trial studied patients over 70 with T1, N0, ER positive breast cancer. Radiotherapy reduced the local recurrence rate from 4% to 1% at five years (P<0.001) with no demonstrable survival benefit.

Are there any contraindications to breast radiotherapy?

Absolute

- Pregnancy

- Previous radiotherapy in this area e.g. mantle radiotherapy for lymphoma

- Active SLE/scleroderma

- Li-Fraumeni syndrome

Relative

- Technical e.g. kyphoscoliosis

What is the optimal dose and fractionation of breast radiotherapy?

The current UK standard is 40Gy in 15 fractions given over a three week period. This is based on evidence from START A plus B trials which demonstrated improved cosmesis and equivalent local regional control compared with less fractionated regimes.

How is hypofractionated radiotherapy defined and what is a breast 'boost'?

Hypofractionated radiotherapy is a dose per fraction that exceeds 2Gy. Boost is the use of electron energy to further improve local control. Dosage for boost equals 10 Gy in five fractions over one week. Surgeons can help to improve the accuracy of delivering boost radiotherapy with the use of titanium ligaclips to the tumour bed as recommended by national ABS guidelines.

What is the evidence to support boost treatment? What are the disadvantages of boost radiotherapy?

The EORTC boost or no boost trial demonstrated approximately 40% relevant risk reduction across all age groups with boost post BCS with adequate surgical margins. However, the absolute relative risk was greatest in the under 40 age group reducing local recurrence from 23.9% to 13.5% at ten years. Boost radiotherapy however increases rates of moderate to severe breast fibrosis by 15% at ten years (28.1% versus 13.2%).

Is young age (< 40 yrs) the only consideration?

Other relative indications to consider include:

- Radial/posterior margin less than 1 mm that can't be improved surgically
- LVI
- Grade III
- ER/PR negative
- Extensive Intraductal Component
- T3 disease

When should adjuvant radiotherapy commence following completion of surgery or chemotherapy?

Ideally within six weeks of completion of surgery. A large meta-analysis (N=15,000+) demonstrated significantly increased local recurrence rates when radiotherapy was delayed beyond eight weeks from 5.8% to 9.1% at five years. Ideally, radiotherapy should follow three to four weeks following chemotherapy to capitalise on the radio sensitising characteristics of Anthracycline and Taxane chemotherapy.

What are the complications of breast and/or regional radiotherapy?

Early;

- fatigue
- skin erythema/desquamation (Grade 0-4)

Intermediate;

- Radiation pneumonitis (<1%)
- Breast firmness and shrinkage

Late;

- Lymphoedema
- Cardiac toxicity (<1%)
- Angiosarcoma (rare)

What is the evidence for recommending adjuvant radiotherapy following BCS for DCIS?

Three large RCTs (NSBP B17, EORTC and UKCCCR DCIS) demonstrate reduced local recurrence by around 50%. Around half of all local recurrences were invasive cancers. There is no proven survival advantage.

What is the rationale for partial breast irradiation?

Over 90% of local recurrences occur within the index quadrant whether radiotherapy is given or not, therefore implying radiotherapy to the index quadrant alone may be sufficient to achieve sustained local control. Intraoperative single dose radiotherapy can either be given low energy photons (TARGIT A) or electrons (ELIOT). The target technique utilises the Intrabeam system that creates a small high dose region that attenuates clinically beyond 1 cm from the applicator, thereby protecting normal surrounding breast tissue. This technique has recently been approved by NICE.

The TARGIT A trial randomised over 2,000 patients with early breast cancer to whole breast irradiation +/- boost versus single intraoperative partial breast irradiation. At four years follow-up, there was no significant difference in local recurrence or toxicity.

Axilla Management

Can you define the anatomical levels of the axillary lymph nodes?

The anatomical levels of the axillary lymph nodes are defined by their relationship to pectoralis minor. Level1 lymph nodes are inferolateral, level 2 posterior and level 3 superomedial to pectoralis minor. In reality these lymph nodes are in continuity, but the description of levels of axillary nodes is helpful when describing the extent of axillary surgery performed during an axillary clearance.

What is the role of sentinel lymph node biopsy (SLNB) and how is it performed?

SLNB accurately stages the clinically and radiologically node negative axilla and is the UK standard of care. Most commonly dual localisation is performed using blue dye (patent V blue) injected immediately preoperatively and radiolabeled nanocolloid (20 mb technetium 99) injected within 24 hours prior to surgery. They are injected into Sappey's subareolar lymphatic plexus. Radioactive isotope alone is an accepted technique, although blue dye alone SLNB is not recommended.

Is sentinel node biopsy accurate? Do false negative SLNBs directly translate to axillary recurrence?

A recent ASCO systemic review of 8,059 patients undergoing SLNB reported an overall accuracy rate of 95% plus false negative rate of 7.3%.

Several randomised controlled trials have shown axillary recurrence rates of less than 1% following negative SNB with six to ten year follow up. Of those patients with a positive SNB in the Z0011 trial who were randomised to have a "completion axillary clearance", 27.4% had further metastatic disease in non-sentinel nodes. Yet only 0.9% of this group developed axillary recurrence at 6.3 years.

Is this follow up too short to detect axillary recurrence?

The majority of breast and axillary recurrences occur within two years of surgery. NSABP-04 reported a median duration of 14.8 months to axillary recurrence with only 7 of 68 recurrences reported beyond five years.

How do we classify axillary metastases on histology?

- Isolated tumour cells (Pn0) [i+] less than or equal to 0.2 mm
- Micrometastasis (pN1) [Mi] > 0.2mm less than or equal to 2 mm
- Macrometastasis (pN1) [Ma] > 2 mm

Are isolated tumour cells (ITC) clinically significant?

ITC's are regarded as node negative in the majority of UK centres.

Which groups of patients are not suitable for SLNB?

- T4 cancers

- Proven axillary metastasis

- Patients with DCIS undergoing breast conserving surgery (unless clinically mass forming)

- Although the uterine dose of radiolabelled colloid is minimal current ASCO guidelines do not recommend SNB in pregnancy. Blue dye usage is contraindicated due to the risk of foetal staining.

Do all patients with SLNB metastasis require axillary clearance?

This remains an area of great debate. Important factors to consider are the size of metastasis, the type of surgery performed and tumour biology. Various large centres have developed decision-making tools to help guide this process e.g. Memorial-Sloan Kettering Nomogram.

ITCs are regarded as node negative and no specific axillary treatment is indicated.

Increasingly further axillary treatment is not routinely recommended with the finding of one or two micro metastases, particularly if a systemic treatment option is available.

The management of SLNB macrometastasis is the source of greatest contention. The RCT ACOSOG Z0011 concluded 'The routine use of axillary lymph node dissection (ALND) is not justified' in clinically N0 patients undergoing breast conserving treatment with only one or two positive SLNBs. Z0011 demonstrated equivalent axillary recurrence rates and overall survival, whether a completion clearance was performed or not.

The most recent ASCO expert panel systemic review analysed all data up to January 2013. They recommend that clinicians should not recommend ALND for women with early stage breast cancer with one or two SLN micro or macrometastases and who will receive breast conserving surgery with conventionally fractionated whole breast radiotherapy. However, clinicians offer ALND for women with early stage breast cancer with nodal metastases found on SLNB and who will undergo mastectomy.

Current NICE guidelines (2009) still recommend further axillary treatment in the presence of axillary micro and macrometatases. However, an ABS multidisciplinary consensus meeting on axillary lymph node management in 2015 agreed with the ASCO recommendations.

Do you know of any UK based RCTs investigating this subject?

The POSNOC (POsitive Sentinel NOde: adjuvant therapy alone versus adjuvant therapy plus Clearance or axillary radiotherapy) is a pragmatic, randomised, multi-centre, non-inferiority trial that will randomise women with early stage breast cancer and one or two macrometastases to either adjuvant therapy alone or adjuvant therapy and axillary treatment. The primary outcome measure is axillary recurrence at five years. The recruitment target is for 1,900 patients, which began in July 2013 for 45 months. Follow up will be for five years with results published in approximately 2024.

Why has axillary radiotherapy (ART) been included as an axillary treatment option?

The EORTC phase 3 non-inferiority AMAROS trial was designed to answer the hypothesis that ART offers equivalent control and less morbidity than axillary clearance in SNB positive patients.

They concluded ALND plus ART provide excellent and comparable regional control. Axillary recurrence rates were 0.54% versus 1.03% at five years respectively. There were no significant differences in five year survival. Lymphoedema was significantly less common following ART at 1 year (40% ALND, 22% ART($p < 0.0001$)) and five years (28% ALND, 14% ART($p< 0.0001$)).

When would you consider ART instead of ALND? Are there any advantages of ALND?

I would offer ART to those patients undergoing breast conservation in which the decision regarding ACTx has already been made.

Some clinicians argue the additional histological information obtained regarding the nodal burden will influence adjuvant treatment decisions for chemotherapy and/or additional regional irradiation. The AMAROS group reported that this lack of information had no major effect on the adjuvant treatment decisions made.

References/ Further reading:

Lyman GH et al. Sentinel Lymph Node Biopsy for Patients With Early-Stage Breast Cancer: American Society of Clinical Oncology Clinical Practice Guideline Update. J Clin Oncol 2014:32(13);1365-1386.

National Institute for Health and Clinical Excellence. Early and locally advanced breast cancer: Diagnosis and treatment. 2009 NICE clinical guideline 80 guidance. nice.org.uk/cg80

Association of Breast Surgery Trustees 16th March 2015. Association of Breast Surgery Consensus Statement: Management of the Malignant Axilla in Early Breast Cancer. http://www.associationofbreastsurgery.org.uk/media/48727/axilla_abs_consensus_statement_16_3_15.pdf

Breast Infection and Associated Conditions

A 35 year old lady is admitted with a painful tender red left breast swelling and associated pyrexia. She reports no prior breast symptoms. She is a smoker, though otherwise in good health. How would you manage this?

The clinical picture described is in keeping with non-lactational breast infection. On clinical assessment any areas of fluctuance would need to be identified to locate any possible underlying abscess. The area of surrounding cellulitis should also be marked. If systemically unwell, she would need to be commenced on IV antibiotics and IV fluids. If a collection is clinically palpable then this can be aspirated under local anaesthesia. If no collection is clinically palpable then an ultrasound scan of the breast would have to be arranged with a view to aspirating any collection.

If the patient is systemically unwell with a fluctuant swelling then this should be drained as per any abscess, ideally sending a sample of frank pus for culture and sensitivities. If facilities for image guided drainage are not available, then this should be surgically drained. A small incision is sufficient to drain pus and minimise scarring, packing is rarely required. Any areas of necrotic tissue should be debrided. When the systemic disturbance has resolved with associated clinical improvement the patient could be switched to oral antibiotics and discharged. However it is essential that the patient is followed up to ensure complete resolution.

How do you classify breast infections and how does this affect treatment?

Breast infections are classified into either lactational, non-lactational or post surgical. Lactational mastitis where the breast is inflamed and red occurs in 10% of women who are breastfeeding; up to half of these can have associated infection. This is usually during the first month or weaning. It is caused by *S. aureus* infection introduced to the duct system from cracking of the nipple. Most cases are mild and are managed in the community with oral antibiotics and patients are encouraged to continue breast feeding if possible or express milk on the affected side. Severe cases require admission for IV antibiotics and drainage of any collection. Antibiotic use may vary according to local microbiology protocols but a suitable choice would be Flucloxacillin. Alternatives could be Clarithromycin or Clindamycin in more severe case if penicillin allergic.

Non lactational breast infection is more common in patients who smoke or who are diabetic. Patients may have recurrent episodes of inflammation +/- infection due to this known as periductal mastitis. Pathogens are typically mixed involving *S. aureus* and anaerobes. Suitable antibiotics could include Co-Amoxiclav or Clarithromycin and Metronidazole if penicillin allergic. All breast infections would require subsequent follow up to ensure clinical resolution. If there are persisting changes then further imaging and assessment would be required.

Post surgical infections can develop in the immediate post operative period or several weeks later after the wound may have appeared to have initially healed without complication. In the immediate postoperative phase this is due to skin flora and anaerobes. If however there is an implant inserted, organisms can include Staphylococcal species (including coagulase negative Staph), gram negative bacteria and anaerobes. Seromas are likely to be present with associated infection and these should be aspirated and cultured prior to commencing antibiotics.

Antibiotics are best guided by local microbiology protocols and management of these cases is best dealt with by a specialist breast surgeon. Complications generally arise from tissue ischemia and necrosis. Early open debridement, cavity irrigation, controlled drainage and exchanging an implant for a tissue expander may help save the skin envelope. Should this fail, the implant and any biological/prosthetic mesh used would have to be removed.

What follow up would you provide?

Following discharge on the appropriate antibiotics, clinical follow up is initially required to assess for resolution of symptoms and clinical signs. If there is complete resolution, then no further follow up is required, though a mammogram should be performed for all patients over 35 after resolution of any inflammatory changes. Any concern of a residual collection would require repeat breast ultrasound and further aspiration or drainage if necessary. Any residual solid mass would require further imaging and triple assessment as for any new breast lump. Often interval imaging and follow up may be required to assess for resolution.

Despite various courses of antibiotics, there is still persisting redness of the breast and the tissue feels firm. The patient is otherwise systemically well. Do you have any concerns regarding this?

Although this may still be in keeping with the initial presentation of breast infection, alternative causes must be considered. This may be a chronic inflammatory mass as a result of prolonged antibiotic treatment (antibioma) but the possibility of an inflammatory breast cancer should be considered. Even if there are no suspicious features on imaging, a biopsy of the abnormal area should be performed.

Histology has confirmed a high grade ductal cancer which is triple receptor negative. What would be the next step in management?

Histology has confirmed the diagnosis of an inflammatory breast cancer. Initially staging investigations would need to be performed. If the axilla had not previously been assessed then this would require clinical and radiological assessment initially with ultrasound and tissue biopsy of any abnormal appearing nodes. This may imply locoregional disease. A CT scan of the chest, abdomen and pelvis would also need to be performed along with bone scintigraphy to assess for distant disease. An MRI scan of both breasts would also be considered to further assess the size of the primary breast cancer, as a mammogram has low sensitivity in this age group and situation, given oedema of the tissue.

As the tumour is triple receptor negative, neo-adjuvant chemotherapy would be considered. Prior to treatment the site of biopsy confirming the cancer should also be marked with a radiological clip so the response to treatment can be assessed with interval imaging. Following completion of chemotherapy, surgical options for both the breast and axilla would be considered taking response of treatment into account. There may also be a need for subsequent adjuvant radiotherapy. Whilst undergoing treatment, consideration of a familial predisposition and appropriate referral to a geneticist should also be considered given the patient's young age and triple negative receptor status.

Breast Screening

What are the criteria for a successful screening programme?

Principles for screening were first defined in 1968 by Wilson and Jungner for the World Health Organisation:

- The condition being screened for should be an important health problem.

- The natural history of the condition should be well understood.

- There should be a recognisable early stage.

- Treatment at an early stage should be of more benefit than at a later stage.

- A suitable test should be available for the early stage.

- The test should be acceptable to the population.

- There should be adequate facilities for the diagnosis and treatment of abnormalities detected.

- Intervals for repeating the test should be determined by the natural history of the disease.

- The chance of both physical and psychological harm should be less than the chance of benefit.

- The cost of the screening programme should be balanced against the benefits.

What trials formed the basis for the NHS Breast Screening Programme?

The Forrest report was commissioned by the Minister for Health and performed by Professor Sir Patrick Forrest in 1985, to assess the available evidence on mammographic screening for breast cancer and to make recommendations for UK practice. It analysed the findings of the available breast cancer screening trials and formed the majority of its recommendations based on 2 trials, the US HIP trial and the Swedish two-county trial. These 2 RCTs, comparing breast screening with a control population of unscreened women, demonstrated a 30% reduction in breast cancer mortality in screened women aged over 50. Neither the Forrest report nor the 2 trials on which it was based made any assessment of the harms of breast screening. Based on these, the NHS BSP was established in 1987 and began inviting women aged 50-64 for screening by single-view mammography every 3 years in 1988.

Why is it recommended that breast screening should take place every 3 years?

Initially, the time interval for screening was selected based on the Swedish two-county trial as a similar mortality benefit was demonstrated as that shown in trials also reviewed in the Forrest report with shorter screening intervals.

The Breast Screening Frequency Trial Group published a multicentre UK RCT in 2002 comparing 3 annual screens with the standard triennial screen. Approximately 76,000 women attending for their prevalent screen were included, with the primary endpoint predicted breast cancer deaths based on pathological features. They found that while the group who underwent annual screening had significantly smaller tumours, there was no significant difference in predicted breast cancer death. They concluded that shortening of the screening interval was not justified. Follow up for actual mortality in these patients is ongoing.

What is the rationale behind the age range selected for breast cancer screening?

The Forrest Report concluded that the effectiveness of breast cancer screening was demonstrated only for women aged 50 and over. Poor response rates in the over 65s limited the population benefit in this age group. The initial age range selected was therefore 50-64.

The UK Age Trial randomised 160,000 women aged 39-41 to annual mammography until 48 or no screening. They demonstrated a non-significant reduction in breast cancer mortality at 10 years. This is likely due to limitations of mammography in pre-menopausal women with dense breast tissue and a decreased breast cancer incidence in this age group. Increased accuracy of digital mammography in dense breasts may make screening of younger women feasible in the future.

Extended follow up of the Swedish two-county trial published in 2002 showed an ongoing mortality benefit for women aged 50-70. Earlier data from other RCTs demonstrating lower mortality benefit over 65 may have been unreliable due to the inclusion of breast cancer related deaths secondary to breast cancer diagnoses preceding the commencement of screening for these women. The upper age limit was increased to 70 in 2001.

For women to benefit from screening their life expectancy should be at least 10 years, a reasonable presumption below 70. Over 70 this is less reliable and the evidence for mortality benefit is less clear. Screening in this age group may be appropriate on an individual rather than population basis, and for this reason women over 70 may self refer.

Currently the NHS BSP is being extended to women aged 47 to 49, and 71 to 73. This is expected to be complete by 2016 and the outcomes are subject to an ongoing trial.

What is overdiagnosis and overtreatment?

Overdiagnosis is the diagnosis of 'disease' that would never cause a symptom or death in that patient's lifetime. Overtreatment is unnecessary medical treatment, such as treatment of a condition that would be self-limiting, or more extensive treatment than would be required to treat a medical condition. It is commonly a consequence of overtreatment.

What is the evidence for harm of breast screening?

Gøtzsche and Nielsen performed a Cochrane review of 8 RCTs including approximately 600,000 women in 2011, specifically to balance the harms of breast screening with the benefits. They found a lower reduction in breast cancer mortality of 15% with a 10% false positive rate over 10 years and 30% overdiagnosis. They concluded that for every 2,000 women screened for 10 years, one life would be prolonged, 10 women would be overtreated, and 200 would experience psychological distress due to false positives.

Raftery performed an updated analysis of the Forrest report in 2011 to include harms of breast screening, to address the claims made by Gøtzsche and Nielsen. They utilised quality adjusted life years (QALY) balancing the reduction in breast cancer mortality against the loss of quality of life from false positives, overdiagnosis and surgery. They found that harms offset gains up to 10 years, but thereafter the gains increased. It is therefore possible that more harm than good is done before 10 years.

The Marmot Report, an independent review of breast screening chaired by Professor Sir Michael Marmot in 2012, concluded that breast screening resulted in a 20% absolute mortality benefit. This means that 1 death is prevented for every 235 women invited for screening or 180 women screened for 20 years, which translates to 1,300 lives saved per year in the UK. However, they estimated that for each death prevented, 3 women were overdiagnosed, which meant that each woman aged 50-52 invited to screening had a 1% risk of overdiagnosis in 20 years of screening. The panel concluded that breast screening should continue but women should receive more information to allow them to make an informed decision.

What is the evidence regarding the use of MRI scanning for screening high risk women?

The MARIBS trial (MAgnetic Resonance Imaging for Breast Screening) compared MRI with mammographic breast screening in women at high risk of a BRCA gene mutation. At 5 years, MRI was shown to be more sensitive although both were similarly specific. The authors recommended that annual screening with MRI and mammography would detect most cancers in this group of patients.

References/ Further Reading:

Wilson Jungner. Principles and practice of screening for disease. Geneva: WHO; 1968

Forrest P. Breast Cancer Screening. Report to the Health Ministers of England, Wales, Scotland and Northern Ireland by a working group chaired by Professor Sir Patrick Forrest. HMSO 1986.

Shapiro S, Venet W, Strax P, Venet, Roeser. Ten-to-fourteen year effect of screening on breast cancer mortality. J Natl Cancer Inst 1982;69:349–55.

The Breast Screening Frequency Trial Group. The frequency of breast cancer screening: results from the UKCCCR Randomised Trial. Eur J Cancer 2002:38;1458–1464.

Moss SM, Cuckle H, Evans A, Johns L, Waller M, Bobrow L, for the Trial Management Group. Effect of mammographic screening from age 40 years on breast cancer mortality at 10 years' follow-up: a randomised controlled trial. The Lancet 2006;368:2053–60.

Nyström L, Andersson I, Bjurstam N, Frisell J, Nordenskjöld B, Rutqvist LE. Long-term effects of mammography screening: updated overview of the Swedish randomised trials. Lancet 2002;359(9310):909–919.

Gøtzsche PC, Nielsen M. Screening for breast cancer with mammography. Cochrane Database Syst Rev 2009;4:CD001877.

Raftery J, Chorozoglou M. Possible net harms of breast cancer screening: updated modelling of Forrest report. BMJ 2011:343;d7627

Marmot MG, Altman DG, Cameron DA, Dewar JA, Thompson SG, Wilcox M, and The Independent UK Panel On Breast Cancer Screening. The Benefits and Harms of Breast Cancer Screening: An Independent Review. Br J Cancer 2013:108(11);2205-2240.

Hereditary Breast Cancer

How do we define the levels of risk for hereditary breast cancer and how does this help us guide patient management?

Low risk patients have a risk of breast cancer equivalent to the general population, which is a lifetime risk of less than 17% and a risk of less than 3% of developing breast cancer between the ages of 40 and 49. These patients can be safely managed in primary care.

Moderate risk patients have a lifetime risk of breast cancer of 17%-30% and a risk of 3%-8% of developing breast cancer between the ages of 40 and 49. These patients warrant a referral to secondary care for further assessment of their family history but do not normally require referral to a specialist genetics clinic.

High risk patients have a lifetime risk of breast cancer of more than 30% and a risk of over 8% of developing breast cancer between the ages of 40 and 49. These patients have a greater than 20% chance of a BRCA1, BRCA2 or TP53 gene fault and should therefore be referred to a specialist genetics department for further assessment.

What conditions are known to confer an increased risk of breast cancer?

BRCA1 gene mutations are associated with a 60%-80% lifetime risk of breast cancer and a 40%-50% risk of ovarian cancer. Men who are positive for this gene mutation have a 1%-2% risk of breast cancer and twice the background risk of prostate cancer. There is also twice the background risk of pancreatic cancer.

BRCA2 gene mutations are associated with a 40%-85% lifetime risk of breast cancer and a 10%-25% risk of ovarian cancer. Men who are positive for this gene mutation have a 6% risk of breast cancer and 33% risk of developing prostate cancer by the age of 65. There is also three to four times the background risk of pancreatic cancer.

BRCA gene mutations are also associated with an increased risk of melanoma, colon and haematological malignancies.

Other conditions associated with an increased risk of breast cancer include Li Fraumeni syndrome (TP53), Peutz-Jeghers syndrome (STK11), Cowden (PTEN) and familial diffuse gastric cancer (E-Cadherin)

How common is hereditary breast cancer?

Breast cancer is common, with approximately one in eight women affected during their lifetime. The majority of breast cancers are sporadic, with only 4%-5% of breast cancers presenting over the age of 30 thought to have genetic cause. Below the age of 30 this rises to 1 in 4. The risk of developing a hereditary breast cancer depends primarily on the number of relatives who have developed breast, ovarian or a related cancer, and the age at which these relatives developed breast cancer.

How would you assess a patient's risk for a hereditary breast cancer in secondary care?

To assess a woman's risk of hereditary breast cancer I would take a focused history concentrating on her family history of breast and ovarian cancer in first, second and third degree relatives, including their age at diagnosis, presence of bilateral disease and male breast cancers. To increase the accuracy of the family history I would encourage the patient to discuss this with other family members if possible, and to complete a family history questionnaire.

In the presence of a positive family history, I would specifically enquire about features associated with an increased chance of familial breast cancer, including Jewish ancestry, sarcomas before the age of 45, gliomas or childhood adrenal cortical carcinomas, multiple cancers at a young age, or a paternal history of four of more relatives diagnosed below 60.

If available, I would utilise carrier probability scoring such as BOADICEA or the Manchester scoring system to quantify risk. Based on my assessment I would determine whether the patient met the criteria for referral to a specialist genetics clinic.

Which patients would you refer for assessment in a specialist genetics clinic?

I would consider a patient for referral to a specialist genetics clinic after performing a full assessment of their risk for a hereditary breast cancer. In line with the NICE guidelines the patients who meet the criteria for referral are those with:

- At least one affected first degree relative and a total of two first or second degree relatives diagnosed before an average age of 50, three before an average age of 60 or four at any age. Bilateral cancers count as two relatives.

- One relative with ovarian cancer any age and one first or second degree relative diagnosed with breast cancer before 50, two diagnosed before an average age of 60 or another with ovarian cancer at any age.

- One male relative with breast cancer at any age and at least one first or second degree relative diagnosed with breast cancer before 50 or two diagnosed before an average age of 60.

- A formal risk assessment estimating a 10% chance of a gene mutation in the family, more than an 8% risk in 10 years or more than a 30% lifetime risk of breast cancer.

Patients falling outside these criteria but with families including a history of triple negative cancers below the age of 40 or other features associated with an increased chance of familial breast cancer (listed above) should be discussed, as they may warrant referral.

What are the current NICE guidelines regarding surveillance of high risk patients?

The strategy for surveillance of high risk patients depends on whether they are known to have a gene mutation, or whether they are assessed to have a high risk of breast cancer based on their family history.

Women who are known to have a BRCA mutation are recommended to have annual mammography between the ages of 40 and 69, and annual MRI scanning between the ages of 30 and 49. Women who are known TP53 gene carriers should not have mammography as they are at risk of radiation induced breast cancers. They should have annual MRI screening between the ages of 20 and 49.

Women who have been classified as high risk based on their family history have screening determined by their risk of a BRCA or TP53 gene mutation. If they have a greater than 30% chance of a BRCA gene mutation, annual MRI screening is identical to known gene carriers. Annual mammography is recommended between the ages of 40 and 59, following which they should enter the National Breast Screening Programme. The recommendations for women assessed as having a greater than 30% chance of a TP53 mutation are the same as known gene carriers, with the exception that they should have 3 yearly mammographic screening from the age of 50 as part of the National Breast Screening Programme.

Women at high risk of breast cancer, but assessed to have a risk of 30% or less of being a BRCA or TP53 gene carrier, should have annual mammography between the ages of 40 and 59 years, following which they should enter the National Breast Screening Programme.

Annual mammography can be considered at a younger age provided the woman is at least 30 years old, is not a TP53 gene carrier, and does not have an estimated risk of more than 30% of being a TP53 gene carrier.

You are reviewing a fit and well 31 year old patient in your clinic who is concerned that she has an increased risk of breast cancer. Her mother had breast cancer aged 35, a maternal aunt had bilateral breast cancer aged 37 and her maternal grandmother had ovarian cancer aged 54. How will you assess this woman's risk and what would be your management plan?

This woman has a high risk family history. If available, I would utilise carrier probability scoring such as BOADICEA or the Manchester scoring system to quantify risk, however with 3 affected family members, including one with bilateral breast cancer, one with ovarian cancer, and 3 breast cancers diagnosed below 40 years of age she meets the NICE guidelines for referral to a specialist genetics clinic to discuss her risks and options, which may include genetic testing after suitable counselling.

Your patient has now been referred back to you from the genetics department as she has been found to have a BRCA 1 gene mutation. She is requesting bilateral prophylactic mastectomy. How would you counsel this woman?

The key issues I would make clear to her regarding bilateral risk reduction surgery are:

- It reduces the risk of breast cancer by approximately 95%. It is a risk-reducing not risk-removing operation.

- Her individual benefit will depend on the degree of risk conferred by her specific gene mutation taken in conjunction with any other risk factors, including the fact that breast cancer incidence increases with age.

- There are alternatives to prophylactic surgery, including enhanced screening and chemoprevention.

- Bilateral oophorectomy, which can be considered to reduce the risk of ovarian cancer once her family is complete, independently reduces the risk of breast cancer with a proven mortality benefit in BRCA1 gene carriers.

- There is a possibility of breast cancer being diagnosed histologically following risk-reducing surgery.

- It is not a rapid process, taking between six and twelve months, to allow her:

  - Time to discuss and consider both immediate and delayed breast reconstructive options.

  - Pre-operative psychological counselling, including psychosocial and sexual consequences of bilateral mastectomy.

  - Access to support groups and / or contact with women who have undergone risk reduction surgery.

Following this process I would offer her further appointments to discuss her options, before listing for surgery in line with her wishes.

Would there be any difference in your counselling or management if this patient had not been found to carry the BRCA 1 gene but was requesting prophylactic risk-reducing surgery based on her high risk family history?

In line with the NICE guidelines, all women considering bilateral risk-reducing mastectomy with no definite gene mutation should have attempted verification of their family history. If this is not possible, agreement by a multidisciplinary team should be sought before proceeding with bilateral risk-reducing mastectomy. In all other aspects the counselling process is the same.

Your patient has a breast MRI performed while she is considering prophylactic surgery. This detects a 15mm lesion in the right breast which is visible on mammogram and USS. After biopsy under USS guidance, it is confirmed to be a triple negative grade 3 invasive ductal carcinoma. The axilla is normal on USS. How would this change your management?

The priority is surgical and oncological treatment of the known breast cancer. With a 15mm cancer she can be offered breast conserving surgery (BCS) and radiotherapy or mastectomy, although she should be informed that because she is a BRCA1 gene carrier her risk of ipsilateral breast cancer recurrence is higher following BCS than in patients with sporadic breast cancers, and higher than BRCA carriers who undergo mastectomy. However this is not translated to an effect on survival. The tumour biology means that she will be offered adjuvant chemotherapy.

If she still wishes to consider contralateral prophylactic surgery it is important to stress the following:

- Her outcome will be determined by the known breast cancer and not by the possible risk of a contralateral breast cancer.

- Any subsequent breast cancer is likely to be detected at earlier stage due to annual mammography following diagnosis, in addition to ongoing mammographic and MRI surveillance, in line with the NICE guidelines for BRCA gene carriers.

- A significant number of breast cancers recur as distant metastases, which will not be impacted by prophylactic surgery.

- Any surgery carries the risk of complications which may delay and therefore reduce the effectiveness of potentially lifesaving adjuvant treatment. More complex surgery, such as contralateral risk-reducing surgery, increases the chance of complications.

- The urgency implicit in a cancer diagnosis means that the time for psychological counselling and support in decision-making will be curtailed.

- For these reasons it is usually preferable to defer contralateral surgery until after completion of adjuvant treatment.

Reference/ Further Reading:

National Institute for Health and Clinical Excellence. Familial breast cancer: Classification and care of people at risk of familial breast cancer and management of breast cancer and related risks in people with a family history of breast cancer. 2013 NICE clinical guideline 164 guidance.nice.org.uk/cg164

Histological Subtypes of Breast Cancer

What histological subtypes of invasive breast cancer do you know?

The most common type of breast cancer, making up approximately 80% of all breast cancer diagnoses, is invasive ductal carcinoma, also known as invasive breast carcinoma NST (no special type), because it does not show specific histological differentiating features. It arises within the breast ducts, invading into the surrounding breast tissue, and is often associated with DCIS. Mammography classically reveals a spiculated mass, sometimes within an area of microcalcification.

Breast cancers classed as a special type include invasive lobular carcinoma and other rarer types of breast cancer. Invasive lobular cancer arises in the breast lobules, invading into the surrounding breast tissue, and is the histological diagnosis in approximately 5%-10% of cases. It can be harder to diagnose because it may not form a definite mass, and is often mammographically occult or under-represented. It is also associated with an increased incidence of bilaterality and multifocality.

Which histological subtypes of breast cancer have a more favourable prognosis?

Tubular, cribriform and mucinous carcinomas are typically ER positive cancers with a particularly good prognosis. Tubular and cribriform cancers have similar low-grade nuclear features. Most mucinous cancers are characteristically of the luminal A molecular subtype. Pure mucinous carcinomas have an excellent prognosis, but the outcome for mixed mucinous carcinomas is similar to NST tumours.

Which histological subtypes are associated with a less favourable prognosis?

Carcinomas with apocrine differentiation and metaplastic cancers are typically triple negative breast cancers with a less favourable prognosis than other histological subtypes. Apocrine differentiation is usually associated with NST ductal cancers but can be present in other histological subtypes. For this reason they therefore are usually described according to their primary invasive type. Metaplastic cancers form a heterogeneous group and therefore a descriptive classification is used. They can be either low or high grade cancers. They typically show a worse prognosis than other forms of triple-negative breast cancers.

What are the clinical and pathological features suggestive of an inflammatory breast cancer?

Inflammatory carcinoma is an aggressive form of breast carcinoma that can be diagnosed in the presence of characteristic clinical or histopathological features. The classical clinical presentation is one of rapid breast enlargement and skin changes, including redness, oedema, and peau d'orange, involving more than a third of the breast. Often there is a diffuse firmness rather than a discrete palpable mass. The typical histopathological finding is the presence of numerous lymphatic tumour cell emboli in the breast skin.

What can you tell me about molecular subtypes of breast cancer, and why is this subtyping important?

The importance of tumour biology to predict prognosis and treatment response in breast cancer is emerging. Gene expression profiling has identified distinct molecular subtypes – luminal A, luminal B, HER2 positive and basal-like, with differing clinical features, treatment response and prognosis. Immunohistochemical analysis of ER, PR, and HER2 provides an approximation of these molecular subtypes. ER and PR positive, HER2 negative cancers are most likely luminal A. ER and PR positive, HER2 positive cancers are most likely luminal B. Hormone receptor negative, HER2 positive are most likely HER2 type. Triple negative cancers are most likely basal-like.

Biomarkers not routinely identified such as cytokeratins, EGFR, and Ki67, increase the accuracy of molecular subtyping. Accurate assessment of molecular subtype is important because certain subtypes may respond differentially to adjuvant treatment. For example, Luminal A cancers respond well to endocrine therapy, whereas basal-like cancers are sensitive to platinum-based chemotherapy. This may become increasingly important as treatments targeting specific molecular subtypes, such as PARP inhibitors, are developed.

What are the typical histological features associated with breast cancers in BRCA gene carriers?

BRCA1 gene carriers typically present with high grade triple negative cancers with less in situ disease and a molecular profile similar to basal-like cancers in approximately 80% of cases. The chance of finding a BRCA1 gene fault in a patient with a triple negative cancer is approximately 10%-15%. The current NICE guidelines (2013) suggest that patients presenting with triple negative cancers under the age of 40 should be considered for genetic testing to look for a BRCA1 mutation.

BRCA2 associated breast cancers show more similarity to sporadic cancers, commonly being lower grade and ER positive with more in situ disease.

What role do molecular profiling gene expression tests play in breast cancer management?

Two molecular tests, OncotypeDX and Mammaprint, have been retrospectively validated in previous large scale prospective adjuvant therapy RCTs such as those undertaken by NSABP. OncotypeDX is a 21 gene signature RT-PCR-based assay performed on formalin-fixed paraffin embedded tissue. It is reported as a 'recurrence score' that correlates with prognostic outcome, and response to endocrine and chemotherapies. Mammaprint uses microarray analysis of 70 genes in fresh frozen tissue to identify patients with good and poor prognostic signatures. Both of these tests are commercially available and utilised in the selection of patients with borderline indications for chemotherapy to identify those who would benefit from adjuvant treatment, while avoiding toxic side effects if the chance of benefit is small. Prospective RCTs currently underway, TAILORx and RxPONDER trials evaluating OncotypeDX and the MINDACT trial evaluating Mammaprint, hope to quantify their clinical significance, but the results are several years away.

OncotypeDX has been recommended for use by NICE to help make decisions about adjuvant chemotherapy in some patients with ER positive, lymph node negative, and HER2 negative early breast cancer. However current funding issues mean that use is not widespread.

References/ Further reading:

National Institute for Health and Clinical Excellence. Familial breast cancer: Classification and care of people at risk of familial breast cancer and management of breast cancer and related risks in people with a family history of breast cancer. 2013 NICE clinical guideline 164 guidance.nice.org.uk/cg164

Zujewski JA, Kamin L. "http://www.ncbi.nlm.nih.gov/pubmed/18922117" Trial assessing individualized options for treatment for breast cancer: the TAILORx trial. Future Oncol 2008;4(5):603-10.

Gonzalez-Angulo AM, Barlow WE, Gralow JR, et al. A randomized phase III clinical trial of standard adjuvant endocrine therapy +/-chemotherapy in patients (pts) with 1-3 positive nodes, hormone receptor (HR)-positive and HER2-negative breast cancer with recurrence score (RS) of 25 or less: SWOG S1007 [abstract]. Cancer Res 2011;24(Suppl 3):Abstract OT1-03-01.

National Institute for Health and Clinical Excellence. Gene expression profiling and expanded immunohistochemistry tests for guiding adjuvant chemotherapy decisions in early breast cancer management: MammaPrint, Oncotype DX, IHC4 and Mammostrat. 2013 NICE diagnostics guideline 10 guidance.nice.org.uk/dg10

Immediate Reconstruction

A 48 year old lady has had her first screening mammogram which has shown 60mm of microcalcifications in the left breast. This appears to be away from the nipple and chest wall. She is asymptomatic and is otherwise fit and well. She wears a size 34B bra. No lesion is palpable and the lesion is occult on ultrasound. How would you proceed?

A vacuum assisted stereotactic guided biopsy would be performed in the first instance. This would usually be with a 10-11G needle, but if inconclusive this may need to be repeated with a larger bore needle (e.g. 7G)

Biopsy has confirmed the microcalcifications to be low/intermediate grade DCIS. What are the treatment options?

Given the size of the lesion relative to the size of the breast, breast conserving surgery is not appropriate. Mastectomy would be recommended. However, as adjuvant radiotherapy is unlikely in this situation, a skin sparing mastectomy, with or without nipple preservation, and immediate reconstruction would be an alternative to simple mastectomy. In either case a sentinel lymph node biopsy should also be performed at the same time as mastectomy.

When would you not preserve the nipple-areolar complex (NAC)?

If the micro-calcification extends to within 2cm of the nipple base, excision of the nipple is generally recommended to avoid a close surgical margin. If the nipple is preserved, the mastectomy specimen should be clearly orientated to denote the overlying nipple position e.g. with a silk loop. Whenever a nipple is preserved the patient must be informed that a small amount of ductal tissue will be left behind and that this incurs a very small chance of cancer recurrence in the future. In borderline cases, the patient may accept an attempt at nipple preservation in the knowledge that it may be necessary to partially excise the NAC under local anaesthetic should the margins be inadequate. In any case the entire NAC does not need to be sacrificed, only a central ellipse centred on the nipple. The remaining areolar skin provides a good base for a future nipple reconstruction and/or areolar tattooing.

After appropriate counselling she has opted for an immediate implant based reconstruction. What are the benefits of immediate reconstruction?

Immediate breast reconstruction preserves the skin envelope, with or without the NAC, and this provides the surgeon with the optimal blueprint on which to base their reconstruction. This offers the potential for a single stage reconstruction which can be advantageous to both the patient and the health care provider in reducing hospital admissions. In addition, the patient does not suffer the loss of body image and the inevitable asymmetry simple mastectomy incurs.

Are you implying patients undergoing Immediate Breast Reconstruction (IBR) are more satisfied than Delayed Breast Reconstruction (DBR)?

No, in fact the National Mastectomy and Breast Reconstruction Audit (NMBRA) reported that patients undergoing DBR reported the highest satisfaction rates of all. However, IBR provides the opportunity to preserve the skin envelope and even the best DBRs cannot improve on that.

What are the key principles in marking the patient and choice of incision?

The patient must be marked pre-operatively in the upright position with a high quality marker. Strict attention to the footprint of the breast is essential to achieve a high quality reconstruction, both in marking pre-operatively and performing the mastectomy itself. In particular preservation of the infra-mammary and lateral mammary folds are key manoeuvres.

Incision choice is determined by a number of variables including size of the breast, patient co-morbidities, surgical preference and whether the NAC is being preserved or not. In cases of NAC preservation peripheral incisions in the IMF or lateral mammary fold (allowing good access to the axilla) are preferable. However these incisions provide more challenging access, particularly in a larger or more ptotic breast. In the larger breast a partial peri-areolar incision with a small radial extension may be more appropriate. Care must be taken not to extend too far around the NAC border as this will increase the risk of NAC necrosis. Ultimately the choice of incision must not compromise the ability of the surgeon to perform a high quality mastectomy.

Are there any potential disadvantages to IBR?

Simple mastectomy is a reproducible and standard technique with a predictable and low rate of complications. IBR involves greater operative duration and technical expertise. The type and rate of complications varies significantly depending on the type of reconstructive technique, however all IBR carry greater risk of complications than mastectomy alone. Therefore there is a potential for a significant complication that may delay subsequent adjuvant treatments and compromise their oncological efficacy. Patient selection and patient education are key components of a successful reconstructive journey.

What advantages and disadvantages does an implant-based technique have?

Implant based reconstructions are the most common type of immediate reconstruction currently being performed in the UK. They avoid donor-site morbidity and do not preclude any future autologous reconstructive options. Donor site complications were also reported in up to 11% of cases in the NMBRA. Length of hospital stay, subsequent recovery and post-operative pain are all superior compared to autologous reconstruction.

Disadvantages of implant based reconstructions include that they often fail to recreate breast ptosis and thus are more suitable for reconstructing smaller, non-ptotic breasts or in bilateral reconstruction cases. Patients are more likely to develop progressive asymmetry as the normal breast becomes more ptotic with time. There are also the complications associated with implants (capsular contracture, rupture, rotation) with up to half of patients requiring revisional procedures within the first 10 years according to the US core study data. The most common indication for revisionary surgery is capsular contracture. The most devastating complication is infection and subsequent explantation which was reported at 9% within 3 months in the NMBRA.

What implants are commonly used in breast reconstruction?

Implants are either fixed volume or adjustable volume. Adjustable volume implants are either pure tissue expanders which are temporary e.g. Allergan style 133, or hybrid permanent expanders e.g. Allergan style 150, which can provide a definitive solution through a fixed volume silicone compartment and adjacent adjustable saline compartment. Fixed volume implants are either 'anatomical' or 'round' in shape.

How would you categorise approaches to immediate implant based breast reconstruction?

Implant based reconstruction is either 1 stage or 2 stage. One stage reconstruction can only be performed in IBR in the context of a carefully dissected healthy skin envelope where there is no intention to increase breast volume. Two stage reconstruction whereby the initial tissue expander is subsequently replaced with a definitive implant is appropriate if there are any concerns over the skin envelope viability, surgeon preference or if the patient wishes to increase their breast volume. One stage reconstruction avoids committing every patient to a second operation. Two stage reconstruction offers the opportunity to make any minor adjustments to the pocket to improve the aesthetic outcome.

What techniques of immediate implant based reconstruction are you aware of?

Complete submuscular implant coverage is less commonly performed in the advent of biological and synthetic scaffolds. Controlling the implant position is difficult and dissection of serratus anterior or rectus abdominis pockets results in increased post-operative pain. Partial sub-pectoral coverage using a dual plane technique remains a popular technique as it avoids the potential complications of using internal scaffolds. However, care must be taken to respect the breast footprint, maintain a good quality envelope and carefully suture the infero-lateral edge of pectoralis major to the skin envelope to limit its retraction.

An inferiorly based de-epithelialised dermal flap is an appropriate technique in medium-large ptotic breasts. This provides immediately well-vascularised tissue coverage of the lower pole of the implant beneath a wise pattern type scar.

If a dermal flap technique is not appropriate, various biological and synthetic matrices have been developed to act as an internal sling for the lower and lateral aspects of the implant. These can provide excellent short and midterm results. There is a relative lack of truly long term data to inform whether these matrices alter the natural history of implant breast reconstruction such that long term patient satisfaction is achieved. These products have a high initial cost and there is a learning curve associated with their use in order to avoid such complications as prolonged seroma and/or infection. Meticulous patient selection, surgical technique and aggressive intervention to prevent escalation of complications are essential.

What peri-operative factors could you take into account to minimise potential morbidity in this case?

To minimise infection risk, I would screen all patients for MRSA and MSSA prior to admission. If there was evidence of another concomitant infection of other body systems, postponing surgery should be considered until this was treated. I would also plan to give a single intravenous dose of antibiotics on induction.

Inadequate peri-operative analgesia was another significant finding of the NMBRA with 20% of patients reporting severe pain in the first 24 hours after surgery. This can be reduced with use of regional anaesthetic blocks (intrapleural, paravertebral, interpectoral) and the use of short term (<48 hrs) indwelling catheters, which provide a sustained dose of local anaesthesia. This can reduce the dependency on opioid analgesia and aid post-operative mobilisation reducing thromboembolic risk.

What are the relative and absolute contraindications to immediate breast reconstruction?*

There are few absolute contraindications to breast reconstruction, the main one being patient choice. However, careful patient selection and the choice of method are crucial to reconstructive outcome.

Relative contraindications include smoking, diabetes, obesity, need for adjuvant treatment (especially postmastectomy radiotherapy), advanced age and the presence of advanced disease. Where you draw the line depends on the context, including number of relative contraindications, co-morbidities, method of reconstruction under consideration and patient expectations. For example, most would consider it contraindicated to perform an immediate Deep Inferior Epigastric Perforator (DIEP) flap reconstruction in a smoker with a BMI of 45 and poorly controlled diabetes, with a triple negative cancer requiring adjuvant chemotherapy. However, a fit healthy smoker with no other contraindications could be appropriately counselled regarding the increased risk of complications following implant-based reconstruction.

In the presence of relative contraindications, patient counselling is crucial to ensure they have realistic expectations regarding what can be achieved, their chance of complications and the impact of a potential delay in adjuvant treatment. The option of simple mastectomy followed by delayed reconstruction once they have completed adjuvant treatment should be discussed, particularly where modification of risk factors in the intervening time period (e.g stopping smoking, losing weight) may reduce the chance of complications and thereby increase the chance of a successful reconstruction.

Be prepared to justify what YOU would do

Incidental Finding of Breast Lesion

You have requested a CT colonography as an outpatient for a 65year old lady with change in bowel habit. No other symptoms were reported. There were no significant intra-abdominal findings but a soft tissue density was reported in the lower left breast. How would you proceed?

Although asymptomatic this patient will require triple assessment in a breast clinic. After taking an appropriate history particularly assessing for previous symptoms, imaging performed (both in clinics and on previous screening mammograms) will determine whether this is a new finding. CT images are inadequate and initially bilateral 2 view mammograms (cranio-caudal and mediolateral oblique views) and ultrasound of the left breast would be performed. If the lesion was clinically and/or radiologically indeterminate or suspicious then a core biopsy would be performed, ideally under image guidance. If the lesion was clinically and/or radiologically suspicious then ultrasound scanning of the axilla should also be performed with aspiration cytology or tissue biopsy of any abnormal appearing node(s).

Clinical assessment was normal. Ultrasound of the left breast and axilla was unremarkable. Mammograms of the left breast however have shown a 3cm suspicious calcified area in the lower outer quadrant of the left breast. Mammogram of the right breast was normal. How would you proceed?

As the suspicious area is clinically impalpable and not visible on ultrasound, a stereotactic core biopsy would need to be performed. A vacuum-assisted biopsy technique could also be utilised to obtain a greater volume of tissue sampling for analysis. Following biopsy a radiological marker clip would also be inserted into the sampled area to aid future localisation or monitoring.

Biopsy has confirmed intermediate grade DCIS. What is DCIS and what treatment options are available?

Ductal Carcinoma in situ (DCIS) is pre-invasive breast cancer. Malignant epithelial cells remain confined within an intact basement membrane. The majority of DCIS (>90%) is impalpable and asymptomatic, being detected by breast screening or as an incidental finding. Symptomatic DCIS can present as a mass, with nipple discharge or Paget's disease (eczematous changes) of the nipple. Low and intermediate grade DCIS develop and progress in a different pattern to high grade DCIS and are viewed as separate entities. The natural history of DCIS is still not completely understood. The majority of cases of high grade DCIS will develop into invasive ductal cancer over a shorter timeframe (2-3 years). A minority of cases of low and intermediate grade DCIS will progress to invasive cancer thought this may take several decades. It would be uncommon for low grade DCIS to progress to high grade DCIS. Given the risk of progression to invasive disease surgical excision is currently recommended for DCIS. A prospective UK wide audit of screen detected DCIS (Sloane project) has been running for more than 10 years to help our understanding of this condition.

Breast conserving surgery is the treatment of choice for DCIS if lesions are small (<4cm) relative to the size of the breast. Poorer cosmetic outcomes result when more than 20% of breast volume is resected. Therapeutic mammoplasty (a modified type of breast reduction) can be offered in larger breasted women and may allow breast conserving surgery for slightly larger lesions. As in this case impalpable DCIS is usually localised with radiological guided wire placement prior to surgery. A mammogram of the specimen is also performed immediately following excision to help ensure complete removal. Alternative techniques using radioisotope localisation have also been developed.

When would you consider axillary surgery?

Axillary surgery for DCIS in the absence of any invasive disease is not usually performed for breast conserving surgery; however there are instances when sentinel lymph node biopsy (SLNB) would be considered. The main instance is when mastectomy is the surgical choice as SLNB cannot be subsequently performed if an invasive focus is confirmed on final histology. A mastectomy would be considered for extensive DCIS or by patient choice if they were unable to accept the risk of the need for a second breast operation if excision and margins (aim for 1-2mm) were incomplete.

If microinvasion (invasion <1mm) is confirmed on core biopsy or the DCIS presents as a mass then there is a higher likelihood for invasive disease being confirmed on final histology. In these instances SLNB would be strongly considered, and if not performed concomitantly with wide local excision the patient would be made aware of the potential need for a subsequent SLNB procedure to stage the axilla. An invasive focus is also more likely to be discovered in symptomatic DCIS.

When would adjuvant therapies be recommended?

Adjuvant radiotherapy would be considered following breast conserving surgery for high grade DCIS usually around 6 weeks after surgery. Although this has been proven to reduce local recurrence and the development of ipsilateral invasive cancer, there is no effect on overall survival. Radiotherapy would also be considered if the histological feature of comedo necrosis was present, or following discussion in MDT if margins could not be surgically improved for larger areas of low/intermediate grade DCIS. Radiotherapy following mastectomy for DCIS is currently not recommended in the absence of any invasive disease.

The current evidence does not support the use of adjuvant endocrine therapy for DCIS outside a trial setting in UK practice. IBIS II is a recently reported international double blind randomised placebo-controlled trial (n=4000) in assessing the use of Anastrazole in post menopausal women deemed at high risk of breast cancer. This included patients with prior DCIS. After 5 years the number of breast cancers developed in the Anastrazole treatment group was less than half of that in the placebo group.

There is no role for chemotherapy in DCIS. The Van Nuys Prognostic Index has been previously linked as an algorithm for predicting the likelihood of recurrence. The parameters included tumour size, margin width and certain histological features. However this was a US retrospective study and is not directly applicable to our practice as the majority of large tumours which recurred would have undergone a mastectomy in the UK.

Management of Indeterminate Breast Lesions

What do you understand by the term 'B3 lesion'?

B3 breast lesions are indeterminate lesions with uncertain malignant potential. They are often detected during breast screening and include:

- Papillary lesions

- Radial scars and complex sclerosing lesions

- Classic lobular neoplasia, including lobular carcinoma in situ (LCIS) and atypical lobular hyperplasia (ALH)

- Atypical ductal hyperplasia (ADH)

- Flat epithelial atypia (FEA)

- Phyllodes tumour / cellular fibroepithelial lesions

These cases should be discussed in the MDT with correlation between imaging and pathological findings before planning further diagnostic or therapeutic interventions.

What indeterminate breast lesions are associated with an increased risk of breast cancer?

- LCIS – relative risk 7

- ALH – relative risk uncertain but less than LCIS

- ADH – relative risk 4-5

- Usual type ductal hyperplasia (UDH) – relative risk 1.5-2

- Columnar cell lesions – relative risk 1.5

- FEA – uncertain significance, possibly a precursor to low grade DCIS

- Multiple papillomas – relative risk 2-5, depending on the presence of atypia

- Radial scars / complex sclerosing lesions – relative risk 1.5

What is lobular carcinoma in situ and how should it be managed?

In contrast to DCIS, classical LCIS is not a malignant precursor lesion, but it is associated with a seven-fold increased incidence of invasive breast cancer in both breasts. This translates to an annual risk of breast cancer of 1%. According to the 2009 ABS guidelines, LCIS should be excised by VACB or open surgical biopsy for definitive diagnosis and to rule out the presence of invasive cancer. There is no need for a margin. Following this the patient should undergo annual mammography for 5 years. Patient data should be entered into the Sloane project.

If the pathological diagnosis is pleomorphic rather than classical LCIS, this is considered a B5 lesion, as it behaves in a similar manner to DCIS. These lesions should be treated as DCIS with therapeutic excision.

A 63 year old fit and well lady is recalled from the National Breast Screening Programme with 10mm of indeterminate microcalcification in the right breast (M3). There are no significant features in her history and clinical examination and USS is unremarkable. She underwent core biopsy under stereotactic guidance and the histology has confirmed the presence of atypical ductal hyperplasia (B3). How are you going to manage her?

The diagnostic differentiation between ADH and DCIS is quantitative only, with ADH being diagnosed in the presence of epithelial hyperplasia in up to 2 ducts and less than 2mm in size. Therefore the lesion should be completely excised, preferably by VACB, to ensure that this lesion is not DCIS which would require surgical treatment. At the time of VACB excision a clip should be left in situ to aid localisation if the lesion was found to be DCIS.

If the diagnosis of ADH was confirmed I would explain to her that this confers an increased risk of breast cancer, with a relative risk of three to five times that of the general population. She will require surveillance with annual mammography for 5 years.

A 57 year old lady presents to the one stop breast clinic with unilateral blood stained nipple discharge. There are no significant features in her history and, apart from the presence of discharge, clinical examination is unremarkable. Mammography is normal but there is a 10mm well circumscribed intraductal lesion suggestive of a papilloma seen on USS (U3). Describe the next steps in your management.

She requires completion of triple assessment with USS guided core biopsy or VACB. If the papilloma is unequivocally benign she will not require further treatment. However, it may not be possible to get a definitive diagnosis with core biopsy and in these circumstances excision is recommended with either VACB or open surgical biopsy to rule out the presence of ADH or DCIS which can be present in papillomas. If VACB is performed a clip should be left in situ to aid localisation in case she requires further surgery.

Reference

Association of Breast Surgery at BASO 2009. Surgical guidelines for the management of breast cancer. Eur J Surg Oncol 2009;35(Suppl 1):1-22.

Metastatic Disease Presenting as Abdominal Pain

A 70 year old lady is admitted with generalised abdominal pain, nausea and back pain. She has a history of breast cancer 15 years ago in which she underwent a right mastectomy and nodal clearance. She took Tamoxifen for 5 years and has long been discharged from follow up. How would you manage this?

Although there are several possible causes for her abdominal pain, I am concerned that this may represent hypercalcaemia of malignancy. This would be confirmed on serum electrolytes performed after initially resuscitating the patient with oxygen and fluids. Cardiac monitoring would also need to be instigated for ECG changes (increased PR interval, shortened QT interval and flattened or inverted T waves) or arrhythmias.

Management of acute hypercalcaemia (>3.0 mmol/L) is predominantly with fluid rehydration. Central venous pressure monitoring may be required in a critical care setting to prevent fluid overload. Furosemide can be added to aid the calcium diuresis.

How would you confirm this diagnosis?

Clinical assessment may show signs of locoregional recurrence. CA 15-3 levels may also be raised. However, the patient would need to be staged with a CT of the chest, abdomen and pelvis and an isotope bone scan. MRI of the spine and plain X-ray views may also need to be considered if initial imaging is inconclusive and needs further correlation. If possible the original histology result and confirmation of prior adjuvant therapies would help to determine management.

Staging investigations have shown multiple osteolytic areas in the thoracic vertebrae suspicious of metastases. No visceral abnormalities have been detected and both clinically and radiologically there are no signs of local recurrence. Details of her original cancer histology cannot be located. CA 15-3 is raised (>200). How would you proceed?

Despite the clinical suspicions of bone metastases, CT guided bone biopsy would aid confirmation of the diagnosis, particularly if there was no other visceral lesion to biopsy. Bisphosphonates should be commenced. They help further reduce skeletal complications by inhibiting osteoclast activity, resulting in reduced bone resorption and reducing the likelihood of pathological fractures. They also reduce bone pain palliating symptoms alongside other analgesics. Pamidronate (90mg) and Zolendronic acid (4mg) are intravenous preparations given in 4 weekly intervals. Clodronate and Ibandronate are oral bisphosphonates that have similar effectiveness though gastrointestinal disturbance is more common with oral preparations. Patients are advised to take them with a full glass of fluid and remain upright immediately after to minimise the disturbance.

What other complications are associated with bisphosphonates?

Bisphosphonates can cause renal impairment through various mechanisms including focal glomerulosclerosis. Due to this, renal function should be monitored during treatment and temporarily discontinued if the renal function deteriorates.

Jaw osteonecrosis is an uncommon complication of bisphosphonates usually affecting the mandible. This is more likely following dental extraction and it is advised that therapy is suspended prior to and after any planned dental procedure. Treatment of osteonecrosis is generally conservative with infection management, pain control and debridement of necrotic bone where feasible. Increasing age and duration of treatment are also factors that can increase the likelihood of osteonecrosis.

Bone biopsy has confirmed metastatic cancer which is ER (7/8), PgR (8/8) and Herceptin (HER2) receptor negative. What other management options are available?

Specific targeted endocrine therapy can be commenced as the metastases are both Oestrogen and Progesterone receptor sensitive. This would initially be in the form of an aromatase inhibitor, usually Letrozole, 2.5mg daily. Bone mineral density would also need to be assessed with a DEXA (dual energy X-ray absorption) scan to assess for osteopaenia or osteoporosis. This is a recognised side effect of aromatase inhibitors. Appropriate bone health can be aided with calcium and vitamin D supplementation. If however osteoporosis is already established then Tamoxifen 20mg daily would be a suitable alternative, to minimise the risk of a subsequent osteoporotic fracture.

Palliative radiotherapy can also be considered either as single or multiple fractions in areas not responding to treatment or analgesics. Spinal stabilisation is considered in selected cases or if there are signs of nerve root or spinal cord compression. Given systemic therapy can be provided with endocrine manipulation, palliative chemotherapy would not be initially considered unless there was no response to treatment or there was evidence of disease progression with visceral metastases.

Neoadjuvant Chemotherapy

What is neo adjuvant treatment and when is it indicated?

It is the use of therapeutic systemic agents prior to operative surgery. In the context of breast cancer, it typically takes the form of chemotherapy (NCTx) or endocrine (NEx) treatment.

NCTx is first line management for inflammatory breast cancer (Stage T4d). NCTx may be indicated in locally advanced or inoperable tumours whereby downstaging may facilitate breast conserving surgery (BCS). NCTx may also convert a node positive axilla to a node negative axilla. The type of axillary surgery performed in this situation is uncertain.

How important is tumour biology?

Tumour biology is crucial. The diagnosis of invasive cancer including ER, PR and HER2 status should be established pre-operatively via image guided core biopsy.

Grade 3 triple receptor negative breast cancer typically responds well to cytotoxic chemotherapy despite a poorer prognosis overall. HER2 positive cancers typically respond well to chemotherapy plus targeted biological treatments (e.g. Trastuzumab) given the inherent traits of increased proliferation and inadequate DNA repair capabilities.

Pathological complete response (pCR) is more likely in triple negative tumours e.g. in 1,118 patients receiving Anthracycline Taxane chemotherapy, pCR rates were 22% versus 11% in triple negative and non triple negative patients respectively.

Which cancers are not suitable for neo-adjuvant treatment?

NEx

- ER/PR negative tumours
- ER/PR positive, HER2 positive cancers which are relatively hormone resistant
- For pre-menopausal patients NCTx is preferred

NCTx

- Invasive lobular cancers are relatively chemo resistant
- Grade I/II, ER/PR positive, HER2 negative i.e. luminal A cancers. Luminal B cancers with higher proliferation may still respond well to NCTx.

What is Pathological Complete Response (pCR)? Why is this important?

This is diagnosed when there is no histopathological evidence of invasive or non invasive cancer in the resected breast tissue or axillary lymph nodes (ITCs are disregarded).

pCR is regarded as a surrogate end point for improved disease free survival and overall survival, particularly in ER negative and/or HER2 positive patients. This subset of patients tends to have a very favourable outcome. However the majority of triple receptor negative cancers undergoing NCTx will not achieve pCR. This translates to a poorer prognosis overall, reflecting the underlying heterogeneity present within this disease subtype. Less than complete pathological response in ER positive patients is more difficult to interpret as they will still receive endocrine treatment.

What is combination therapy in the context of HER2 positive disease?

Combination therapy represents the addition of a targeted biological agent (e.g. Trazumatab) to cytotoxic chemotherapy. Several large studies (NEOSPHERE) have demonstrated huge increases in pCR rates with the addition of a targeted biological agent.

What is the HER2 receptor and how does overexpression alter cellular function?

It is a protein that is a member of the type 1 growth factor receptor and tyrosine kinase family. HER2 positivity (overexpression) alters cellular function by:

- Increased growth/proliferation
- Decreased differentiation
- Increased cell survival
- Increased motility
- Increased neo-angiogenesis
- Reduced oestrogen dependency and insensitivity to hormonal blockade

How does targeted treatment differ from chemotherapy?

Chemotherapy affects all cells based on the assumption that cancerous cells have an impaired capacity to sustain injury and regenerate relative to normal cells. Targeted treatments target abnormal cancer cells in a specific manner, thereby sparing non-cancerous cells.

How does Trastuzumab work?

Various mechanisms of action have been described, including:

- inhibition of signal transduction pathways (e.g. the RAS-MAPK pathway and the PI3K-AKT-mTOR pathway)
- blocking of cleavage of the extracellular domain
- endocytosis and degradation of the receptor
- inhibition of angiogenesis

- inhibition of DNA damage repair
- immune-mediated response

Do you know of any other biological agents used in breast cancer?

Pertuzumab inhibits HER2 forming dimer pairs resulting in a dense blockade of HER signalling. Trastuzumab and Pertuzumab bind to different regions of the HER receptor, thus in combination this results in synergistic activity and increased pCR.

What preparation is required prior to commencing NCTx?

- If T3 or node positive, CT chest, abdomen and pelvis +/- bone scan
- Baseline MRI to be repeated mid treatment and at the end of treatment to assess radiological response
- Marker clip should be inserted at the commencement of NCTx in case of
- complete radiological response
- Standard investigations to assess patient fitness e.g. MUGA scan

When should surgery be planned and when should SLNB be performed?

Breast cancer resection is usually planned 3-4 weeks following the last cycle of chemotherapy.

In the context of a clinically and radiologically node negative patient, sentinel node biopsy can be performed before or after NCTx as per ASCO guidelines. There is no universal consensus regarding what is a hotly debated topic. SLNB post-NCTx offers the potential to avoid axillary clearance in those patients who undergo pCR. However, dual localisation is advised to minimise the risk of a false negative SNB, as false negative rates are recognised to be higher following NCTx.

In those patients in whom a positive SNB requires axillary treatment, this can take the form of axillary radiotherapy, thereby achieving equivalent local control with less morbidity (AMAROS). This is a particularly attractive option in those patients due to receive whole breast irradiation.

How would you manage the axilla in a patient who had proven axillary metastasis at the time of diagnosis but who has undergone NCTx and has achieved a complete radiological response?

The standard of care would be to perform formal axillary clearance post NCTx. Some surgeons would advocate a more limited axillary dissection if the initial axillary nodal burden was felt to be low.

In a patient who has achieved a complete radiological response thereby facilitating BCS, how much tissue should be removed at wide local excision?

Wide local excision will be wire guided, centred on the marker clip. There are no national guidelines advising on volume of resection and a common sense approach is required. There is no point attempting wide local excision if the tumour response to NCTx appears poor. Similarly, there is no point resecting the original size of the cancer if the radiological response is significant. A representative well orientated specimen will allow the pathologist to assess the degree of response.

How does the pattern of tumour response vary between NCTx and NEx treatment?

Whilst the pattern of response can vary within these treatments, in general NEx results in concentric shrinkage of the tumour, whereas NCTx can result in a more diffuse patchy response in the absence of pCR. NEx generally takes longer to demonstrate effect.

Can you name an accepted NCTx regimen and what adjuvant treatments are required subsequently?

An Anthracycline and Taxane regimen is usually used. HER2 positive patients will continue on Herceptin. All hormone sensitive cancers will require endocrine treatment. Adjuvant whole breast irradiation is indicated in all patients undergoing BCS. Post mastectomy radiotherapy is dependent on pre-NCTx tumour size (≥ 5 cm), tumour position (< 1 mm to chest wall), degree of nodal burden (≥ 4 involved nodes) or any patient diagnosed with inflammatory breast cancer.

Can you describe the T section of the TNM tumour classification for breast cancer?

The T section relates to tumour size and relation to local structures.

- TiS = DCIS
- T1 = tumour 2 cm or less
- T2 = > 2 cm < 5 cm
- T3 = > 5 cm
- T4a = chest wall involvement
- T4b = skin involvement
- T4c = chest wall and skin involvement
- T4d = inflammatory cancer

References

Krag DN, Anderson SJ, Julian TB et al. Sentinel-lymph-node resection compared with conventional axillary-lymph-node dissection in clinically node-negative patients with breast cancer: overall survival findings from the NSABP B-32 randomised phase 3 trial. *Lancet Oncol* 2010; **11**(10): 927-933

Veronesi U, Paganelli G, Viale G et al. A randomized comparison of sentinel-node biopsy with routine axillary dissection in breast cancer. *N Engl J Med* 2003; **349**:546-53

Mansel RE, Fallowfield L, Kissin M et al. Randomised multicentre trial of sentinel node biopsy versus standard axillary treatment in operable breast cancer: The ALMANAC Trial. *J Natl Cancer Inst* 2006; **98**:599-609

Giuliano AE, Hunt KK, Ballman KV, et al. Axillary dissection vs no axillary dissection in women with invasive breast cancer and sentinel node metastasis: a randomised clinical trial. *JAMA* 2011;**305**:569-75

Baildam A, Bishop H, Boland G et al. Oncoplastic breast surgery--a guide to good practice. Association of Breast Surgery at BASO; Association of Breast Surgery at BAPRAS; Training Interface Group in Breast Surgery. *Eur J Surg Oncol.* 2007;33 Suppl 1:S1-23.

https://www.nice.org.uk/guidance/CG164 [accessed 01/10/14] Familial breast cancer: Classification and care of people at risk of familial breast cancer and management of breast cancer and related risks in people with a family history of breast cancer

http://www.bapras.org.uk/downloaddoc.asp?id=899 [accessed 01/10/14] Oncoplastic Breast Reconstruction Guidelines for Best Practice

http://data.gov.uk/dataset/national-mastectomy-and-breast-reconstruction-audit [accessed 01/10/14] National Mastectomy and Breast Reconstruction Audit, Fourth Annual Report - 2011

COLORECTAL SURGERY

**Alan Horgan Mike Lim Sonia Lockwood
Sudakhar Mangam Alexander Phillips Irshad Shaikh**

Contents

Anal Cancer

A 45 year old man presents with a history of anal pain and bleeding. He reports occasional pruritus, and no incontinence. This has been getting progressively worse over the last six months. Digital rectal examination in clinic is painful with suggestion of a mass just palpable. The patient would not tolerate proctoscopy or rigid sigmoidoscopy. How would you further investigate this patient?

Given the suggestion of a mass, examination under anaesthesia (EUA) would be the most useful next step. Clinical examination to exclude inguinal lymphadenopathy should be done. EUA would allow assessment of the mass and an opportunity to biopsy the mass. I would also perform a colonoscopy to exclude synchronous or metachronous lesions and request an urgent staging CT Scan (chest, abdomen and pelvis) for distant disease. Local staging should be done either with MRI or endoanal ultrasound depending on expertise.

Examination under GA reveals a 1cm plaque-like irregular lesion 4cm from the anal verge. Colonoscopy was otherwise unremarkable. The biopsy reported this as high grade AIN III. What are the treatment options?

In this patient there is a 1cm lesion. It is possible that a sampling error has occurred and that a carcinoma may coexist. Complete local excision can be done to obtain accurate histology, and if there is no invasive component, observation with regular 6 monthly follow-up. The natural history of the disease is unclear to warrant radical surgery. Topical imiquimod or infrared photocoagulation therapy is recommended for large areas of field change and certainly works for AIN 1 and II. Localised areas may be excised but anal stenosis may occur. All cases of AIN require regular mapping biopsies or high resolution anoscopy with acetic acid. Extensive areas should make one think of the immunosuppressed patient and can be difficult to cure. Curative excision may require wide debridement and should be done with a defunctioning colostomy and skin grafting to facilitate healing.

What is Bowen's disease?

This is another name for intraepithelial squamous cell carcinoma in situ. Many patients with Bowen's disease will have or are at risk of developing one or more primary internal malignancies, or will develop a primary cancer of the skin. Other terms include anal intraepithelial lesion (AIN), anal dysplasia and squamous intraepithelial lesion. AIN is graded from I to III which corresponds to the depth of invasion of dysplasia, with each grade representing a further one third involvement.

What are the risk factors for anal cancers?

Up to 90% of cases can be attributed to HPV particularly HPV-16 and HPV-18. The two of them account for approximately 70% of cervical cancers, and a

similar or higher proportion of anal cancers. Smoking increases the risk fourfold
– the underlying cause is unclear although this may be due to it interfering with
apoptosis or leading to a level of immunosuppression. HIV infection, and patients
receiving immunosuppressants are also at increased risk.

How would you stage a squamous cell carcinoma of the anal canal?

This is based on size of the tumour and lymph node involvement and should
involve MRI to determine the extent of the disease. Lymph node involvement
correlates with the size of the tumour. It is extremely low in tumours under 2cm in
size and occurs in up to 25% of tumours between 2cm and 5cm and two thirds of
tumours greater than 5cm.

AJCC classification-

T1< 2cm
T2 2-5cm
T3 >5cm
T4 Tumour invading deep structures (vagina, urethra, bladder, not sphincter).

Regional lymph nodes (N)	
NX	Regional lymph nodes cannot be assessed
N0	No regional lymph node metastasis
N1	Metastasis in perirectal lymph node(s)
N2	Metastasis in unilateral internal iliac and/or inguinal lymph node(s)
N3	Metastasis in perirectal and inguinal lymph nodes and/or bilateral internal iliac and/or inguinal lymph nodes
Distant metastasis (M)	
M0	No distant metastasis
M1	Distant metastasis

What treatment options are available for proven squamous cell carcinoma of the anal canal?

First line treatment is usually chemoradiotherapy which negates the requirement
for radical surgery. Chemoradiotherapy follows the Modified Nigro regimen
(5FU Mitomycin C and 50Gy DXT). There is an 80% cure rate following this
regimen. This also has the advantage of preserving sphincter function, although
some patients may report post treatment incontinence. Salvage abdominoperineal
resection is reserved for recurrence or persistent disease, particularly those with
bulky T4 disease where it may be difficult to achieve a complete pathological
response.

What would you consider doing and telling a patient with locally advanced T4 squamous cell carcinoma that you would not necessarily do in a patient with early disease?

First, the patient may need a defunctioning colostomy or ileostomy prior to commencement of chemoradiotherapy. Radiotherapy induced large bowel obstruction can occur, particularly in those with pre-existing difficulty with rectal evacuation. A subgroup of patients can also develop severe incontinence and fistula with treatment.

Secondly (as mentioned above) extensive disease may require salvage surgery and a permanent colostomy. Third, any perineal surgery after curative irradiation can be technically challenging and is almost always associated with poor healing. There is some evidence to suggest that the resultant defect heals better with the use of myocutaneous flaps (the most popular being the vertical rectus abdominis) when compared with primary closure. However, dehiscence can still occur, perhaps to a lesser degree.

The same patient has palpable lymph nodes in the right groin. What is the implication of inguinal lymph node involvement and how would you manage it?

This may be present in up to 25% of patients presenting with anal cancers. However, lymphadenopathy may be reactive inflammatory rather than metastatic. MRI and PET-CT may give you an idea morphologically and physiologically but really an FNA for cytology is needed to be 100 per cent accurate. If positive for metastasis, the prognosis is less good and alteration to the radiotherapy field to include the right inguinal region is needed.

Anal Pain

You are reviewing a 24 year old female in clinic who is complaining of a 3 month history of severe anal pain after defaecation. She has noticed the passage of a small amount of fresh blood particularly on wiping. She gives a life long history of constipation. What is the most likely diagnosis and what might you find on examination?

This lady has given a good history of an anal fissure. Anal fissures present in the midline and should be visible in the midline posteriorly or anteriorly and can be identified on gentle parting of the buttocks. Per rectal examination and proctoscopy is rarely possible. Atypical fissures seen elsewhere on the anal verge should raise the suspicion of Crohn's disease, sexually transmitted diseases e.g. gonorrhoea, chlamydia or syphilis or indeed anal cancer. Nicorandil has been associated with unusual anal ulcerations. If there are other worrying symptoms and features, an urgent EUA should be arranged.

You confirm an anal fissure. How would you treat this patient and how successful are you likely to be?

First, I would recommend dietary modification, perianal hygiene advice and stool bulking agents or softeners. Second, I would also commence treatment with either topical GTN 0.2% or topical diltiazem 2%. I favour the latter as it results in less headache and is associated with better patient compliance. Topical treatments have a success rate of between 60% to 70%. The patient needs to be warned that even in those who achieve healing, recurrence may occur in half of all patients. Success rates of topical treatment are dependent on the type of fissure (higher for acute rather than chronic) and patient compliance.

What is the underlying pathophysiology for chronic anal fissures?

The exact etiology of anal fissures is unknown, but the initiating factor is thought to be trauma from the passage of a particularly hard or painful bowel movement. Studies have identified at least one abnormality in the internal anal sphincter of many anal fissure patients. Common abnormalities are hypertonicity and hypertrophy of the internal anal sphincter, leading to elevated anal canal and sphincter resting pressures.

The posterior anal commissure is the most poorly perfused part of the anal canal. In patients with hypertrophied internal anal sphincters, this delicate blood supply is further compromised, thus rendering the posterior midline of the anal canal relatively ischaemic, accounting for poor spontaneous healing, even after many months.

You review this lady in a further clinic and the diltiazem has had little impact. What other options are available?

If topical treatment has been unsuccessful the next treatment would be to carry out an EUA and botulinum toxin (type A) injection. This involves injection of approximately 40-50 international units of botox directly into the internal anal sphincter at two sites equidistant from the fissure. Success rates of up to 90% are quoted for uncomplicated fissures.

What risks should you consent the patient for?

Patients should be warned that there is a risk of urgency and incontinence. This is usually flatus, however faecal incontinence has also been reported. Any incontinence is usually transient but may persist for up to 6 weeks post injection. This can be in the range of 5% to 10% for incontinence of flatus and is less for faecal incontinence. Other significant complication/risks include perianal sepsis and failure/fissure recurrence.

If botox fails to work in this lady, how would you then proceed?

One option is to repeat the administration of botox (with a higher dose i.e 60-80 international units) particularly if the patient had partial response or transient response to the first treatment. A biopsy of the area should also be considered if the fissure is in a position other than the midline (and also in older patients) to exclude malignancy or inflammatory bowel conditions.

If she continues to fail to respond I would consider performing ano-rectal physiology to confirm that she has high resting pressures (secondary to hypertonicity and hypertrophy of the internal sphincters). In patients with low or normal sphincter pressures, it is likely that the fissure is secondary to something else. More importantly, patients with low pressures do not do well with any sphincterotomy, be it chemical or surgical. Sphincterotomies are particularly dangerous in young women who are of a child bearing age. Any damage to sphincters after a surgical sphincterotomy is irreversible and is likely to be compounded by childbirth. If she fails to respond to botox administration, I would consider a fissurectomy with Y-V cutaneous advancement flap. This should be done by a colorectal surgeon.

When would you consider a sphincterotomy and how would you do one? Is it always successful?

A lateral internal sphincterotomy is usually reserved for male patients. On the rare occasion, a lateral sphincterotomy may be considered as a last resort in females who are post partum and have high resting pressures on anorectal physiology. All patients who have a sphincterotomy should have clear documentation regarding risk/benefits. I would limit the sphincterotomy to the height of the fissure and I would perform it at a site away from the fissure under direct visualisation of the internal sphincter. A sharp blade and Eissenhammer retractor is usually necessary.

Lateral sphincterotomy has a recurrence or non-healing rate of between 1%-6%. Although lateral internal sphincterotomy heals and relieves symptoms of chronic anal fissure in nearly all patients, incontinence can occur. Most episodes are indeed minor and transient but significant incontinence is higher in females and may be permanent in 6%-8% of cases. In a review of four prospective randomized controlled trials, Shao et al concluded that surgery, specifically lateral internal sphincterotomy, is more effective than botox treatment for healing chronic anal fissures. In their analysis of the studies, which involved a total of 279 patients, the investigators found that the absolute benefit increase rate was 23% for the surgical patients in comparison with the botox-treated patients. However, minor anal incontinence occurred more frequently with lateral internal sphincterotomy than it did with botox.

References

Shao WJ, Li GC, Zhang ZK. Systematic review and meta-analysis of randomized controlled trials comparing botulinum toxin injection with lateral internal sphincterotomy for chronic anal fissure. *Int J Colorectal Dis.* Mar 6 2009

Nelson RL, Thomas K, Morgan J, Jones A. Non surgical therapy for anal fissure. Cochrane Database Syst Rev. 2012 Feb 15;2:CD003431.

Colon Cancer

You are seeing a new referral from a GP – a normally fit and healthy 40 year old man with a 6 month history of generalised crampy abdominal pain. His GP has done routine bloods and he has an Hb of 11.6, MCV 76, CRP 18. There is no family history of bowel complaints. How will you investigate this gentleman?

The bloods reveal a microcytic anaemia which may be related to iron deficiency and chronic GI blood loss. I would check his haematinics and iron levels. There are numerous causes for GI blood loss and the differential diagnosis includes inflammatory bowel disease (Crohn's or UC), colorectal cancer, coeliac disease or infective colitis. A full history and examination should be carried out, focusing on any change of bowel habit or passage of blood PR. Given the history of lower GI symptoms a colonoscopy would be the first investigation of choice. However if this was entirely normal an OGD should be considered with D2 biopsies to exclude coeliac disease, or a small bowel study or MRE to rule out Crohn's disease. A faecal calprotectin test could also be considered.

Colonoscopy reveals an impassable ascending colonic lesion, which appears to be an adenocarcinoma. What further investigations should be arranged and what would you tell the patient?

After the endoscopy and any sedation has worn off it should be explained (also to any next of kin) that a suspicious growth has been identified which has been biopsied. Ideally I would have the cancer nurse specialist present as well. It is more than likely that this is a cancer. Further investigations need to be carried out, but as it appears to be causing obstructing symptoms (the crampy pains) surgical resection may be required imminently.

A staging CT chest, abdomen and pelvis should be urgently performed. This gentleman should also be discussed at a specialist colorectal MDT once the results are available, and the outcome discussed with the patient as soon as possible.

What operation would you perform, and what complications would you counsel the patient about?

A laparoscopic right hemicolectomy would be the procedure of choice. Possible complications include general surgical complications such as bleeding, infection and deep venous thrombosis and pulmonary embolism. Complications specific to this procedure include anastomotic leak, stoma formation and ureteric, vascular or visceral injury. Patients should be counselled on the risk of conversion to open resection.

Histology shows a poorly differentiated mucinous adenocarcinoma. There is invasion just beyond the muscularis propria, and 0 out of 40 lymph nodes are involved. There is no vascular or lymphatic invasion. There is florid and extensive perineural invasion. At what stage is this tumour?

T3 N0 Mx.(Duke's B). Stage II colorectal cancer.

Primary tumour (T)	
TX	Primary tumour cannot be assessed
T0	No evidence of primary tumour
Tis	Carcinoma in situ: intraepithelial or invasion of lamina propria
T1	Tumour invades submucosa
T2	Tumour invades muscularis propria
T3	Tumour invades through the muscularis propria into the pericolorectal tissues
T4a	Tumour penetrates to the surface of the visceral peritoneum
T4b	Tumour directly invades or is adherent to other organs or structures
Regional lymph nodes (N)	
NX	Regional lymph nodes cannot be assessed
N0	No regional lymph node metastasis
N1	Metastasis in 1-3 regional lymph nodes
N2	Metastasis in 4 or more lymph nodes
Distant metastasis (M)	
M0	No distant metastasis
M1	Distant metastasis

Stage	TNM Status
I	T1-2, N0,M0
II	T3-4, N0,M0
III	ANY N1 STAGE
IV	ANY M1 STAGE

Does this patient need chemotherapy?

This histology needs to be discussed at an MDT. However, there are no lymph nodes involved, which is a good prognostic factor, but the fact that it is poorly differentiated and has evidence of perineural invasion and the patient's young age would suggest that chemotherapy should be considered and the risk benefits discussed with the patient. Some would regard impending obstruction as a poor prognostic feature too. Adjuvantonline.com can be used to help gauge the benefit of chemotherapy.

The patient is anxious about having chemotherapy and wants to know what drugs to expect and what the side effects are, especially regarding hair loss. What do you inform him?

Adjuvant chemotherapy is for six months, although the SCOT trial (Short Course Oncology Therapy) has just finished recruiting (November 2013) to determine if treatment can be shortened to 3 months without impact on outcome. Standard treatment is 8 cycles of intravenous oxaliplatin and 5-fluorouracil (5-FU). Capecitabine is an oral 5-FU equivalent (XELOX/FOLFOX/CAPOX). The oxaliplatin is given as an infusion at the start of each cycle and the patient is commenced on two weeks of capecitabine tablets twice daily followed by a rest week.

There are a number of side effects that can be experienced with this regimen. Most patients however, do not lose their hair. The most common are lethargy, diarrhoea or constipation. Oxaliplatin is also associated with a heightened sensitivity to cold, which can be problematic in cold climates and can make eating cold food and drinks uncomfortable.

What follow up investigations will this patient need?

Most centres will have their own follow up protocols, as yet there is no consensus about a specific follow-up regime. Most centres would recommend a combination of CEA measurements, endoscopic surveillance and CT imaging at suitable intervals, usually for the first 5 years after curative surgery. The results of the FACS (follow-up after colorectal surgery, published January 2014) trial demonstrated that identification of recurrences were three-fold higher with intensive follow-up, but identification did not lead to statistical difference on cancer survival. In terms of numbers needed to treat, one would have to follow-up 15-20 patients intensively to identify a patient who may undergo potentially curative resection of metastasis. This raises issues of cost-effectiveness.

Additionally, this patient should be referred for genetic counselling given his age to determine subsequent surveillance protocol after the standard colorectal cancer follow up has ceased and to determine risk to siblings and offspring.

Colonoscopy and Polyps

You are performing a colonoscopy list and are asked to consent the patient for the procedure. What are the important things to consider?

After identifying the correct patient the indication for the procedure should be checked and also that the patient has received the appropriate bowel preparation. Specifically to this procedure the important consideration is the risk of perforation, which is usually quoted as around 1/2000 for a colonoscopy. Risk increases if any intervention or biopsies are required. This may necessitate a stay in hospital or even surgical intervention. Other risks include bleeding and abdominal discomfort. Sedation and its associated risks should also be discussed.

Briefly outline how you would perform the procedure?

I would confirm whether the patient wants intravenous sedation or would prefer to use entonox. They would be positioned in the left lateral position and having administered the appropriate sedation I would inform that I was going to perform a PR prior to introducing the endoscope. The basic technique for navigating the colon is to use torque as far as possible to try and minimise looping. I would note any abnormalities and aim to carry out any biopsies on withdrawal. Confirmation that I had intubated the caecum is from identification of the appendiceal orifice and triradiate fold, and also by transillumination. Withdrawal of the scope should take approximately 10 minutes to aid identification of any abnormalities.

How do you classify colonic polyps?

These can be largely classified into three broad subheadings:

Epithelial

Adenoma: tubular / tubulovillous / villous

Metaplastic polyp

Mesodermal

Lipoma

Leiomyoma

Haemangioma

Other rare tumours

Hamartoma

Juvenile polyps: the commonest polyp in children

Peutz-Jeghers polyp

In the above patient, as well as observing sigmoid diverticular disease, you remove a 7mm tubulovillous adenoma from the sigmoid colon. What follow-up, if any, should this patient have?

Patients found to have an adenoma at colonoscopy are graded as being low, intermediate or high risk. This patient would be regarded as being low risk as the criteria stipulates 1-2 adenomas less than 1cm. In this cohort BSG guidelines would suggest either no follow up or a further colonoscopy in 5 years. If the latter course is followed they should be discharged after repeat colonoscopy if there is no evidence of any further polyps. Other factors to consider are age, comorbidities and accuracy and completeness of the procedure.

What is the management of intermediate and high risk patients?

Intermediate risk patients are defined as 3-4 small adenomas (<1cm) or one adenoma >1cm in size. These should have further surveillance at three year intervals with follow-up stopped after two negative colonoscopies. High risk patients are regarded as those with 5 or more adenomas or three or more with at least one >1cm, these should have annual follow up and will be regarded as intermediate risk after a negative colonoscopy.

You are called to see this patient 30 minutes after the procedure as he is complaining of severe abdominal pain, he has a distended abdomen and is tachycardic. How would you proceed?

This patient may have a perforation secondary to the colonoscopy - he needs appropriate resuscitation with fluids, oxygen, analgesia and antibiotics. Examination and erect CXR or CT may confirm the diagnosis. A laparoscopic resection should then be discussed with the patient. Depending on the state of the bowel and site of perforation, it would be reasonable to carry out a primary repair (small defect and healthy tissue) or a resection and anastomosis (big defect and unhealthy tissue) as there should be minimal contamination thanks to the bowel preparation required for the colonoscopy.

The next male patient is 18 years old and has been referred in for a flexible sigmoidoscopy as he has been having painless rectal bleeding for the last 3 months. You see over 20 polyps in his rectum and they all appear adenomatous. What are your thoughts?

I would be concerned about him having familial adenomatous polyposis (FAP). I would arrange for him to have an upper GI endoscopy, full colonoscopy and genetic assessment. Patients with FAP have a tendency towards polyp formation throughout the entire GI tract and may also have extra-colonic manifestations: ectoderm (eye and brain), mesoderm (dental, bone, desmoids) and endoderm (adrenal, thyroid, biliary).

He appears to have no other family members with this problem. He is concerned about the implications of your findings. What do you say?

I would tell him that he requires more testing and I would refer him on to a geneticist. Genetic testing identifies the defective gene 95 percent of the time. Although FAP tends to be familial, up to 15 per cent of cases are sporadic. The faulty gene is located on chromosome 5 and inheritance is autosomal dominant. This means that he has a one in two chance of passing his gene on to any of his children. If he has FAP, then he requires endoscopic surveillance. As he has established polyps already, he requires yearly colonoscopy. He also requires upper GI endoscopy (with a side viewing endoscope to assess the ampulla) every two years.

He wants to know why you have to keep performing endoscopies?

The risk of colorectal cancer is extremely high in patients with FAP. Almost all patients with FAP eventually develop a cancer. Most patients are encouraged to have surgery before reaching 30 years. Colonic surveillance begins in the teens and use of aspirin/COX-2 inhibition/sulindac may slow progression.

Surgical options for the colon include:

a) Subtotal colectomy with ileorectal anastomosis (favoured if they have rectal sparing or are older at time of presentation). Results in fewer problems with bladder and bowel function, erections and ejaculations are maintained but this requires commitment on the individual to stick with biannual surveillance of the rectum

b) Proctocolectomy with end ileostomy formation

c) Restorative proctocolectomy with ileoanal pouch

On the upper GI side, polyps develop with similar frequency within the duodenum. Spigelman's classification allows for the determination of surveillance frequency from annually to five yearly. The score is the summation of polyp size, number, type and presence of dysplasia. If the calculated score is >9, one may have to consider a pylorus preserving pancreatico-duodenectomy.

What is Peutz-Jeghers syndrome?

This is a polyposis syndrome inherited in an autosomal dominant fashion associated with a mutation in the tumour suppressor gene STK11 on chromosome 19. It is characterised by numerous hamartomotous polyps in the stomach, small intestine, and colon. These are benign with low malignant potential. Patients also may have spots containing melanin on the skin and mucous membranes, especially of the lips and gums. Patients may suffer from intussusception often before the age of 18. They have a lifetime risk of all cancers of approximately 85%, and 60% for GI cancer.

References

W S Atkin, B P Saunders Surveillance guidelines after removal of colorectal adenomatous polyps Gut 2002;51:v6-v9 doi:10.1136/gut.51.suppl_5.v6

Adenoma surveillance: http://www.cancerscreening.nhs.uk/bowel/publications/nhsbcsp-guidance-note-1.pdf

Crohn's Disease

You are on a post-take ward round reviewing a 25 year old lady complaining of generalised crampy abdominal pain for three months. She has lost 3kg in weight and denies any other bowel symptoms. Examination reveals a fullness in the right iliac fossa. How would you proceed?

This history suggests ileocolic Crohn's disease, although other possibilities exist including an appendix mass, ileocaecal tuberculosis or even a malignancy (which is unlikely given the patient's age). A CT scan should be performed to confirm the diagnosis along with blood tests to look for evidence of anaemia and an inflammatory process (FBC/U&E/CRP).

The CT scan suggests a likely diagnosis of ileocolic Crohn's disease. There is thickening of the terminal ileum and collapsed proximal colon with an obvious phlegmon. How would you manage this?

The CT suggests Crohn's and there may be a degree of obstruction - although this is not clinically apparent at the moment. Further tests may be necessary such as faecal calprotectin, MRE and sigmoidoscopy. Colonoscopy is dangerous in someone with 'impending' obstruction because of the need for bowel preparation. Although the case should be discussed and managed jointly with a consultant gastroenterologist there is a general reluctance for treatment to be commenced without histological confirmation of inflammatory bowel disease. Treatment with steroids can be commenced provided intra abdominal sepsis has been ruled out, and the patient should be monitored very closely.

The patient asks you what is the likelihood that she will need surgery?

The crampy abdominal pain suggests intermittent obstruction, which would be an indication that surgery is likely to be required, although the impact of the steroids remains to be seen. This would help with acute inflammation but not with any chronic stricture that may have developed. Even if she does not require surgery on this occasion there is an 80% chance she will require a resection within the next five years. After an initial resection there is a further 25% chance of a further resection being required in the next five years, which rises to approximately 40% at 10 years.

The patient would like to know what Crohn's disease is and whether it would affect her for the rest of her life? Can she do anything to reduce her chance of recurrence?

Crohn's is defined as chronic transmural inflammation of the bowel wall that may affect the gastrointestinal tract anywhere from mouth to anus. Rectal involvement is rare although perianal disease is not uncommon. There is a rise in the incidence of Crohn's disease worldwide for unknown reasons although ulcerative colitis remains the more common of the two. The majority of patients with Crohn's disease lead a fairly normal life but 20%-30% have severe restrictions of their working ability. The commonest age group to be affected is between 30 and 40 years of age, with men affected more commonly than women. The condition is rare in Asia and Africa and is predominantly a disease of the West.

The exact pathogenesis is unclear but the condition is characterised by an exaggerated inflammatory response at the mucosal level. There is interplay between genetic and environmental factors with a variety of mechanisms proposed. DNA from patients with Crohn's has isolated *Mycobacterium paratuberculosis,* measles and *Listeria monocytogenes.* This would suggest that these infective pathogens might play a role in the pathogenesis. The NOD2/CARD15 gene on the IBD1 locus of chromosome 16 has been implicated as proof of a genetic component of the disease.

The patient should be advised to stop smoking and encouraged to seek cessation advice. Smoking has been shown to be harmful and significantly increases the risk of relapse.

The patient has noted an exacerbation of mouth ulcers, dyspepsia and rashes on her legs preceding her current admission. Are you surprised by this?

No. Crohn's disease affects the entire gastrointestinal tract and has numerous extra-intestinal manifestations. The extra-intestinal manifestations of Crohn's are divided according to the affected system as well as whether or not they are related to disease activity.

Disease activity related:

- Erythema nodosum
- Pyoderma gangreonosum: usually multiple lesions that may affect not only the leg but also scars and stoma sites
- Arthropathy: usually affects a single large joint during exacerbations, but small joints may be affected otherwise
- Uveitis
- Iritis

Non-disease activity related:

- Ankylosing spondylitis: seen in 5% of Crohn's patients and is usually HLA-B27 positive
- Primary sclerosing cholangitis

In terms of distribution, the terminal ileum is most commonly affected (30%-50%). Other areas include small bowel (30%-35%), colon (25%-30%), perianal Crohn's (>50%) and gastroduodenal (5%). Crohn's can also be classified according to the Montreal classification: Age (A1 under 17, A2: 17 to 40 to A3: above 40), Location (L1 ileal, L2 colonic, L3 both, L4 upper GI) Behaviour (B1: non-strictured non-penetrating, B2: strictured, B3: penetrating, P: perianal)

How would you assess response to treatment in this lady?

Response to steroids in this lady would be done clinically. Symptom improvement, vital signs with clinical examination and haematological parameters such as haemoglobin, white cell count and CRP would indicate whether the patient is responding to treatment. There are also research tools such as the Crohn's Disease Activity and Harvey-Bradshaw Indices that can be used to assess for a response.

Despite 48 hours of intravenous steroids, your patient is failing to improve. On the ward round this morning she is noted to be pyrexial and tachycardic. The pain that was confined to area over the mass yesterday appears to be more generalised today. What would you do?

There has been a change of her clinical condition from yesterday. I am concerned that the phlegmon has now progressed to an abscess or worse, perforated. Intravenous steroids can mask clinical signs and dampen the immune response to sepsis – so this patient could be very sick and may become even more unwell over the next few hours. I would consider the use of antibiotics now, and arrange for her to have urgent repeat imaging.

The repeat CT scan shows free air and a large collection around the phlegmon. The distal small bowel is intimately involved with this phlegmon/abscess. The patient has been transferred to the high dependency unit and wants to know what you will do next? If surgery is indicated what will you do?

She requires a laparotomy, washout and resection of the diseased small bowel. Small bowel resection should be as conservative as possible because surgery is never curative. However, leaving diseased bowel behind in a sick septic patient is also unwise. Patients with untreated Crohn's disease die of sepsis, liver failure and thromboembolism.

I would be very reluctant to re-anastomose her. She is likely to be nutritionally depleted with a low albumin, and this, along with contamination, and immunosuppression due to steroid use, would make this high risk. The lady would be better served with an ileostomy and allowed to recover before considering restoring intestinal continuity in the future.

What are the macroscopic and microscopic pathological features you would expect to find within the resected specimen?

Macroscopic: Skin lesions, mesenteric fat wrapping and strictures may be seen which can vary from 1 cm to 30 cms. There may be associated proximal dilatation and distal collapsed segments. An inflammatory mass/phlegmon with or without fistulation to adjacent organs may occur. There may also be mesenteric lymphadenopathy and local perforation with abscess formation may be evident. On opening a specimen you may see oedematous mucosa with intervening linear ulcers on the mesenteric side of the lumen, giving rise to a cobblestone appearance. Deep fissuring may arise from the ulcerations that extend through the bowel wall.

Microscopic: Non-caseating granuloma is one of the pathological hallmarks of Crohn's disease. Mucosal lymphoid aggregates, transmural inflammation with thickening of the muscularis propria and muscularis mucosa. Further, chronic inflammatory infiltration (lymphocytes) and histiocytic cell proliferation may be seen. Preservation of goblet cell mucin – mucin depletion is a feature of UC.

How easy is it to distinguish UC from Crohn's disease on pathology?

Sometimes it is very difficult even for experienced GI pathologists to differentiate between the two. Approximately 10%-15% of cases are termed indeterminate colitis for this very reason. Over the course of time the clinical pattern of the disease may declare itself thereby changing the diagnosis from one to another.

Your patient has recovered from her surgery and wishes to know if there are any drugs to prevent recurrence when she has restoration of intestinal continuity?

While steroids can be used to treat an acute flare of Crohn's it is not recommended for long term prevention due to its side effects. Budesonide has fewer side effects as its release is pH dependent. Once absorbed into the portal circulation 90% of the drug undergoes first-pass metabolism. Thus only 10% is systemically absorbed thereby reducing systemic side effects. However, this is still not recommended for prevention of recurrence.

5-aminosalicylic preparations and thiopurines (azathioprine and 6-mercaptopurine) have been shown to reduce recurrence of Crohn's but the benefit is small, duration of treatment is long and side-effects can be rather prohibitive. Azathioprine requires close monitoring and serum TPMT – transpurine methyl transferase levels should be checked as 5% of individuals have a deficiency of this enzyme, which normally acts to metabolise azathioprine. Toxic levels can develop in patients with such a deficiency. A FBC and LFT should also be done as a baseline to assess neutrophil count and liver enzyme status.

Biologic treatment with anti-tumour necrosis factor antibodies are on the rise. Two randomised studies (with infliximab and adalumimab respectively) have shown benefit in reducing endoscopic recurrence. Follow-up was short and recurrence appeared upon cessation of treatment. The benefit of using these drugs has to be balanced against the risk. These include:

a) Anaphylaxis

b) Loss of efficacy because of the development of antibodies

c) Reactivation of tuberculosis and hepatitis

d) Rare but lethal: Development of lymphoma and skin malignancies

Finally, your patient wishes to get pregnant soon. Does Crohn's affect fertility rate and should she stop any of her medication to prevent harm to the baby?

In short, unless she has had pelvic surgery, there should be no reduction to her fecundity. Untreated active disease can also affect her ability to conceive so any active disease should be controlled with medication.

5-ASA based preparations are safe to be continued in females (but not males due to sperm alteration which is reversible after 2 months of cessation), and likewise corticosteroids and thiopurines are safe throughout pregnancy. Data on the new biologics are lacking, but results from recent studies indicate that they are safe. Metronidazole may not be safe after the first trimester and methotrexate is teratogenic. This drug must be discontinued at least 3 months prior to conceiving.

Diverticular Disease

You are reviewing a 58 year old lady in outpatient clinic who has been complaining of intermittent left iliac fossa pain for the last year and a change in bowel habit. What are your concerns and how would you investigate this lady?

Although her symptoms may be from diverticular disesase there is a concern she may have an underlying colorectal cancer. The differential diagnosis would also include inflammatory bowel disease (UC or Crohn's), ischaemic colitis and tubo-ovarian pathology. Further exploration of the history in respect of the change in bowel habit, any weight loss, passage of blood and family history of bowel cancer should be elicited. As well as taking bloods to investigate for anaemia, an urgent outpatient colonoscopy should be arranged.

At colonoscopy there is no evidence of malignancy but the lady appears to have severe diverticular disease in the sigmoid colon. How would you explain these findings to the patient?

This patient should be reassured that the cause of her discomfort is benign and there is no evidence of cancer, and that colonoscopy is the gold standard for identifying bowel cancer provided the preparation has worked well. The finding of diverticular disease - a benign "pouching of the bowel" - should be explained and the need to achieve a regular bowel habit reiterated. Interestingly, a high fibre diet is no longer thought to prevent diverticulosis. The patient should be given written information / advice leaflet on discharge.

The patient re-presents two months later. She has localised left iliac fossa tenderness and is pyrexial. She is commenced on antibiotics and a CT demonstrates a 7cm x 10cm x 5cm pelvic collection. What would be your management?

The clinical and radiological features suggest perforated diverticulitis with abscess formation. Subsequent management is dependent on the clinical status of the patient. Management options include radiological drainage or laparoscopic washout and placement of pelvic drains if the patient is clinically stable. Radiological drainage can be performed under ultrasound or CT guidance. Remember to check coagulation profile in the presence of sepsis, prior to any intervention. Pus should be sent for MC&S. However, if the patient is septic and unstable a laparoscopic or open sigmoid resection maybe required.

What is the Hinchey Classification?

This is a classification used to grade levels of diverticular perforation:

Hinchey I – localised pericolic abscess

Hinchey II - pelvic abscess

Hinchey III - purulent peritonitis

Hinchey IV - faeculent peritonitis

The Hinchey classification is useful as it guides surgeons as to how conservative they can be. Recent studies have shown with anything up to a Hinchey III, a laparoscopic wash-out is a safe procedure, avoiding the need for a laparotomy and stoma formation.

What are the treatment options for a patient with perforated diverticular disease and generalised peritonitis?

This patient would need appropriate resuscitation, antibiotic treatment and urgent anaesthetic review. Conventional thinking would be to carry out a Hartmann's procedure for perforated diverticular disease. However, there are some who would advocate carrying out an initial diagnostic laparoscopy. In patients with purulent peritonitis rather than faeculent (Hinchey III rather than IV) and no obvious perforation, lavage and placement of abdominal drains has shown to be feasible with low short term recurrence (Myers et al). Some would also advocate a resection and primary anastomosis because of the high incidence of a permanent stoma (30%).

On balance, patients with perforated faeculent peritonitis are usually elderly and very sick and there is nothing to be gained by risking an anastomosis.

Her husband wishes to see you to discuss her previous management. According to the GP, she has had two previous admissions with abdominal pain and surgery should have been considered earlier. What do you say?

I would reassure him that the GP acted sensibly as symptomatic diverticulitis tends to respond to antibiotics. Surgery is clearly indicated for diverticular disease when symptomatic fistulation or perforation is present. Surgery is not to be taken lightly and is far from ideal. There is a significant risk of anastomotic leakage and permanent stoma rate in these patients. Moreover, diverticulosis and subsequent inflammation can recur adjacent to the resected bowel or even proximal to it. Surgery should therefore be reserved for those with repeated admissions, or those who have significant stenosis due to recurrent inflammation and stricture formation to 1) improve bowel function and 2) exclude concurrent sinister pathology.

Further reading

Toorenvliet, B.R., Swank, H., Schoones, J.W., Hamming, J.F. and Bemelman, W.A. Laparoscopic peritoneal lavage for perforated colonic diverticulitis: a systematic review. *Colorectal Disease* 12(9):862-7, 2010 Sep

Myers et al BJS 2008 Myers E, Hurley M, O'Sullivan GC, Kavanagh D, Wilson I, Winter DC. Laparoscopic peritoneal lavage for generalised peritonitis due to perforated diverticulitis. BR J Surg, 2008 Jan;95(1):97-101.

Early Rectal Cancer

You are reviewing an 80 year old lady who has undergone recent flexible sigmoidoscopy for PR bleeding. This demonstrated a 1.5cm mid-rectal polyp which was biopsied and has shown adenocarcinoma. What further investigations are required?

This lady needs to be fully staged which includes CT of chest abdomen and pelvis, MRI and endoanal ultrasound if available. Provided she is fit enough a completion colonoscopy or CT colonography should also be carried out.

What is the value of an endoanal ultrasound?

This is the best method for determining the depth of invasion of the tumour with an accuracy of 90%. It has a better specificity and similar sensitivity as MRI for T staging. Furthermore it allows lymph node assessment and has an accuracy of 80%.

What is the most important factor in determining the risk of malignancy of a polyp?

Size is the most important consideration with nearly 40% of those greater than 10mm having evidence of malignant transformation. The risk increases to nearly 80% in patients with polyps greater than 40mm.

Staging demonstrates no evidence of disease spread. Completion colonoscopy is normal and endoanal ultrasound demonstrates a T1 lesion. What are the treatment options?

The gold-standard treatment would be an anterior resection. The risk of concurrent lymph node metastasis is dependent on a) size of tumour, b) depth of submucosal invasion, c) presence of extramural and lymphovascular invasion and d) grade of tumour. Local excision deals with the primary lesion but not the potential of lymph node metastasis within the mesorectum. I would compare the risk from definitive surgery (and quality of life) versus the risk of recurrent disease and need for surveillance after local excision. Simple transanal excision, TAMIS (transanal minimally invasive surgery) or TEMS (transanal endoscopic microsurgery) are all possible and are dependent on the height and position of the lesion together with local expertise. All treatments should be discussed at an MDT and with the patient to determine their view.

At what stage of disease is TEMS regarded suitable?

Currently the ACPGBI recommends that local excision is appropriate for pT1 cancers which are graded well or moderately differentiated, and less than 3cm in diameter. TEMS may also be employed for selected T2 tumours in patients who are very frail. However, lymph node positivity is much higher in this T2 group of patients. TEMS for T3 tumours is a bad idea. Proponents of TEMS argue that those patients with more advanced tumours who undergo local excision followed by salvage radical surgery are not harmed. Published series do not show any increase in adverse outcomes compared with those who underwent radical surgery as their primary treatment.

What is the Kikuchi classification?

This is a classification for sessile polyps and is divided into three components dependent on the depth of invasion of the submucosa of a T1 tumour. These are classified SM1-3 and correspond to the superficial, intermediate and deep thirds of the submucosa. The purpose of this is to correlate depth of invasion with likelihood of lymph node involvement. There is a 1% -2% risk of lymph node involvement in SM1 tumours, 8% in SM2 and 23% in SM3.

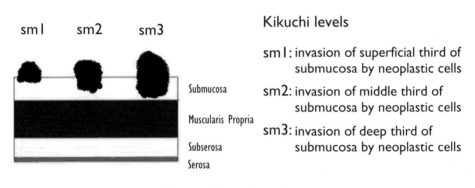

Taken from www.learncolorectalsurgery.com

What is the difference between the Kikuchi classification and the Haggitt level?

The former is used to classify sessile polyps while the latter is used for pedunculated polyps. The Haggitt classification runs from 0 to 4:-

0= Non invasive carcinoma in situ- ie intramucosal

1= Carcinoma invading through to the submucosa but confined to the head of the polyp

2= Carcinoma confined to the level of the neck of the polyp

3= Carcinoma invading the stalk of the polyp

4= Carcinoma invading into the submucosa of the bowel wall below the stalk but not into the muscularis propria

Thus, stages 0-3 of the Haggitt level equate to SM1 of the Kikuchi level

Is there any role of radiotherapy for patients who have had a TEMS procedure for a lesion with adverse features?

Theoretically, radiotherapy to the pelvis would deal with lymph node involvement within the mesorectum and local excision with the primary, and the combination of local surgery and radiotherapy would be potentially curative and preserve organ function. This is the focus of the TREC trial which is a randomised trial comparing local excision after short course preoperative radiotherapy with traditionally radical surgery in patients with T2 lesions without any other poor prognostic features. Most patients these days would be persuaded to radical surgery if local excision had poor prognostic features, however, a subset of very frail patients could be offered radiotherapy.

Reference

Bach S, et al A predictive model for local recurrence after transanal endoscopic microsurgery for rectal cancer *British Journal of Surgery* 2009; 96: 280–290

Enterocutaneous Fistulae

A 65 year old male undergoes an emergency laparotomy for strangulated small bowel in a parastomal hernia. He underwent a small bowel resection and repair of the parastomal hernia. His recovery was uneventful and he was discharged home on day 5 post op. He represents to the hospital on day 10 with leakage of small bowel content through the midline laparotomy wound. A diagnosis of enterocutaneous fistula is made. He is apyrexial and systemically well and does not have peritonitis.

What do you think is the aetiology of this fistula?

Although the majority of enterocutaneous fistulae develop secondary to surgery for inflammatory bowel disease or adhesiolysis they occasionally occur due to anastomotic breakdown, as in this case. This is more common in the emergency setting as well as malnutrition and previous radiotherapy. Enterocutaneous fistulae may develop spontaneously in Crohn's disease or diverticular disease.

Would you manage this patient with an operation and will you keep him nil by mouth?

In short, I may operate on him but not immediately. In terms of keeping him nil by mouth, it depends on a few factors.

The management of any patient with a fistula is divided into three phases. 1) Resuscitation, 2) Restitution and finally 3) Rehabilitation. Following resuscitation patients should be managed according to the 'SNAP' algorithm as part of the restitution phase.

Sepsis: Uncontrolled sepsis remains the major cause of mortality in these patients. In the presence of clinical evidence of sepsis, broad spectrum antibiotics should be commenced. Septic foci need to be identified using CT scanning. Remember the presence of contrast from other investigations may distort CT images so try and perform CT first. Once identified these foci are drained by percutaneous drainage using CT or USS guidance. Collections are sent to microbiology for urgent culture and sensitivities. Exploratory laparotomy must be avoided at all cost for fear of further damage to already fragile small bowel and is only indicated in patients with generalised peritonitis. Less is more in these patients!

Nutrition and fluid balance: The volume of the fistula dictates the means of nutritional and fluid support. Enteric support requires the presence of approximately 120 cm of functioning small bowel. If the predicted site of fistulation is proximal then volume is likely to be high. Skin care is important to the patient's well being. This is best achieved through involvement of stoma nurse therapists. Application of various skin-protective preparations to avoid skin maceration, cellulitis and cutaneous necrosis is useful. The effluent must be collected and measured as part of a strict fluid balance chart. Fistula volume can be reduced with proton pump inhibitors (check that effluent pH is >6 secondary to reduced gastric secretions), loperamide melts (up to 96mgs/24 period) and codeine phosphate (60mgs qds).

As a rule if it is less than 500mls/24hr period, then patients can eat and drink enterally and do not need to be nil by mouth. The use of isotonic oral fluids when palatable will help to minimise fistula output. If it is between 1-2L/24hr period, there are mixed views about the best treatment. Some would advocate allowing enteral intake with IV supplementation to replace fluid loss, however others would suggest this may prolong healing of the fistula and that parenteral nutrition should be used. If it is greater than 2L/24hr period, then patients usually require both parenteral nutrition and IV fluids. Adequate nutritional support is necessary to allow spontaneous closure of the fistula. Wherever possible enteric nutrition is encouraged with some suggesting that it has a trophic effect on the bowel mucosa and preserves immune function thus reducing bacterial translocation although bacterial translocation is probably a normal occurrence which only becomes apparent in patients where the normal mechanisms for dealing with this are compromised. TPN, when required, should be administered via a dedicated feeding line. In addition to volume replacement, attention to calories (amino acids, triglycerides and carbohydrates), electrolytes, vitamins, and trace elements, is necessary on a regular basis.

Anatomy: As opposed to sepsis and nutrition, there is no rush to delineate anatomy. This requires close collaboration with gastrointestinal radiologists. Often CT is adequate but sometimes contrast small bowel follow-through or contrast enemas (fistulograms) are necessary to exclude distal obstruction.

Plan procedure: As a rule, if the above is addressed and a fistula has not reduced its output significantly by a 4–5-week period it is unlikely that the fistula will close spontaneously. This raises the question as to when it is next best to operate.

When would you consider a re-laparotomy? Are there any practical guidelines?

In short, the longer you leave it the easier the operation becomes. I would leave it for about 6 months if possible. This is largely because the adhesions mellow and the abdominal cavity re-peritonealises whereby sites of fistulation begin to develop small bowel spouts. Patients should not be malnourished and if possible should cope with discharge back to their home for a period of rehabilitation. In patients who have persistent sepsis (intra-abdominal or line related), distal obstruction or active disease not amenable to medical control, surgery may have to be expedited.

What technical aspects of the re-laparotomy do you have to consider before performing the definitive operation?

Bowel: Careful adhesiolysis must be done to minimise the number of enterotomies. In patients with multiple repair sites and tenuous bowel (eg previous radiotherapy) a proximal defunctioning stoma (despite its high output and electrolyte issues) may be considered to avoid further intra-abdominal catastrophe should any of the suture lines fail. Place omentum over the bowel so that it is protected ventrally.

<u>Fascia</u>: The majority of patients with straightforward fistulae can be closed primarily without problems. In those with complex fistulae, some patients also have a concurrent laparostomy, incisional hernia and poor abdominal wall domain. Closure of the fascial defect is best done without the use of any mesh. A component separation technique to release the rectus sheath is useful to gain 5cms on each side, but larger defects may require a bridging technique with use of a biological mesh. Protection of small bowel is the key, as long as there is omentum and minimally reacting mesh over bowel, it is out of harm's way.

<u>Skin:</u> The quality of skin can be poor in individuals with laparostomies. Full thickness skin grafts can be employed by those with plastic expertise but epithelialisation and imbibition can be difficult after closure of fascia. Often the use of a VAC dressing is necessary, but this must be used cautiously in those with mesh and poorly protected bowel. VAC induced re-fistulation is probably over reported in the literature, as use for short periods with minimal negative pressure are safe in my experience.

Further reading

Pritts TA, Fischer DA, Fischer JE. Postoperative enterocutaneous fistula. http://www.ncbi.nlm.nih.gov/books/NBK6914/

Faecal Incontinence

A 28 year old lady six months post partum has been referred to the outpatient clinic with faecal incontinence. How would you proceed?

I would take a detailed history of her symptoms including incontinence for flatus, liquid or solid faeces, whether passive or on straining, the frequency, urgency and the consistency of stools. I would enquire of any associated bleeding or mucus discharge or a history of urinary incontinence. I would also take a detailed past medical history of trauma, inflammatory bowel disease, chronic diarrhoea, rectal prolapse, fistula in ano, anal fissures, haemorrhoids and surgical history especially perineal. History of neurological and congenital problems is vital as is detailed obstetric history.

How would you investigate this patient?

I would start with a general physical examination as well as abdominal and neurological examination. I would then do a digital rectal examination and rigid sigmoidoscopy.

What would you assess on digital rectal examination?

I would initially look for any signs of perianal lesions including anal fissure, fistulae, scars, perianal excoriation. I would then assess the degree of perineal descent by asking the patient to bear down. I would assess the resting anal pressure (internal anal sphincter), and then ask the patient to squeeze to assess the voluntary squeeze pressure (external anal sphincter). I would then do a bi-digital exam of the external sphincter in a relaxed state to assess any defects. I would then ask again to contract to assess the puborectalis sling. I would look for any rectocele as well as internal rectal intussusception. In the process I would rule out any mass lesions in the anal canal and rectum. It is sometimes possible to assess for any enterocele or sigmoidocele. I would complete the examination with a proctoscopy and rigid sigmoidoscopy. Per Vaginal examination may be valuable in some cases.

What other investigations would you like to order?

I would request a colonoscopy to rule out any significant colonic pathology. We then obtain a full anorectal physiology assessment. These include endo-anal ultrasound to image the sphincters, anorectal manometry, defecating proctogram (if obstructive defection is suspected), rectal compliance.

What are the treatment options?

Treatment options comprising conservative treatment include biofeedback and physiotherapy. Surgical options include sacral nerve stimulation, sphincter repairs and sphincter augmentation procedures and artificial sphincters.

What are the basic principles of sphincter repairs?

Direct repair of the damaged sphincter, plication and augmenting or replacing the sphincter muscle may be performed. Care must be taken to avoid too much lateral dissection to mobilise the sphincter as it can damage the neurovascular bundle to the external sphincter. A stoma is not routinely required.

Can you describe the procedure?

The patient is prepped in lithotomy position. We approach the sphincter through a transverse curvilinear incision anteriorly in the skin between the anal verge and the vaginal introitus. The skin flap is raised and the external sphincter is identified and dissected. The incision may need to be extended laterally, but care must be taken not to extend it too far. In my experience the distinction between the external and internal sphincter in such cases is difficult due to scarring, but on occasions the plane can be separated. The external sphincter would be bulky as it is dissected more laterally. The external sphincter when dissected is teased off the recto-vaginal septum. Dissection in the recto-vaginal septum is carried to identify the levator muscles, which also need plication stitches.

If the external sphincter is completely divided then the two ends need to be apposed, if associated with excessive scarring, then the division through scar tissue is advocated. I would suture together the two ends of the external sphincter with interrupted 2-0 PDS with an overlapping 2-layer technique.

Reference

Brown SR1, Wadhawan H, Nelson RL. Surgery for faecal incontinence in adults. Cochrane Database Syst Rev. 2013 Jul 2;7:

Familial Adenomatous Polyposis (FAP)

You are about to see a 25 year old lady with Gardner's syndrome who has had a restorative proctocolectomy and now has an end ileostomy.

What is Gardner's syndrome?

Familial adenomatous polyposis when associated with desmoid tumours.

Why would she have had a restorative proctocolectomy?

Restorative proctocolectomy is usually offered as a prophylactic operation before cancer develops. The other options are colectomy with ileo rectal anastomosis (IRA) (dependent on the status of the rectal polyps) and total proctocolectomy with end ileostomy.

What is meant by pouch failure and rate?

Pouch failure may be defined as the clinical situation when the pouch needs to be excised or a permanent diversion needs to be created. Early failure rate ranges from 5% -10%, but longer term failure rate has been quoted at 10% at 10 years. The most common reason for pouch failure is pelvic sepsis (50%), followed by poor function and pouchitis.

How would you follow up a patient with desmoid tumours ?

A variety of approaches are used depending on the size and complication due to desmoid tumours. This include watch and wait, surgery, radiotherapy, anti-oestrogens, NSAIDs and chemotherapy.

CT scan is the common modality of investigation. However MRI is a better choice and more useful to evaluate recurrence.

How would you deal with desmoids intraperitoneal/extraperitoneal ?

Surgery is the last resort for desmoid tumours especially intraperitoneal lesions. They are best left alone unless causing a complication. There is evidence that surgery may be useful for extraperitoneal desmoids but the recurrence rate is high. When managed conservatively intraabdominal desmoids need regular follow up and an abdominal ultrasound scan to rule out ureteric obstruction.

What follow up would you organise for patients with FAP?

All patients would require yearly follow up. I would carry out clinical examination with digital rectal examination and flexible sigmoidoscopy at least every 12 months for patients who had RPC or IRA.

I would also organize an OGD to rule out duodenal malignancy between 1 and 5 years depending on the severity of duodenal polyposis.

What is the incidence of duodenal polyposis in FAP?

More than 90% of patients have duodenal polyps, but this is severe in only 10%. Malignancy has been reported in about 5%.

Why would a patient with FAP undergo a duodenal resection?

The reason for surgery may be that she now has a very high/large polyp load in the duodenum causing obstruction or there may be evidence of malignancy.

What are the options for duodenal polyps?

Close surveillance and monitoring, endoscopic therapy especially argon plasma coagulation. (Endoscopic polypectomy is associated with high recurrence rate). Pancreatico-duodenectomy is advocated usually in patients with invasive cancer.

Reference

A Companion to specialist surgical practice: Colorectal Surgery, 4th edition. Penna C, Bataille N, Baladur P et al. Surgical treatment of severe duodenal polyposis in familial adenomatous polyposis. British Journal of Surgery 1998;85:665-8

Haemorrhoids

You are reviewing a 40 year old lady who complains of painful haemorrhoids.

How may haemorrhoids present?

The commonest symptom of haemorrhoids is rectal bleeding. Patients may describe a palpable lump, usually noticed after defecation, that can be reduced by the patient or reduces spontaneously. Other symptoms include perianal discomfort, pruritis ani and mucus discharge. Haemorrhoids cause pain when they thrombose.

What is the classification of haemorrhoids?

They are usually classified as first degree to fourth degree:-

First degree: these bleed but do not prolapse. They are not visible on inspection of the anus and are not palpable on PR but can be visualised on proctoscopy. They slide below the dentate line on straining.

Second degree: these prolapse through the anal margin but reduce spontaneously.

Third degree: these prolapse and require manual reduction.

Fourth degree: are prolapsed and irreducible.

They can also be classed as internal or external haemorrhoids.

Internal haemorrhoids originate from the anorectal mucosa above the dentate line. These are the classic piles classified as above.

External haemorrhoids occur at the anal-skin margin. These originate from below the dentate line and are covered with sensate epithelium.

What are anal skin tags?

Anal skin tags are excess skin growths that usually occur at the anal opening, where the inside of the anorectal canal joins with the outside of the body. They are not contagious and are very common, often found in connection with other anal conditions. Anal skin tags usually occur as a result of an inflammatory lesion, anal injury or trauma.

What are the complications of prolapsed haemorrhoids?

Ulceration and bleeding

Thrombosis – of the submucous veins causing pain

What are the treatment options for thrombosed external haemorrhoids?

These may be extremely painful with a peak at 48-72 hours. Conservative treatment may be employed which involves stool softeners, the use of local anaesthetic gel, and ice packs. Rarely do patients require a haemorrhoidectomy in the acute setting.

The above patient has never tried any treatment for her haemorrhoids. How would you proceed?

First line treatment is usually provided in the primary care setting. This includes suppositories, stool softeners and dietary advice. Anusol with hydrocortisone will help with perianal symptoms or pruritus and should be trialled for seven to ten days.

Any rectal bleeding should be investigated with flexible sigmoidoscopy (especially in those aged over 35 years) to rule out colorectal malignancy or inflammatory bowel disease. Banding is successful in up to 70% of patients with grade I / II haemorrhoids and can be performed either in the outpatient clinic or at endoscopy.

Surgical management is indicated in recurrent disease (ie bleeding), Grade IV haemorrhoids, and haemorrhoids with a large external component. The surgical options include:

HALO

Stapled haemorrhoidectomy

Formal surgical haemorrhoidectomy

What are the surgical indications for formal haemorrhoidectomy of internal haemorrhoids?

- Refractory to usual treatment
- Significantly prolapsing haemorrhoids
- Large external haemorrhoids

What is a stapled haemorrhoidopexy?

Stapled haemorrhoidopexy or PPH (procedure for prolapsed haemorrhoids) is used to treat third and fourth degree haemorrhoids rather than formal resectional haemorrhoidectomy. It may also be used in patients with less severe haemorrhoids who have failed conservative treatment.

It involves the use of a circular stapler that excises a strip of mucosa from the anal canal which draws the haemorrhoid cushions proximally.

What other surgical options are available for treatment of haemorrhoids?

A conventional open surgical resection can be performed which may be a Milligan-Morgan or Ferguson procedure. The difference between them is that the wounds are left open in the former. Both procedures are regarded as being more painful than PPH and lead to a slower return to normal activities.

A HALO and RAR (haemorrhoid artery ligation operation and rectoanal repair) may also be performed. This involves using an ultrasound probe to identify the arteries and ligate. This is theoretically pain free as the ligation is performed above the dentate line. In patients with larger haemorrhoids the rectoanal repair may also be carried out which involves further sutures to "hitch" the haemorrhoids more proximally.

What are the late complications of open haemorrhoidectomy?

Secondary bleeding

Incontinence

Anal fissure

Anal stricture/stenosis

How do you proceed if you suspect anal stenosis?

I would like to obtain a history of previous surgery and establish the symptoms such as constipation, increasing use of laxative, pipe stem type of stools, bleeding and perianal pain.

Then I would perform a rectal examination. If examination is difficult, I will examine the anus under anaesthesia.

On digital examination thickening of the lumen may be felt. If the lumen is large enough to insert the finger into the anal canal, the type of stenosis is established, i.e. annular or tubular. Biopsy is obtained to rule out malignant process or inflammatory bowel disease.

Examination under anaesthesia of the anus and a gentle dilatation with graded Hegar's dilators may be performed. Post operatively regular dilations with bougies (St Mark's dilators) are advised.

What are the causes of anal stenosis?

Congenital: atresia

Benign: post haemorrhoidectomy, Crohn's disease, sexually transmitted disease

Malignant: anal cancer, rectal cancer

How do you treat post haemorrhoidectomy anal stenosis?

Examination under anaesthesia and anal dilatation

Post operatively the patient may have to self-dilate with St Mark's dilators

What are the surgical options for severe anal stenosis?

V-Y plasty. Inverse House Flap. Y-V plasty

There are several procedures available, and it is expected that you know one of the procedures. You may be asked to draw a diagram.

Obstructed Defecation

You are referred a 70 year old lady with incontinence of faeces over the past six months. This lady has a history of intermittent faecal leakage for about twenty years and had sphincter repair surgery six years ago. Her incontinence improved after the repair but gradually she had been having problems with evacuation.

What further history would you obtain?

I would take a detailed history of her symptoms including incontinence for flatus/ liquid or solid faeces, whether passive or on straining, the frequency, urgency, and consistency of stools, associated bleeding or mucus discharge as well as history of urinary incontinence. I would also take a detailed past medical history of trauma, inflammatory bowel disease, rectal prolapse, fistula in ano, anal fissures, haemorrhoids etc. and surgical history. History of neurological and congenital problems is also vital. I would also take a detailed obstetric history.

What do you understand by the term obstructed defecation?

Obstructed defecation is a syndrome of difficulty in rectal evacuation characterised by sense of incomplete evacuation, straining, prolonged or recurrent attempts to evacuate and in extreme cases digital evacuation or vaginal digitation to achieve evacuation.

This lady also has a feeling of incomplete evacuation. What investigations would you request?

I would initially organise either a colonoscopy or barium enema to rule out any colonic lesions. Thereafter I would organise anorectal physiology including manometry, rectal compliance, colonic transit studies, endoanal ultrasound and defecating proctogram.

What will a defecating proctogram tell you? Is it truly physiological?

A defecating proctogram is carried out in a laboratory with equipment, understandably the patient will not be defecating normally and hence I do not think this is exactly physiological. However under the circumstances, it needs an expert to correlate the findings of the defecating proctogram with clinical data and examination.

Would you do an endo anal ultrasound?

Yes. But opinions differ. As she had previously had a sphincter repair, it would be informative to know the status of the sphincter.

How will you manage this patient with obstructed defecation?

After careful interpretation of the results of the investigations, I would have a frank discussion with this lady and explain the options. It is important to manage the expectations of the patients as the options are limited and a complete cure of her symptoms is not possible. In the biofeedback unit we recommend a course of escalating conservative treatment with support from incontinence nurse specialists in the community. We recommend post evacuation glycerine suppositories along with non-straining techniques of evacuation. She may also benefit from pelvic floor exercises as well as in some cases transanal rectal irrigation (Peristeen).

Surgical management is the last resort and is tailored for individual patients. There are a number of procedures both perineal and laparoscopic with varying success rates.

What do you see in this image?

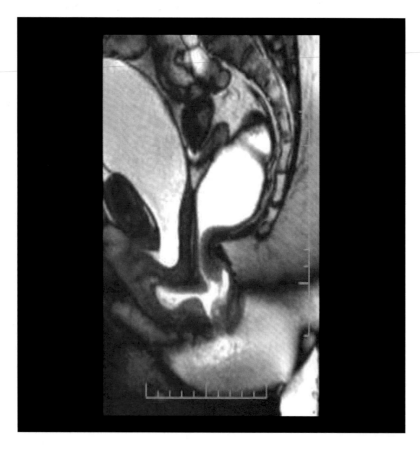

Defecation proctogram showing a rectocele.

How would you treat this condition?

I will examine this patient, obtain a history to identify the problem and confirm results of investigations.

If this patient has obstructive defecation the initial treatment would be conservative treatment. This includes dietary manipulation and biofeedback treatment.

What are the surgical options?

Rectocele repair by: Transvaginal, perineal, transanal and transabdominal approaches.

The procedure is generally performed by coloproctologists or gynaecologists.

A range of techniques are employed including suture plication, mesh reinforcement, rectovaginal septum reinforcement or resection of rectum.

STARR (stapled transanal rectal resection. This procedure entails resection of the rectum with a linear and circular stapler).

The results of the STARR procedure from German registry showed significant improvement in the obstructed defecation score (ODS) over 6 and 12 months. However 21% of patients had complications including: staple line complications (minor bleeding, infection, or partial dehiscence; 7.1%), major bleeding (2.9%), and postsurgical stenosis (2.1%). Also a new onset faecal urgency was noted in 23% of patients and about 3% of patients had faecal incontinence. So they concluded that even though it is associated with improvement in the ODS score, the STARR procedure is associated with complications in 1 in 5 patients and new onset faecal urgency.

Reference

Schwandner O, Fürst A; German STARR Registry Study Group.Assessing the safety, effectiveness, and quality of life after the STARR procedure for obstructed defecation: results of the German STARR registry. Langenbecks Arch Surg. 2010 Jun;395(5):505-13.

Parastomal Hernia

A 70 year old man presents with a parastomal hernia around an end ileostomy following a failed restorative proctocolectomy. The hernia is painful and very difficult to manage due to its size.

How will you investigate this further?

I would take a full history and examine the patient. I would organise a CT scan of the abdomen and pelvis to characterize the defect (especially in a large defect, recurrent hernia and very obese patients), and contents of the hernia sac as well as to rule out any other abdominal wall defects.

What are the problems associated with parastomal herniae?

Poor fitting of stoma appliance causing leakage

Pressure related peristomal skin injury

Bowel obstruction, abdominal pain

Psychological effects

What is the incidence of parastomal hernia?

End ileostomy – up to 28%

End colostomy – up to 48%

Loop ileostomy – up to 6%

Loop colostomy – up to 30%

Loop ileostomy is associated with the lowest risk of parastomal hernia due to the temporary nature of the stoma.

How would you repair a parastomal hernia?

The options include

1) Consider a reversal of the stoma where possible

2) Primary suture repair (high recurrence)

3) Mesh repair with synthetic or biologic mesh (still has a high recurrence rate)

4) Re-site it on the same quadrant or opposite side of the abdomen

In my practice I would do an open repair of the parastomal hernia using the Sugarbaker technique. If the sheath is very weak, then I would re-site the stoma with mesh repair of the hernia. Laparoscopic techniques are available but should only be done by those with extensive experience and training.

How do you do an open repair of a parastomal hernia?

I would do a midline laparotomy, dissect the hernial sac intraperitoneally, and close the defect snug to the stoma with interrupted 1 nylon. I would then use a coated dual layer mesh (prolene mesh with no adhesive layer towards the side of the bowel) to suture over the defect with the ileum entering lateral to the mesh. This technique is known as Sugarbaker's technique. Other open repair techniques include primary suture repair, onlay, sublay or intra peritoneal mesh repair.

What are the other options for parastomal hernia repair?

Laparoscopic repair is an intraperitoneal repair similar to Sugarbaker's technique or keyhole technique. Laparoscopic repair is best reserved for when fewer adhesions are expected and the defect is smaller.

What is the recurrence rate?

Parastomal hernia repairs are associated with a range of recurrence rates due to variations in technique, size of hernia, follow up assessment and duration.

Primary suture repair recurrence can be up to 70%

Mesh repairs are associated with recurrence rate of 7% -17%

Intraperitoneal mesh repairs are associated with recurrence rate of 7% -15%

Laparoscopic repairs are associated with a recurrence rate up to 12%

How would you treat a recurrent parastomal hernia?

If the previous repair was primary suture repair, a mesh can be used

If the previous repair was open only or sublay, then intraperitoneal repair can be used

Re-site the stoma with prophylactic mesh placement

Pilonidal Disease

You are reviewing a 22 year old man who was admitted with an abscess in the natal cleft. His GP has been giving him antibiotics for five days with little effect. What is your diagnosis and how will you manage it?

This is a pilonidal abscess. Examination of patients without an acute abscess may reveal the presence of hairs or dimples in the sacrococcygeal area. Initial management would be an incision and drainage of the abscess and removal of any hair. The incision should be made off the midline. Pits may be visible on inspection, which will confirm the diagnosis. This patient should then be reviewed in outpatients to discuss if definitive treatment is required.

How successful is simple incision and drainage of a pilonidal abscess?

Incision and drainage alone not only leads to good symptom relief but may be definitive itself in 50% of patients. In patients with recurrent symptoms of acute abscesses or persistent discharge an elective surgical procedure should be performed to remove the sinus tracts.

LA incision and drainage is rarely performed. Local anaesthetic is not effective in the presence of pus, and the cavity is always larger than the superficial appearance.

Who is mainly affected by pilonidal disease?

This inflammatory condition of the natal cleft mainly affects young adolescents. There is a male preponderance.

What aetiological factors have been described?

The pilonidal disease is an acquired problem. Risk factors include:

- Deep hirsute natal cleft
- Buttock friction causing local trauma
- Prolonged sitting
- Obesity
- Increased sweating
- Hormonal imbalance

How does pilonidal disease usually present?

Pilonidal disease can present as either an acute abscess or as a chronic ongoing discharge from the natal cleft. Acute presentation accounts for approximately 80% of patients.

What surgical options are available for treatment of chronic pilonidal disease?

Laying open technique with curettage: excision may be carried out with primary closure but this is not advocated if there is any evidence of persistent infection.

Wide excision with marsupilisation of wound edges.

Wide excision and flap based reconstruction- commonly a Karydakis procedure. This involves making an off-centre excision keeping the scar from the midline and aims to also flatten the natal cleft. This has a recurrence rate of approximately 5%. The Bascom procedure involves excision of the midline pits with a lateral incision to allow off midline drainage of any underlying abscess.

What is the reason for keeping the closure off the midline?

This is to minimise the impact of shearing forces which can lead to wound breakdown and persistent wound problems.

For recurrent pilonidal disease or tracts with multiple lateral extensions what reconstruction techniques are available?

A Limberg (rhomboid) flap may be used which is a random pattern flap utilising simple geometry to close soft tissue defects by taking advantage of laxity in the adjacent tissues. Excision is completed as a rhomboid, with sides of equal length, two angles of 60 degrees and two angles of 120 degrees. The flap is designed by extending the incision from one of the 120 degree angles, the same length as the sides of rhomboid, and a further incision parallel to the side of the rhomboid. As such, four possible flaps can be designed, two on each side of the defect. The tissues are elevated and transposed into the defect, with direct closure of the donor site. Variations of the rhomboid flap include the "square peg round hole" and the Dufourmentel flap.

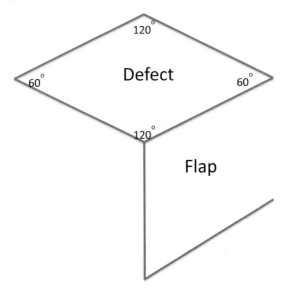

Pouchitis

You are reviewing a 30 year old lady in clinic on whom you have performed a restorative proctocolectomy for ulcerative colitis. She is now complaining of bloody diarrhoea and urgency with opening her bowels approximately 20 times per day. What is your diagnosis and how would you manage this?

This lady is most likely suffering from pouchitis. Initial treatment should include a two week course of oral antibiotics (metronidazole or ciprofloxacin). In the majority of patients there will be symptomatic improvement. If symptoms do not resolve then combination antibiotic treatment may be employed. If there is a relapse of symptoms maintenance ciprofloxacin with probiotics may be used.

How can pouchitis be assessed?

A complete assessment requires clinical, endoscopic and histological evaluation.

If symptoms fail to improve with this treatment what would be the next step?

Other possible causes (eg Crohn's disease, cuffitis) will need to be excluded. A longer course of metronidazole may be used, however caution should be employed due to the risk of peripheral neuropathy with longer term use.

If the symptoms continue, further options would include the use of steroids (budesonide), immunomodulators, 5-ASA or as a last result defunctioning ileostomy or pouch excision with end ileostomy.

Are you aware of any objective scoring measures?

The three principal methods are:

1) St Mark's Triad: (diarrhoea, endoscopic changes and histological changes)

2) The pouchitis disease activity index (PDAI) (Includes frequency, bleeding, urgency, fever, endoscopic criteria and histological criteria)

3) The Heidelberg pouchitis activity score (Clinical components: frequency, bleeding and urgency. Endoscopic components: oedema, friability, granularity, erythema, flattening of mucosal surface, ulcers. A degree of acute or chronic histological inflammation)

What possible aetiologies for developing pouchitis are you aware of?

Potential aetiologies include faecal stasis, ischaemia, bacterial overgrowth, and altered immunoregulation. The latter is supported by the extraintestinal manifestations that may be seen with pouchitis, increased lymphocyte and inflammatory cytokines and interleukin 1 receptor antagonist gene allele 2, which has been used as a predictor of pouchitis.

Rectal Cancer

A normally fit and healthy 60 year old man has been diagnosed with a mid-rectal adenocarcinoma. It has been staged as T3N1. What are your treatment options?

I would like to know if an MRI scan has demonstrated a clear circumferential resection margin (CRM). Patients with T3N1 disease may still have a negative CRM if the tumour is located posteriorly (bulkier mesorectum) and lymph nodes with suspicious morphology are greater than 2mm away from the mesorectal plane. If the CRM is not threatened then one option is to proceed directly to surgery in the form of a low anterior resection. If the CRM was threatened or involved, then initial treatment with long course chemoradiotherapy (LC-CRT) would be delivered in an attempt to downstage the tumour and facilitate a negative CRM prior to surgery. Most centres would restage the patient after LC-CRT prior to surgery. After surgery, if the resected specimens confirmed it to be node positive, post-operative chemotherapy would be considered. This should be discussed at the MDT and treatment options discussed with the patient.

Rectal cancer is interesting because of a) the mesorectum morphology, b) the bony confines of the pelvis and c) the potential of tumour involvement in adjacent structures and the pelvic floor/ sphincter complex - particularly in those with lower tumours.

When you review the patient pre LC-CRT, he is very anxious about the possibility of a stoma as part of his surgery. What will you tell him?

This patient needs to be counselled about the possibility of a temporary loop ileostomy. Although the tumour is mid-rectum, and therefore amenable to a low anastomosis, this procedure can be technically challenging and he is likely to require chemotherapy post surgery. Any complications e.g an anastomotic leak, will lead to a delay in commencement of adjuvant treatment. A loop ileostomy does not reduce the likelihood of a leak but it reduces the sequelae of any leak should it occur. The anastomosis can often be salvaged and further revisits to theatre are avoided. Moreover, the reversal of ileostomy is a straightforward procedure, although the risk of an anastomotic leak is not negligible. This can be done after completion of chemotherapy and when the anastomosis has been evaluated by a water soluble contrast enema.

He then asks you if this will be a "keyhole" procedure?

NICE guidelines recommend that laparoscopic surgery should be offered as an alternative to open surgery if the resection is deemed suitable for both methods. The oncological aspects of laparoscopic surgery are not inferior in expert hands. The operative time may be longer but the postoperative recovery is a little quicker. In obese men with bulky disease and a very narrow pelvis, laparoscopic surgery is extremely difficult.

He completes LC-CRT over a 5 week period and undergoes restaging scans just before surgery after another 2 months. He feels much better and his rectal bleeding has stopped. The CT remains reassuring and the lesion is no longer seen on post treatment MRI scans. What would you do?

This is an interesting scenario. Complete pathological response to LC-CRT is not unusual. The Brazilian series from Habr-Gama reveal a complete response in up to 40 per cent of patients, particularly if the interval from completion of treatment to time of surgery is extended. This raises the issue of how best to select patients for this type of treatment and how to survey them for a failure (incomplete response) or recurrence after a complete response. The Brazilians recommend a schedule of clinical, endoscopic and radiological surveillance but there remains an element of scepticism about whether waiting represents a window of lost opportunity for curative intent. The issue of LC-CRT and delay for rectal cancer is being investigated in several trials at the moment. On balance, I would discuss the evidence and need for any surgery with my patient. Certainly, the risk of surgery has to be balanced against any potential gain achieved by removing residual disease.

What is the role of preoperative radiotherapy in rectal surgery?

In the UK, radiotherapy is used preoperatively in two forms. This is either short course or long course (in conjunction with chemotherapy). Short course preoperative radiotherapy (SCPRT) reduces local recurrence rates from difficult or poor surgery. Long course chemoradiotherapy (LC-CRT) is given to 'downstage' bad disease and to facilitate a negative circumferential resection margin along the 'holy' TME plane.

SCPRT (25 Gy in 5 daily fractions over 1 week) is followed by surgery within 1-2 weeks. Any delay results in misery both for the surgeon (technically challenging because of oedema and bleeding) and the patient (complications). It reduces local recurrence by half from 10% to 5%. However, there is no obvious improvement to overall survival. SCPRT results in higher risk of impotence, and poorer bowel function from damage to nerves. In those who have an APER, perineal wound problems were noted. These trials showed the benefit of SCPRT

1) Swedish trial (1997): Preop SCRT followed by surgery better than surgery alone

2) Dutch trial (2005): Preop SCRT followed by TME surgery better than TME surgery alone

3) CR07 (2006): Preop SCRT better than selective postop CRT

LC-CRT (45-50 Gy in 25 daily fractions over 5 weeks) is followed by surgery after 6-10 weeks. Local recurrence falls from 20% to 10%. There is no improvement in survival once again. The patient is more likely to suffer from diarrhoea with LC-CRT when compared with SCPRT. Neither of the trials below enforced TME surgery so broad conclusions have been drawn about local recurrence rates.

1) EORTC trial (2005): LC-CRT better than SCRT

2) FFCD trial (2005): As above

What is a 'total mesorectal excision' and the Quirke's score?

TME is now the standard for anterior resection procedures. It was popularised by Professor Heald and involves excision of the complete rectum along with its surrounding lymphatics in a package surrounded by the mesorectal fascia to produce a better oncological outcome. The adequacy of surgical resection of rectal cancer would be determined by a pathologically determined grading of the mesorectum - the so-called total mesorectal excision score (TME score or Quirke's score). Scores ranged from 1–3 with 3 being a perfect specimen.

So, when would you consider an abdomino-perineal resection for a patient with rectal cancer?

Essentially, in patients with low rectal tumours that are involving the sphincter complex, or patients with very bulky tumours where it would not be possible to obtain a clear margin should the sphincters be preserved. Patients with poor sphincter function would be another group of patients that may not benefit from a restorative procedure. The vogue for sphincter preservation surgery is returning (once again), and in selected patients with low tumours, surgery along the intersphincteric planes together with removal of the tumour and involved internal sphincters can be done. The colon is hand sewn or stapled to the external sphincters complex. Continence must not be preserved at the expense of oncological outcome.

What do you understand about an extra-levator abdominoperineal excision then?

The procedure was first popularised by Professor Holm (Karolinska Institute, Sweden). His technique halves the number of intraoperative perforations of specimens (20% to 10%) and halves the rate of CRM positivity (50% to 20%) in resected specimens. This is thought to be secondary to the removal of a larger volume of 'normal' tissue and avoidance of 'waisting' of the specimen. His technique recommends that the perineal portion of the procedure is done in the prone position. Prone APER confers the above chiefly by providing a better view of the lower pelvis by a) removal of the coccyx, b) portions of the levator muscle and c) a more comfortable dissection by the operator and assistant. Quirke scores to assess the quality of mesorectal excision have been modified for APER to incorporate circumferential component of levator muscles. 3: good (has levator), 2: moderate (has no levator), 1: poor.

This technique results in a larger perineal defect and a higher rate of perineal complications (40% instead of 20%). It remains unknown how best to close this defect. Options include input from plastic surgeons with concurrent use of myocutaneous flaps (commonly a Vertical Rectus Abdominis Myocutaneous flap) and/or biologic meshes.

References

Green BLI, Marshall HC, Collinson F, Quirke P, Guillou P, Jayne DG, Brown JM Long-term follow-up of the Medical Research Council CLASICC trial of conventional versus laparoscopically assisted resection in colorectal cancer. Br J Surg. 2013 Jan;100(1):75-82.

Sebag-Montefiore DI, Stephens RJ, Steele R, Monson J, Grieve R, Khanna S, Quirke P, Couture J, de Metz C, Myint AS, Bessell E, Griffiths G, Thompson LC, Parmar M. Preoperative radiotherapy versus selective postoperative chemoradiotherapy in patients with rectal cancer (MRC CR07 and NCIC-CTG C016): a multicentre, randomised trial. Lancet. 2009 Mar 7;373(9666):811-20.

Habr-Gama A, Sabbaga J, Gama-Rodrigues J, São Julião GP, Proscurshim I, Bailão Aguilar P, Nadalin W, Perez RO. Watch and wait approach following extended neoadjuvant chemoradiation for distal rectal cancer: are we getting closer to anal cancer management? Dis Colon Rectum. 2013 Oct;56(10):1109-17

Rectal Prolapse

You have been referred a 45 year old patient from the medical wards who the nurses feel has a rectal prolapse. What are the risk factors for this?

It is frequently found in elderly female patients, and is associated with multiple vaginal deliveries. It is also seen in those with mental health problems particularly those suffering from chronic constipation and straining. It occasionally also affects infants.

How would you investigate this patient?

A number of factors need to be investigated. First one must assess how much of a problem the current condition is for the patient and her carers. As she has been admitted, we need to understand her level of function and the reason for her admission. All co-morbidities will impact on the surgical risk. Surgery will be the only effective way of ensuring significant resolution of the symptoms. Finally, an examination to ensure there is no other underlying pathology, and a flexible sigmoidoscopy should be carried out to exclude an underlying neoplastic process. You must be confident of visualising the prolapse yourself. If you cannot confirm its presence then you must either order a proctogram to facilitate its presence or perform an examination under anaesthetic to access its magnitude. It would also be worth considering anorectal manometry and pudendal nerve testing, which may predict function and continence after surgery.

She is highly symptomatic from the prolapse. It is about 5 cms in size and it bleeds whenever she gets constipated. What operative procedure will you offer her?

Prolapse surgery can be divided into abdominal and perineal procedures. Abdominal procedures can be done open or laparoscopically. All abdominal procedures involve a rectopexy of some description but those with constipation may also benefit from a concurrent resection. Perineal procedures can be done under a spinal/epidural but abdominal procedures all require a general anaesthetic. Perineal procedures are thought to have a higher recurrence rate (40%-50% on long term follow-up) compared with abdominal procedures (10%-20% on long term follow-up). It is important to reiterate the importance of maintaining a regular bowel habit and avoiding the need for straining.

For a perineal approach, I favour an Altemeier procedure. This involves a resection of the prolapse and a low anastomosis. Recurrence rates are lower than with a Delorme procedure but it does require the patient to have a low anastomosis. For an abdominal approach I favour a laparosopic (if possible) ventral mesh rectopexy and I try to avoid a concurrent resection for fear of mesh contamination should an anastomotic leak occur.

Two years after your rectal prolapse operation, she returns to your clinic with a proctogram ordered by her GP. Although she has no prolapse, she has problems with defaecation and the proctogram reveals a rectorectal intussusception. She also has difficulties with urinary incontinence and pelvic floor discomforts. What would you do?

It is likely that we are dealing with a patient who has complex pelvic floor problems. She requires assessment by a pelvic floor specialist and this is often multidisciplinary. I would refer her on to one of my urogynaecology colleagues for an opinion on her anterior and middle compartments. From the posterior compartment point of view, I think it is important to exclude anything sinister to begin with. It has been two years since I last saw her. I would repeat her flexible sigmoidoscopy, send her for anorectal physiology and consider putting her through an MRI proctogram, which would provide me with triple compartment information. With regards to the rectorectal intussuception, this is often very difficult to improve. It is often associated with obstructive defaecation and is associated with radiological findings such as rectoceles, pelvic floor descent and anismus. These findings are often the result of pelvic floor discoordination, rather than the cause of it. The progressive spectrum of these disorders can result in solitary rectal ulcers.

She wishes surgery to be performed, as life is unbearable. What would you do?

A trial of pelvic floor retraining and use of oral, suppositories and/or rectal enemas would be advised. Surgery can sometimes correct the visible anatomical abnormalities but it is unlikely to improve physiology and pelvic floor function. I would do my best to dissuade her against surgery. If she remains keen, then I will warn her of the risks of surgery and manage her expectation accordingly. There are two options for rectal intussuception. This can be done trans-anally (stapled trans-anal rectal resection STARR) or trans-abdominally. A laparoscopic ventral mesh rectopexy minimises pelvic floor descent (due to the rectopexy), reinforces the rectovaginal septum (treats the rectocele) and minimises damage to the pelvic nerves.

ENDOCRINE SURGERY

Titus Cvasciuc Radu Mihai

Contents

Airway Compromise in a Patient with Goitre

A 62 year old lady presents to the emergency department with severe dyspnoea. She is obese (BMI 36), with a history of hypertension and atrial fibrillation. She is taking warfarin daily. On clinical examination she has stridor, hoarseness and a large cervical mass in the anterior triangle of the neck.

What clinical signs are important?

- On inspection: degree of respiratory distress (able to speak in sentences, etc.), presence of stridor, voice changes (suggestive of recurrent laryngeal nerve palsy), signs of superior vena cava obstruction, Pemberton's test, presence of thyroid ophthalmopathy

- On palpation: tracheal shift from midline, character of the mass (e.g. fixed, hard/firm), and presence of local lymphadenopathy

- On percussion: mediastinal dullness (unreliable sign of retrosternal extension of a goitre)

- On auscultation: bruit over the thyroid (rarely encountered, historically described in large overactive thyroids)

What investigations need to be organised at this stage?

- CT neck and chest - to assess the extent of the goitre and the (possible) involvement of surrounding structures

- Flexible laryngoscopy - hoarseness is a symptom of vocal cord paralysis hence laryngoscopy is done to assess airway patency and vocal cord movements

- Fine needle aspiration biopsy (FNAB) – to determine whether the goitre is benign or malignant

CT chest/neck showed a left thyroid mass with deviation of the trachea to the right and extrinsic compression (airway diameter approximately 5 mm), with minimal invasion of the tracheal wall. The left lobe extends approximately 4 cm below the sternal notch and there are multiple thyroid nodules on the right side of the thyroid. In addition, two nodules of 5-10 mm were identified in the right lung.

Preoperative laryngoscopy showed left vocal cord paralysis.

Should warfarin be stopped at this stage?

Fine needle aspiration biopsy can be performed in patients on warfarin. However, warfarin should be stopped on admission, as it is very likely that urgent surgical intervention will be needed.

What further preoperative investigations are needed?

- Thyroid function tests (likely to be normal, but they should be checked)
- Flexible bronchoscopy – if a CT scan raises suspicion of intraluminal invasion of the tumour (if present, it might require tracheal stenting or tracheal resection as part of the radical operation for thyroid cancer – the choice of treatment should be discussed at an MDT)
- Anaesthetic review/discussion: to discuss management of a difficult airway

What are the common causes of preoperative airway obstruction?

Large goitre/retrosternal goitre

Haemorrhage into a nodule/goitre

Invasion of the airway – ie carcinoma

What is the appropriate management in this case?

General anaesthesia, possibly/likely requiring fibre optic awake intubation should be used

A total thyroidectomy - avoiding gross/macroscopic tumour residual, +/- resection of strap muscles should be performed

Central compartment lymph node dissection (high risk patients are likely to have local metastases in level VI-VII lymph nodes even in the presence of normal radiological assessment) is required

Intraoperative nerve monitoring (to assess the function of the left recurrent laryngeal nerve before proceeding with surgery on the right side)

Management of tracheal invasion

Management of recurrent laryngeal nerve invasion

What are the management/surgical options of tracheal invasion?

The options include: "shaving" / window resection / segmental resection and re-anastomosis

What are the concerns in this patient postoperatively?

- Airway compromise (postoperative bleeding/haematoma, recurrent laryngeal nerve palsy)

- Tracheomalacia – very rare, allegedly likely to occur in patients with long-standing tracheal compression leading to destruction of tracheal cartilages and a 'floppy'/collapsible trachea once the goitre is removed – this scenario is seldom recognised in western medical practice

- Hypocalcaemia

Key points

If there is bleeding, try to intubate and return to theatre

Any stridor should precipitate return to theatre or intubation

Act early if airway obstruction/stridor develops

If it is not possible to intubate after 1-2 attempts, the wound should be opened and the situation reassessed within 30 minutes

Insertion of a tracheostomy should be avoided

What adjuvant therapy is needed in this case?

Radioactive iodine therapy is ineffective for gross residual disease or anaplastic carcinoma

External beam radiation therapy – controversial, not curative

The patient should be discussed in an MDT

Carcinoids

A 42 year old female with right iliac fossa pain for 12 hours, associated with nausea, was referred to the emergency department for assessment. She had no fever. She has a raised WBC (12.3 × 10⁹/l/mm3), US abdomen demonstrated no abnormality. A CT scan revealed a 2cm mass in the right iliac fossa suggestive of an inflamed appendix. What is her diagnosis and what treatment is needed?

As per the CT scan she has acute appendicitis and an emergency appendicectomy is needed.

Laparoscopic appendicectomy was performed – a 2 cm mass at the tip of the appendix was seen. There was no evidence of enlarged lymph nodes and no mesenteric invasion was identified. What is the intraoperative diagnosis?

These findings are highly suggestive of an appendiceal carcinoid tumour.

Histology showed 2 cm appendix carcinoid, Ki67 index 7%, low mitotic index. Is any further treatment needed? What are the guidelines for treatment of appendix carcinoids?

Appendiceal carcinoids smaller than 1 cm and located at the tip of the appendix are treated only by appendicectomy. Carcinoids between 1-2 cm are treated by appendicectomy alone if localised at the tip, there is no invasion of mesoappendix and no evidence of lymph node involvement. If there is presence of tumour at the resection margins a right hemi-colectomy is indicated. No further treatment is needed for this case.

Carcinoids larger than 2 cm are treated with a right hemi-colectomy. Right hemi-colectomy may also be indicated if the histology demonstrates poor prognostic factors such as: angioinvasion, and high mitotic Ki67 index.

Cushing's Syndrome - Postoperative Care

A 57 year old lady with long-standing diabetes mellitus controlled with oral sulphonylureas, poorly controlled hypertension and obesity (BMI 35) was referred by her general practitioner with the suspicion of Cushing's syndrome.

How do you demonstrate that her combination of morbidities relate to excess cortisol secretion?

Over-night dexamethasone inhibition test (administration of 0.5 mg Dexa at 23:00 with cortisol measurement at 08:00 the following morning) is used as a screening test to demonstrate inappropriately increased secretion of cortisol. Further biochemical and radiological tests usually organised by endocrinologists aim to differentiate between those with hypercortisolism due to

- ACTH –secreting pituitary adenoma (Cushing disease);

- ectopic ACTH secretion from a malignant tumour or

- ACTH-independent secretion for an adrenal tumour (Cushing syndrome);

She is found to have an inhibited ACTH level, with failure to suppress cortisol following a high dose dexamethasone test. A CT scan demonstrated a 48mm right adrenal tumour. She is referred to the endocrine surgical team for adrenalectomy.

What surgical approach is recommended?

Laparoscopic right adrenalectomy is the ideal approach for such a patient. Retroperitoneoscopic adrenalectomy is yet to be widely available (based on lack of experience of most surgeons with this technique) but might increase in coming years as it is allegedly associated with less postoperative pain and faster recovery and possibly shorter stay.

Open adrenalectomy should be reserved for patients with suspicion of malignancy based on CT appearance or intraoperative findings.

What are your specific concerns in the postoperative period?

- Steroid replacement. There is persistent inhibition of ACTH secretion postoperatively hence the contralateral adrenal gland is unable to produce cortisol in the immediate postoperative period. Patients need hydrocortisone replacement for 3-12 months postoperatively, with a progressive decrease in dose monitored under the care of endocrinologists. Once oral intake is restarted after the operation, oral hydrocortisone is administered in a high dose (e.g. 50 or 40 mg/day divided as 20-20-10 or 20-10-10 mg, decreasing within a couple of weeks towards the physiological maintenance dose of 10-10-5 mg and advice to continue to reduce further within the coming months)

- Thromboembolism prophylaxis (high risk of DVT)

- Management of diabetes (insulin and iv fluids then oral medication when diet is resumed) and hypertension has to be altered as normalising cortisol secretion should lead to improved control of sugar levels and BP (hence some drug doses will have to be readjusted)

Which specific complications are more likely in such patients ?

Chronic hypercortisolism results in obesity, impaired wound healing, easy bruising, increased susceptibility to infections and increased risk of deep vein thrombosis and pulmonary embolism compared to patients undergoing adrenalectomy for other indications.

Hypercalcaemic Crisis

A 52 year old lady is admitted with muscle weakness, bone pains, thirst, dehydration, impaired concentration, memory loss, oliguria, nausea and vomiting. She has a history of depression and anxiety. Past medical history includes hypertension, arrhythmias and constipation. Routine blood tests on admission show hypokalaemia (K 3.2 mmol/l), urea 7mmol/L, creatinine 156 µmol/L, calcium 3.8 mmol/l.

What is her diagnosis ?

Hypercalcaemic crisis (severe hypercalcaemia and acute symptoms)

How would you determine the cause of hypercalcaemia?

Measurements of PTH levels differentiate the two most common causes of hypercalcaemia: malignancy (PTH inhibited) and primary hyperparathyroidism (PTH high or 'inappropriately normal')

For this patient PTH was increased (193 pmol/L), confirming the diagnosis of PHPT.

What is the management for hypercalcaemic crisis focused on?

Rehydration

Evaluate and correct comorbidities

Preparation for surgery

Use of bisphosphonates (Pamidronate) should be delayed until the cause of hypercalcaemia is demonstrated as this drug should be used only in those with malignancy. For patients with PHPT Pamidronate should not be used as urgent parathyroidectomy is the ideal treatment (in these patients there is a high risk of severe hypocalcaemia if Pamidronate was administered preoperatively as the drug blocks the osteoclasts and prevents them from being involved in maintenance of normocalcaemia after successful parathyroidectomy).

What further radiological investigations need to be organised at this stage?

Localisation studies with neck ultrasound and Sestamibi scintigraphy. In addition, CT/MRI of neck and chest could be considered.

The patient was transferred to ITU because of coexisting cardiac and renal comorbidities.

What steps are to be taken in the Intensive Care Unit?

Correct rehydration with intravenous saline to achieve a urine output of 100ml/h

Loop diuretics to produce calciuresis and stimulate diuresis

Regular serum electrolyte imbalance to prevent hypokalaemia and hypomagnesaemia

What other drugs are used in extreme cases?

Bisphosphonates

Dialysis

Calcitonin

Steroids

Are bisphosphonates used in patients waiting for surgery and if yes/no why?

They are not used because of profound and prolonged hypocalcaemia following surgery.

What is the best and most rapid method to restore eucalcemia?

Parathyroid surgery

What rare disease can be associated with elevated serum calcium level (especially over 3 mmol/l) and PTH over 10 times the normal range?

Extreme biochemical abnormalities raise the suspicion of parathyroid cancer (this is an extremely rare tumour)

The patient underwent neck USS (3cm tumour localised at the lower pole of the right thyroid lobe) and Sestamibi scan with positive uptake of a parathyroid tumour at the lower pole of the right lobe of thyroid. The scans were concordant.

What type of operation may be needed?

Minimally invasive open parathyroidectomy (MIP) is offered, usually under general anaesthesia but also possible under local anaesthesia in selected patients.

After correcting the serum calcium levels, addressing comorbidities, preoperative laryngoscopy was performed and the patient was transferred to the operating theatre. A minimally invasive open parathyroidectomy was intended – a parathyroid tumour 3.3 cm, inferior to the right thyroid lobe which was very adherent to the lobe was found. How would you proceed?

If macroscopically suspicious of parathyroid carcinoma, the procedure should be converted to a formal neck exploration and the operation should include an en-block resection of the parathyroid tumour and the thyroid lobe (consideration for local lymph node dissection should be strongly considered).

What laboratory tests are needed postoperatively and what timing?

- Intraoperative PTH monitoring (as the half-life of PTH is only 2-3 minutes, measurement of PTH at 10-20-30 min after excision of the adenoma will prove excision of all hyper functional tissue if PTH is found to drop at least 50% from preoperative values)

- Serum PTH 1 hour after surgery (a substitute for intraoperative PTH monitoring as this is a much cheaper method because it avoids the need for having in theatre a biochemist technician and a kit for intraoperative PTH rapid assay)

- Serum calcium level the next morning after surgery - is expected to drop significantly though might not be yet in the normal range if there was significant preoperative hypercalcaemia

- Serum calcium at 6 weeks, 6 months and 1 year postoperatively. Hypercalcaemia present within 6 months of the operation defines **persistent PHPT**. Hypercalcaemia demonstrated at > 1 year from operation defines **recurrent PHPT**

Phaeochromocytoma

A 32 year old woman presented to A & E with recent shortness of breath, headache, sweating and tachycardia. On examination she was apyrexial, had raised JVP, HR 135/min, BP 220/160 mmHG, ECG showed sinus tachycardia.

What are the common causes of secondary hypertension in young patients?

> Renal artery stenosis

> Endocrine causes: hypercortisolism (Cushing's syndrome), hyperaldosteronism, phaeochromocytoma

The patient reported that symptoms started 6 months previously due to stress induced by the operation her father had just undergone for thyroid cancer. Since then she had numerous attacks of anxiety, panic and tremor. She asked for medication to control these symptoms and a beta-blocker was considered by the GP. What would you prescribe?

I would want to carry out further investigations before considering use of a beta blocker. If this lady has a phaeochromocytoma then beta blockers would be contraindicated as it would induce worsening of hypertension or could cause pulmonary oedema.

What investigations would you organise in order to demonstrate the cause of these acute symptoms?

The following investigations should be carried out:

> 24 hours urinary fractionated metanephrines (to exclude/confirm phaeochromocytoma)

> Thyroid function tests (to exclude/confirm thyrotoxicosis)

> FBC, CRP, blood cultures (sepsis)

> Aldosterone/renin ratio and potassium (hyperaldosteronism)

> Cortisol levels after overnight low dexamethasone (hypercortisolism)

> Renal artery ultrasound (to exclude renal artery stenosis)

If the biochemical tests demonstrate a phaeochromocytoma what imaging tests can be done to localise it?

> CT/MRI scan

> MIBG scan

> FDG with PET scan

What is the treatment for a phaeochromocytoma?

It is imperative that medical management is initiated prior to consideration of surgery. Once medical management has been established, the treatment of choice would be a laparoscopic adrenalectomy.

What is the medical management (pharmacological control)?

Alpha adrenergic blockade followed by beta-blockade. (The combination of phenoxybenzamine and propranolol is preferred by most clinicians but doxazosin and calcium-channel blockers are used in preference in some units.)

What is the preferred surgical treatment?

Laparoscopic adrenalectomy / laparoscopic excision of paragangliomas.

Open adrenalectomy should be reserved for patients with suspicion of malignancy based on radiological or intraoperative findings.

What are the tumours producing excess of catecholamines?

Phaeochromocytoma

Extra adrenal paragangliomas (Majority in the abdomen – organ of Zuckerkandl, or around the renal hilum. Less common in the urinary bladder, mediastinum, head and neck – rarely producing catecholamines)

What are the specific concerns in the postoperative period?

Hypotension – thus volume replacement either through an intravenous or an oral route should be used

Hypoglycaemia is common so regular monitoring of blood glucose should be carried out

Phenoxybenzamine should be stopped postoperatively

Propranolol to be considered for 3 days (usually the half dose)

DVT prophylaxis

What is the significance of her father having been treated for thyroid cancer and what impact would it have on this case?

If the father had papillary thyroid carcinoma this would have no impact on her own case (incidental association).

If the father had medullary thyroid carcinoma it would imply that this is a MEN2 family. The patient should be screened for MTC (measuring serum calcitonin) and the father should be screened for phaeochromocytoma. Both should have genetic screening for RET mutation. Once a mutation is identified all first-degree relatives should also be checked.

Which are the most common genes associated with familial phaeochromocytomas?

RET (MEN 2A, 2B syndrome)

VHL (Von Hippel-Lindau syndrome)

NF1 (neurofibromatosis type 1)

SDHB/SDHD (succinyl dehydrogenase subunit B and D)

What are the characteristics of phaeochromocytoma in patients carrying hereditary gene mutations?

The patients are more likely to be young (under 50 years old)

Multiple/bilateral/extradrenal tumours

Which phaeochromocytomas might be malignant? What are the treatment options?

Malignancy is suspected especially in large phaeochromocytomas, in extradrenal paragangliomas and in those associated with SDHB mutations. Treatment options are:

Alpha and beta blockade followed by excision of tumour or tumour debulking

External beam radiotherapy / chemotherapy

Therapeutic dose of I^{131} MIBG

How would you perform a laparoscopic adrenalectomy?

A transperitoneal approach is preferred by most general surgeons (more familiar with the landmarks) but retroperitoneal adrenalectomy is increasing in popularity for small tumours (<4 cm).

Compared with other types of adrenal tumours, phaeochromocytomas are more friable and bleed easily, hence the tumour cannot be grasped and it should be 'pushed' during the dissection.

Right transperitoneal adrenalectomy:

- 4 ports, subcostal
- liver retractor to lift the liver (it might require division of the triangular ligament to increase the mobility of the liver)
- peritoneum divided under the liver and along the cava (occasionally mobilizing the duodenum is necessary)
- a space ('groove') created between the IVC and the adrenal tumour (retracted laterally)

-   right adrenal vein identified towards the upper pole of the tumour, generally entering the IVC in a posterior position (i.e. not really on the lateral side of the IVC)

-   Harmonic dissection of the tumour from the retroperitoneal space

Left transperitoneal adrenalectomy:

-   3 ports (a fourth might be necessary to retract the spleen)

-   descending colon and splenic flexure mobilized

-   peritoneal reflection along the lateral side of the spleen is divided to mobilise the spleen medially

-   a 'groove' is being created between spleen and pancreas (retracted medially) and the Gerota's fascia (i.e. kidney and adrenal tumour, retracted laterally)

-   Gerota's fascia divided to allow identification of the tumour and of the renal vein

-   Adrenal vein identified, clipped and divided

-   Tumour dissected with Harmonic from the perinephric fat and retroperitoneal space

Post Thyroidectomy Complications

A 38 year old lady with Graves' disease (2 years treatment with carbimazole) is booked for total thyroidectomy. Blood tests were normal, there is no other past medical history. Surgery finished at 3 pm.

The total thyroidectomy was uneventful. No drain was used. The patient was in postoperative recovery for 45 minutes then moved to the ward with a good voice, and no signs of neck swelling.

At 20:00 the patient is restless, anxious, and complains of swallowing difficulties and voice changes. The nurses call you because of concerns related to postoperative bleeding.

Which symptoms / signs are important in postoperative follow up of neck surgery?

- swallowing complaints
- breathing difficulty
- neck swelling
- voice changes (especially if voice was good after surgery)

How do you assess the patient?

You should follow the generic principles:

A airway maintenance

B breathing

C circulation with haemorrhage control

D disability and neurological status

This can become a major airway crisis. On arrival, ensure the bed is elevated and the patient positioned with a slight neck extension. Assess the degree of airway obstruction (ability to speak in sentences, use of accessory muscles, presence of stridor) and associated swallowing difficulties (in severe cases patients cannot swallow saliva). Have oxygen delivered and iv access secured. Call for help from the oncall anaesthetist. If time allows discuss the case with the operating surgeon. If the patient is distressed and the neck swelling easily apparent proceed to opening the sutures (ensuring all layers of the closure are opened, i.e. skin, platysma and strap muscles) – this can be done on the ward or (if feasible) in theatre.

What surgical manoeuvre should be avoided in such scenario?

Tracheostomy – this is totally unnecessary. The first manoeuvre is to open the neck – the release of the haematoma should lead to a decrease in the local venous congestion. Improvement in the laryngeal oedema would make the anaesthetist more likely to succeed with tracheal intubation.

Thyroid Cancer - Speciality Topics

What is the importance of prophylactic central compartment lymph node dissection (CCLND) in patients with thyroid cancer?

Patients with a diagnosis of papillary thyroid cancer demonstrated on fine needle aspiration biopsy undergo preoperative neck imaging with an ultrasound scan (where local expertise exists) or CT/MRI to determine whether there are enlarged lymph nodes in the central compartment (level VI-VII) or lateral neck (levels II-V). Those with clinically or radiologically involved lymph nodes need lymph node dissection. Those with normal scans might be offered prophylactic lymph node dissection based on the established fact that up to 80% of these patients are likely to have microscopic metastases. Such small volume metastatic disease is likely to respond to radioactive iodine ablation. For the last decade the debate has been on whether a prophylactic lymph node dissection provides a better oncological outcome or whether it could be used in order to avoid postoperative radioactive iodine ablation. The jury is out. The international debate focuses now on the feasibility of organising a multi centre randomised trial addressing these questions.

According to American Thyroid Association (ATA) guidelines cases with tumours bigger than 4 cm or with local invasion (T3,T4) may need prophylactic central compartment lymph node dissection (Recommendation rating C).

There is still a debate about prophylactic CCLND in tumours smaller than 4 cm (i.e. T1-T2 tumours).

What is the central compartment?

Level VI (central compartment) is the anatomical area defined by the carotid artery (lateral), trachea (medial), the hyoid bone (proximal) and the manubrium (inferiorly). It can be divided further into level VIa if only lymph nodes anterior to the recurrent laryngeal nerve are dissected or VIb if lymph nodes posterior to the nerve are also dissected.

After surgery a final histological result indicates 5cm left papillary thyroid carcinoma with lymph node metastases in 3 of 11 lymph nodes in the central compartment. What other treatment options are needed for this case?

Radioactive iodine ablation (RAI) is needed to complete surgical treatment. It is administered after withdrawal of liothyronine medication for 7-10 days (in order to achieve a raise in TSH levels necessary to drive the sodium-iodine symporter, a cell membrane pump that exchanges Na with iodine). Alternatively, Thyrogen (human recombinant TSH) is administered as an intramuscular injection 3 days before RAI in order to avoid the hypothyroid symptoms during treatment.

The left recurrent laryngeal nerve was invaded by tumour.   What are the options?

If on preoperative laryngoscopy the vocal cord is paralysed then the RLN can be resected and +/- reanastomosis (if the contralateral nerve is not invaded)

If the ipsilateral vocal cord is intact try to preserve the nerve (even with residual tumour)

Use intraoperative monitoring (IONM) to confirm the functional status of the contralateral nerve before deciding how best to manage the involved RLN

Try to resect as much tumour as possible

Thyrotoxicosis in a Patient Admitted With Acute Cholecystitis

A 37 year old lady presents to A&E with acute right upper quadrant pain, nausea and vomiting. She has no significant past medical history and no drug history. Her heart rate is 125/min, temperature 37.8°C.

What further investigations are needed?

Routine blood tests: FBC (WBC 13×10^9/l), LFTs (ALT 216 IU/L, Alk Phosphatase 476 IU/L, bilirubin 14 ummol/l), amylase – normal)

Abdominal ultrasonography: distended gallbladder with 1 cm stone impacted in infundibulum, 5-6 mm thickened wall, no intraabdominal abnormalities.

During clerking the FY1 notices a fullness in her neck (symmetric, non-tender) and a possible degree of exophthalmia. Should this be investigated further at this point? How ? Why?

In a patient with goitre and severe tachycardia the thyroid status has to be tested (thyroid function tests: this patient had TSH 0.01, free Thyroxine 29.5).

Uncontrolled hyperthyroidism in a patient with acute surgical problems can trigger a *thyrotoxic crisis*, which is associated with severe morbidity and a significant risk of mortality. Control of the thyroid function is imperative before proceeding to urgent surgical treatment.

What other radiological investigations are needed?

MRCP – because of elevated LFTs, to assess for the presence of a CBD stone

Thyroid uptake scan (pertechnetate) – because of thyrotoxic symptoms and suppressed TSH. Determining whether there is increased uptake - bilateral (Graves disease) or unilateral (Plummer's adenoma, toxic thyroid nodule) or lack of any uptake (thyroiditis) - helps decide treatment with antithyroid drugs (if increased uptake) or conservative management (for thyroiditis).

MRCP showed no stones in the CBD and confirmed the presence of gallstones in the gallbladder. The thyroid scan showed diffuse uptake in the thyroid – consistent with Graves' disease.

What management is indicated?

Conservative treatment for acute cholecystitis (antibiotics, iv fluids, fat-free diet)

Correction of hyperthyroidism: carbimazole (if cholecystectomy can be deferred for 4-6 weeks to allow the drugs to be effective) or potassium iodide+propranolol (if thyroid needs to be inhibited rapidly within 7-10 days).

Is cholecystectomy indicated for now?

Cholecystectomy should be postponed until her thyroid function is normalised (surgery can precipitate a thyroid crisis in patients with untreated thyrotoxicosis).

What is thyroid crisis ?

This is a rare, but life-threatening condition. It can be precipitated in a patient with inadequately controlled thyrotoxicosis undergoing thyroid surgery, parturition, severe infection, uncontrolled diabetes, and myocardial infarction.

Clinically: hyperpyrexia, tachycardia, heart failure, agitation, confusion, vomiting, diarrhoea, and coma, shock

Management: These patients need intensive monitoring in an ITU/HDU setting

Treatment : reducing hormone secretion: carbimazole or propylthyouracil (PTU) + high dose iodide (Lugol drops or potassium iodide tablets) / supportive therapy (propranolol, IV fluids, steroids, external cooling) / treating the underlying cause

What would be the timing for surgery ?

Cholecystectomy is advised after 4-6 weeks of treatment.

What important side effects of Carbimazole are important in this case?

Carbimazole is hepatotoxic (it could lead to further increase in LFTs)

What improvements of thyroid hormones are expected after 4-6 weeks of treatment with Carbimazole?

Free thyroxine level should be in normal range, TSH can be still suppressed (it takes a long time to return to normal value after prolonged inhibition during the period of thyrotoxicosis).

TRANSPLANT SURGERY

Tariq Dosani Shridhar Dronamraju Rodrigo Figuerido
Jeremy French Reza Mohammed Motallebzadeh Colin Wilson

Contents

Access for Dialysis

A 65 year old man had a laparoscopic right radical nephrectomy for an RCC 6 years ago. He made a good post-operative recovery with no recurrence. Now his eGFR is 12%(CKD 5). He has been referred to you by nephrologists for future renal supportive management and is attending your clinic for discussion regarding this.

What types of Renal Replacement Therapy are you aware of?

1) Dialysis

  a) Haemodialysis

  b) Peritoneal dialysis

2) Transplantation

What are the different types of vascular access and their advantages/ disadvantages?

A primary arteriovenous (AV) fistula can be created under local anaesthesia in most cases. A complex fistula (with transposition/superficialisation) will need a general anaesthetic. Fistulas frequently take approximately 6 weeks for maturation, but once fully functional are robust and quite resistant to thrombosis and therefore require minimal intervention. Furthermore there is less chance of infection (compared to graft or central line use) thanks to the use of autologous blood vessels.

Arteriovenous grafts (AVGs) will need general or regional anaesthetic for insertion. They can be used quickly within weeks, once the wound has healed, but are more prone to thrombosis especially at the venous end due to intimal hyperplasia. They also have higher rate of intervention (radiologically or surgically) due to a higher thrombosis rate. They are also more susceptible to infection.

Tunnelled neck lines into central veins, which can be done under local anaesthetic, are the least preferred modality for access. These can however be used immediately and therefore are useful in case of emergency. Central venous lines have increased risk of immediate complications such as pneumothorax, haemothorax, bleeding from arterial puncture, air embolism, and thoracic duct injury leading to chylothorax. They are a poor long-term solution due to a high risk of infection and sepsis. Central venous stenosis as a result of long-term cannulation is a well-documented complication. Such stenoses can cause clinical manifestations in their own right, but also reduce the available vascular 'real estate' for access, as downstream vessels will not have sufficient run-off to permit fistula formation from them.

What is the preferred location for a primary AV fistula?

Ideally an AV fistula should be placed in the non-dominant arm and as distal as possible, where an artery and vein can be joined together. The majority of the time the radial artery and cephalic vein at the wrist are used for construction of a primary fistula. Primary fistula formation can also be attempted in the anatomical snuff box if there are suitable vessels.

If there are no suitable veins in the non-dominant arm then the dominant arm or leg can be used. The reason for using the non-dominant arm is to reduce the impact on the patient's functionality in case a complication occurs or if further intervention is required. For an AV fistula, distal location should be utilized as much as possible so that a more proximal site can be used in case of failure of the distal fistula. Furthermore a distal placement reduces the incidence of steal syndrome/peripheral ischaemia.

How will you assess the patient?

The patient's chest, breast and upper arms should be evaluated for the presence of swelling or collateral veins. The arm should be examined for any scars/operation/previous fistulas. In the creation of an AVF both the artery and vein are important and specially directed evaluations of both must be completed.

Pulses should be palpable clinically (radial/ulnar/brachial). Any evidence of digital ischaemia especially in diabetic patients should be noted. The palmar arch should be patent, and can be tested for patency using the Allen test. The size of the artery should be determined using colour flow Doppler. The arterial lumen should be 1.5-2mm or greater in diameter at the point proposed for the anastomosis.

The neck should be assessed for proximal venous stenosis or previous cannulations. A suitable length of cephalic or basilic vein for access for two needles should be palpable on examination. The cephalic vein is ideal for an AVF because it is located on the ventral surface of the forearm and the lateral surface of the upper arm. These features make it an ideal access site with the patient in a sitting position. The patency of veins can be assessed by performing a tap test. Duplex scanning should be performed. Optimum features for the creation of an AVF are a luminal diameter at the point of anastomosis of 2.5 mm or greater, a straight segment of vein, absence of obstruction and continuity with the proximal central veins.

What are the complications of fistula surgery?

- Local bleeding
- Early failure
- Late failure
- Thrombosis
- Infection (10% for AVG, 5% for transposed AVF, 2% for non-transposed AVF)

- Seromas
- Steal syndrome (5%-15% of brachiocephalic AVF, 1-2% of radiocephalic AVF)
- Aneurysms and pseudoaneurysms (3% of AVF, 5% of AVG)
- Venous hypertension
- Heart failure

Bleeding from the anastomosis or dividing vessels can be a complication in the early postoperative period and requires surgical intervention. In the case of a compressing haematoma early exploration is recommended.

What is early failure?

A fistula that is never usable for dialysis or that fails within three months of use is classified as an early failure. Abnormalities such as an artery that is too small for the creation of a functional access and the presence of arterial disease such as atherosclerosis can prevent the development of an adequate AVF or result in its early failure. Another cause of early failure is juxta-anastomotic venous stenosis, which is narrowing in the segment of vein that is immediately adjacent to the anastomosis. It is thought to be due to stretching or torsion of the vein during mobilisation when creating the fistula.

For an AVF to develop and function adequately for hemodialysis there must also be adequate, low resistance blood outflow. Outflow problems include veins that are too small for fistula development, venous fibrosis or stenosis due to past trauma such as venipuncture, and the presence of accessory veins.

What is late failure?

Late fistula failure is defined as failure that occurs after 3 months. The primary causes are venous stenosis and arterial atherosclerotic disease. Treatment of stenosis, by percutaneous angioplasty, before thrombosis can occur, is important and will materially prolong access survival. Although AVFs have one-sixth the thrombosis rate of AVGs, thrombosis is the most common mechanism for late fistula failures. Thrombosis can be due to pre-existing arterial or venous malformations/pathology or technical problems. In the case of technical issues, re-exploration can be attempted but there is however a high incidence of thrombosis in re-explored fistulas due to intimal damage. Formation of a new fistula in a proximal location instead of salvage surgery is likely to be more successful.

What is steal phenomenon?

The steal phenomenon (or physiological steal syndrome) is common to most AVFs/AVGs and is a result of retrograde flow in the artery distal to the AV anastomosis and into the AV access. Dilatation of collateral vessels around the AVF can compensate for diastolic retrograde inflow into the fistula. If the collateral supply is inadequate the patient is likely to suffer distal ischemia/steal syndrome (1-15%) and can complain of rest pain, a cold hand, altered sensation and may develop ulcers or gangrene. Steal syndrome can also be due to a high flow fistula causing reduced arterial pressure and distal blood flow. An upstream arterial stenosis does need to be considered however. Steal syndrome is common in diabetic and elderly patients, and brachial AVFs compared to radial AVFs. Plication (reduction of fistula) or ligation can be curative. Alternative surgical options include the DRIL (distal revascularization and interval ligation) procedure, and the RUDI (revision using distal inflow) procedure, which involves ligation of the fistula at its origin followed by re-establishment of the fistula via bypass from a more distal arterial source (i.e. beyond the brachial artery bifurcation) to the venous limb.

Why may maturation failure occur?

Maturation failure can be due to an underlying proximal venous stenosis, or arterial factors or systemic issues. Diagnosis is made by duplex scanning or performing a fistulogram. Early surgical revision or angioplasty (surgically or radiologically) are therapeutic options.

Why does fistulation dilatation generally occur?

Fistula aneurysmal dilatation can be a problem occurring many months/years following formation. Aneurysmal change in a fistula is generally indicative of antegrade venous stenosis. It may necessitate ligation or plication if impending rupture is an issue or if the skin overlying the aneurysm is compromised.

Is cardiac failure a problem following fistula formation?

High output congestive heart failure can occur from large arteriovenous fistulae. This problem is more common with PTFE grafts and brachial artery fistulae. At least 200mls/minute of flow is required to maintain or achieve adequate dialysis. These high flows can stress the patient's heart especially in patients with existing cardiac compromise. Furthermore, in such patients the fistula will be at a higher risk for occlusion/non-functional or insufficient flow rates.

Is fistula surveillance important?

Regular surveillance should be carried out to predict and prevent access failure. Fistula surveillance is very important as it is literally the lifeline for the renal failure patient. Fistulae should be clinically assessed regularly. A thrill should be detected over the fistula. This assessment can be done by the patient. Patients are educated to report loss/change of thrill immediately. Such events may be an indication of stenosis or thrombosis. Stenosis can also result in change of thrill character or turgidity. Redness, pain and aneurysm are other clinical signs that should be reported. Access flow is also an accurate predictor of fistula and graft dysfunction. For AVGs a blood flow rate less than 600ml/minute and for AVFs a blood flow rate less than 300ml/minute may be an indication for investigation as these flow rates predict imminent thrombosis.

Further reading

The Evidence for vascular surgery. Ed by J Earnshaw and J Murie second edition.

Clinical practice guidelines - vascular access for haemodialysis, UK Renal Association, 5th Edition, 2008-2011, Final Version

Brain Death and Types of Donors

A 47 year old otherwise fit gentleman was involved in an RTA and sustained severe head trauma with a suspected brain stem injury. He is currently in ITU intubated and ventilated. He had registered himself as an organ donor on the NHS organ donor register in the past. He is now being considered for multi-organ donation.

What are the pre-requisites for considering testing for brain stem death?

Prior to checking for brain stem death we need to exclude any reversible cause for brain stem dysfunction by ensuring that

- *There should be no evidence that this state is due to drugs/medication.*

- *Primary hypothermia (<35ºC) as the cause of unconsciousness must have been excluded, and potentially reversible circulatory, metabolic and endocrine disturbances.*

- *Potentially reversible causes of apnoea (dependence on the ventilator), such as muscle relaxants and cervical cord injury, must be excluded.*

How will you confirm brain stem death (brain death) in this individual?

Brain stem death is confirmed clinically by establishing the absence of brain-stem reflexes, which include

- *The pupils are fixed and do not respond to sharp changes in the intensity of light*

- *There is no corneal reflex – care should be taken to avoid damage to the cornea*

- *The oculo-vestibular reflexes are absent. No eye movements are seen during or following the slow injection of at least 50mls of ice cold water over one minute into each external auditory meatus in turn. Clear access to the tympanic membrane must be established by direct inspection and the head should be at 30º to the horizontal plane, unless this positioning is contraindicated by the presence of an unstable spinal injury*

- *No motor responses within the cranial nerve distribution can be elicited by adequate stimulation of any somatic area or by supraorbital pressure*

- *There is no cough reflex response to bronchial stimulation by a suction catheter placed down the trachea to the carina, or gag response to stimulation of the posterior pharynx with a spatula*

- *Apnoea test*

Apnoea Test

The apnoea test should only be considered once brain-stem areflexia has been confirmed. The apnoea test involves inducing a state of moderate hypercarbia and mild acidaemia [$PaCO_2$ is at least 6.0KPa and pH < 7.40 (in patients with COPD $PaCO_2$ of 6.5KPa and pH< 7.40)] by lowering the minute volume ventilation. The patient should then be disconnected from the ventilator and attached to an oxygen flow of 5L/min via an endotracheal catheter and observed for five minutes. If, after five minutes, there has been no spontaneous respiratory response, a presumption of no respiratory centre activity can be documented.

What are the different types of organ donors?

There are three different ways of donating an organ. These are known as:

- donation after brain stem death (DBD donor)
- donation after cardiac death (DCD donor)
- live organ donation

DBD donor: The donor has been confirmed brain stem dead following a severe brain injury. The circulation is supported by artificial ventilation until the donated organs have been removed. DBD donations have a high success rate because the organs are supported by oxygenated blood until they are removed (short warm ischaemia time).

DCD donor: There are 5 (Maastricht) categories:

I- dead on arrival - uncontrolled

II- Failed resuscitation - uncontrolled

III- Awaiting cardiac arrest - controlled

IV-Cardiac arrest in a brain stem dead donor - controlled

V- Unexpected cardiac arrest in a critically ill patient

In the UK, almost all DCD type donors are in intensive care units with severe disease, but who are not brain stem dead (Maastricht category III). In such individuals where continuing medical treatment is futile and there is no chance of recovery, treatment withdrawal is often instigated. If cardiac arrest occurs without significant functional warm ischaemia, defined as 30 minutes or more of hypotension (systolic blood pressure <50mmHg) /hypoxia (haemoglobin oxygen saturation <70%) between the time of treatment withdrawal and cold in situ perfusion, the liver and pancreas may be considered for donation. The kidneys may be considered if asystole occurs within 4 hours.

The time from asystole to the perfusion of the organs with cold preservation solution in situ, including a 5 minute stand-off time, must be kept as short as possible and is recommended to be no longer than 15 minutes. This is to ensure the organs sustain minimum primary warm ischaemia.

Live organ donation: A live organ donation usually involves one family member donating an organ to another family member. The relative is usually blood-related, most commonly a parent, although it could be a partner/son or daughter. Following changes in the law, it is now possible to be an altruistic donor. Altruistic donors are unrelated to the patient but become donors as an act of personal generosity.

What are the contraindications for being an organ donor?

Although it is the responsibility of the recipient surgeon to decide whether to accept an organ, this decision will depend on both donor and recipient factors. Organs from all donors will carry some degree of risk and the risks associated with transplantation must be balanced against the benefits of transplantation and the risks of awaiting a further offer. However there are certain conditions in the donor that preclude them from being an organ donor.

Absolute contraindications to organ donation

- Known or suspected nvCJD and other neurodegenerative diseases associated with infectious agents
- Infections
  - HIV antigen/antibody positive. In exceptional circumstances, a life-preserving donation from an infected donor may be released for clinical use in a recipient who also is infected with HIV, e.g. supra-urgent liver transplant
  - Hepatitis B surface Antigen positive. (Detection of anti-Hep B core antibody with or without anti-Hep B surface antibody is a relative contraindication for liver donation. The potential for hepatitis B transmission demands consideration of appropriate prophylaxis of recipients. Organs from donors with Hepatitis C can be used in Hepatitis C^{+ve} recipients. Confirmed anti-HCV in the absence of detectable HCV RNA does not exclude use of a life-preserving organ donation in cases of severe clinical need)
  - Unidentified causative organism of bacterial meningitis or meningo-encephalitis
  - Human T cell Leukaemia Virus (HTLV)
  - Tuberculosis: active or within first 6 months of treatment
  - Influenza: Lungs and bowel should not be used from donors with confirmed influenza infection
  - Active malaria (patients with a history of travel to a malaria-endemic area, but afebrile at the time of assessment, can be accepted as donors at one year or longer since return to the UK)
  - Fungi: aspergillosis or other systemic fungal infections (not Candida)

- Chagas disease - *Trypanosoma cruzi* infection. Donors who:
- were born in South America or Central America (including Southern Mexico) or;
- whose mothers were born in these countries; or,
- who may have been transfused with blood in these countries; or
- who have lived and/or worked in rural subsistence farming communities in these countries for a continuous period of >4 weeks; should not donate tissues, other than corneas, or organs unless they have been shown by a validated test for *T. cruzi* antibody not to have antibody in their blood.

- CNS tumours
  - Primary cerebral lymphoma
  - All secondary intracranial tumours
- Non CNS tumours
  - Active cancer with spread outside the organ
  - Active haematological malignancy
  - High risk (>10% risk of transmission) donors include those with melanoma (without spread), renal cell cancer <7cm or at stages 2-6, sarcomas treated previously more than 5 years ago, or those with small cell lung cancer
- Age > 90 years

Organ specific contraindications

Each contraindication is specific to the organ listed and does not preclude the donation of any other organ.

Liver

Acute hepatitis (Serum AST or ALT>1000 IU/L if of liver origin)

Cirrhosis

Hepatic artery thrombosis

Portal vein thrombosis

Significant liver steatosis

For DCD donors, asystole time (from cardiac arrest to cold in situ perfusion) > 15 minutes

Kidney

Chronic kidney disease (CKD stage 3B and below, eGFR<45)

Long term dialysis (that is, not acute relating to acute illness)

Renal malignancy (prior kidney tumours of low grade and previously excised would not exclude donation) (primary renal cancers < 5 cm in diameter may be used)

Previous kidney transplant (> 6 months previously)

Pancreas

Age > 55years

Insulin dependent diabetes (excluding ICU associated insulin requirement)

Any history of pancreatic malignancy

Morbid obesity

Bowel

DCD donors

DBD donor age >56 years or > 80kg

Underlying chronic intestinal disease

References:

http://www.organdonation.nhs.uk

http://www.nhs.uk/conditions/organ-donation

A Companion to Specialist Surgical Practice: Transplantation Ed. John L.R. Forsythe; Saunders Elsevier Fifth edition 2013.

Transplantation of organs from deceased donors with cancer or a history of cancer. SaBTO, Advisory Committee on the Safety of Blood, Tissues and Organs. April 2014.

Immunosuppressant Therapy in Organ Transplantation

What drug remains the first line treatment of acute organ rejection?

Glucocorticoids remain the first line of pharmacological treatment of acute allogenic graft rejection in the majority of transplant centres. The most commonly used steroids for transplantation are prednisolone, hydrocortisone, prednisone and methylprednisolone. All these agents have different relative potencies.

What is the mechanism of action of glucocorticoids?

Glucocorticoids suppress antibody and complement binding, upregulate IL-10 expression, and downregulate IL-2, IL-6, and interferon-gamma synthesis in various types of cells (lymphocytes, macrophages, and other antigen-presenting cells such as dendritic cells).

What are the potential side effects of glucocorticoids?

- Impaired glucose tolerance
- Fluid retention
- Hypertension
- Emotional lability / psychosis
- Hyperlipidemia
- Acne
- Buffalo hump
- Cushingoid facies
- Impaired wound healing
- Increased susceptibility to infection
- Cataracts
- Osteopenia

What is cyclosporin? What is its mechanism of action?

Cyclosporin is a calcineurin inhibitor. It was originally derived from a filamentous fungus *Tolypocladium inflatum* Gams in the laboratories of Sandoz in Basel, Switzerland, and acts as a potent immunosuppressive agent. Cyclosporin inhibits T cell activation through a reduction in IL-2 production. This is achieved through binding to cyclophilin which inhibits the phosphatase activity of calcineurin. (Calineurin is a calmodulin-activated serine phosphatase). As a result, calcineurin cannot dephosphorylate the cytoplasmic component of the nuclear factor of activated T cells (NFATc), and thereby the transport of NFATc to the nucleus and the binding of NF-ATc to the nuclear component of the nuclear factor of activated T cells (NFATn). The NFATc–NFATn complex binds to the promoter of the interleukin 2 (IL-2) gene and initiates IL-2 production. Consequently, T cells do not produce IL-2, which is necessary for T-cell activation.

Cyclosporin has shown to block both the Jun N terminal kinase and p38 signalling pathways, which are necessary for activation of AP-1 among other transcription factors.

Why should cyclosporin levels be monitored frequently?

A number of side effects are possible with cyclosporin treatment and these include: nephrotoxicity, hypertension, hyperkalemia, and hypomagnesemia. Neurotoxicity may present as tremors, altered mental status, polyneuropathy, dysarthria, myoclonus, seizures, hallucinations. Hyperlipidemia, gingival hyperplasia, and hirsutism may occur in the longer term. Therefore cyclosporin levels should be monitored daily in the peritransplant period with the awareness that several medications can alter levels significantly.

The pathogenesis of nephrotoxicity appears to be multifactorial and includes promotion of plasma renin activity and intrarenal renin levels, with enhanced release of vasoconstrictors (endothelin and thromboxane) and suppression of vasodilators (prostacyclin and nitric oxide), which induces nephrotoxicity, and increased expression of transforming growth factor beta (a key cytokine associated with interstitial fibrosis).

Are you aware of any other calcineurin inhibitors in common use in transplantation?

Tacrolimus (also known as FK506) was originally described as a salvage therapy for patients in whom cyclosporin failed. It was originally isolated from *Streptomyces tsukubaensis*, given a code FK506 and later named Tacrolimus (acronym for *T*sukuba m*acroli*de *imm*unosuppressant). Tacrolimus exerts its immunosuppressive effect in the same manner as cyclosporin, except that it binds to a different immunophilin, FKBP-12 (FK-binding protein), resulting in inhibition of IL-2 production. It is 100 times more potent than cyclosporin.

How does the efficacy of tacrolimus compare with cyclosporin?

Multiple studies (several RCTs and meta analyses) have confirmed the superiority of tacrolimus over cyclosporin in terms of graft survival, lower rates of acute rejection, and steroid-resistant rejection in the first year. Patients treated with tacrolimus still have up to five times the risk of post-transplant diabetes mellitus compared with patients treated with cyclosporin. The incidence of lymphoproliferative disease is similar between patients taking tacrolimus or cyclosporin.

Tacrolimus is considered as part of the first line therapy after most renal and liver transplants not only because of its potency and decreased episodes of rejection, but also because lower doses of corticosteroids can be used, thus reducing the likelihood of steroid-associated side effects.

What is sirolimus and what are its advantages over calcineurin inhibitors?

Sirolimus is a macrolide antibiotic produced by Streptomyces hygroscopicus and is a potent immunosuppressive agent. It is not a calcineurin inhibitor but blocks a transduction signal from IL-2 receptors (by binding to FKBP12 and inhibiting mTOR, a key regulatory kinase) thus inhibiting T cell proliferation. It is free from nephrotoxicity and neurotoxicity and this is a major advantage over calcineurin inhibitors. Therefore it may be useful in patients who have calcineurin inhibitor toxicity.

Why is sirolimus not used as a first line agent?

The side effect profile of sirolimus is significant and therefore it is rarely used as monotherapy. Hepatic artery thrombosis, delayed wound healing and incisional hernias have been reported, while long term use has been associated with hyperlipidemia, bone marrow suppression, mouth ulcers, skin rashes, albuminuria, and pneumonia.

Another inhibitor of mTOR is everolimus which is a derivative of sirolimus. Due to an increased risk of hepatic artery thrombosis in the early post-transplantation period, it is not used earlier than 30 days after liver transplantation.

What class of agent is mycofenolate mofetil (MMF)?

Along with azathioprine, MMF blocks purine synthesis via inhibition of the enzyme inosine monophosphate dehydrogenase, and abrogates the proliferation of T cells and B cells, as well as the production of antibodies by B cells. MMF is mainly used to reduce or discontinue calcineurin inhibitor dosing in order to reduce toxic side effects. The addition of MMF may also allow steroids to be discontinued.

Azathioprine is not used in the USA but is still used in the UK and is sometimes substituted for MMF in women who are pregnant or of childbearing age, due to increased safety experience with it in pregnancy. The most common serious side-effect of azathioprine is pancytopenia, in particular leucopenia, which increases the risk of acquiring opportunistic infections. MMF is associated with less bone marrow suppression, but up to one third of patients will develop diarrhoea.

What is the rationale of using antibody based therapy for immunosuppression?

T and B cells express specific antigens on their cell surfaces. Antibodies, either polyclonal or monoclonal, to these antigens can be effective at depleting these cells. The names of monoclonal antibodies conventionally contain "muro" if they are from a murine (mouse) source and "xi" or "zu" if they are chimerized or humanized, respectively.

These agents have an important role as induction agents and in the immediate post transplant period and for treating steroid-resistant acute rejection. An example of such an agent is antithymocyte globulin (ATG).

a) Antithymocyte globulins (ATG)

The only preparation used routinely in the UK is rabbit ATG. Muromonab-CD3 (OKT-3), a murine monoclonal antibody, has been withdrawn from use due to its side-effect profile.

ATG is primarily used, together with other immunosuppressive drugs, at the time of transplantation to prevent early allograft rejection, especially if steroid-free immunosuppression is to be used, or they may be used to treat severe rejection episodes or corticosteroid-resistant acute rejection. The antibody-bound cells are phagocytosed in the liver and spleen, resulting in lymphopenia and impaired T-cell responses.

b) IL-2-receptor antagonists

Targeting of the IL-2 receptor has also been used for the induction of immunosuppression. Daclizumab (a humanized monoclonal antibody) and basiliximab (a chimeric monoclonal antibody) reduce the incidence of acute rejection when added to immunosuppressive regimens. Basiliximab is about 10-fold more potent than daclizumab as a blocker of IL-2 stimulated T-cell replication. They act by binding to the alpha subunit of the interleukin-2 receptor on activated lymphocytes and prevent IL-2 mediated responses.

c) Alemtuzumab

Alemtuzumab, a humanized monoclonal antibody against CD52, exerts its effects by causing a profound depletion of T, B and NK cells from the peripheral circulation. It is used as an induction agent in high immunologic risk recipients (highly sensitised and poor HLA match) and in those with a prednisolone-free regimen.

References

Knoll GA, Bell RC. Tacrolimus versus cyclosporin for immunosuppression in renal transplantation: meta-analysis of randomised trials. BMJ 1999;318:1104-7.

McAlister VC, Haddad E, Renouf E, Malthaner RA, Kjaer MS, Gluud LL. Cyclosporin versus tacrolimus as primary immunosuppressant after liver transplantation: a meta-analysis. Am J Transplant. 2006;6(7):1578-85.

Cantarovich D, Giral-Classe M, Hourmant M, et al. Low incidence of kidney rejection after simultaneous kidney-pancreas transplantation after antithymocyte globulin induction and in the absence of corticosteroids: results of a prospective pilot study in 28 consecutive cases. Transplantation 2000;69:1505-8.

Vincenti F, Kirkman R, Light S, et al. Interleukin-2–receptor blockade with daclizumab to prevent acute rejection in renal transplantation. N Engl J Med 1998;338:161-5.

Legal Issues and Ethics of Transplantation

What is the Human Tissue Act?

The Human Tissue Act 2004 provides the framework for regulating the storage and use of human organs and tissue from the living and deceased. It makes consent a fundamental principle underpinning its role. The Act is enforced by the Human Tissue Authority (HTA).

The 2004 Act repeals and replaces earlier legislation, including the Human Tissue Act 1961, the Anatomy Act 1984, and the Human Organ Transplants Act 1989. The 2004 Act does not apply in Scotland; separate legislation, the Human Tissue (Scotland) Act 2006, has been developed and now applies in Scotland.

What are the concerns with regard to prospective living donors?

All living donations must be approved by the HTA before donation can take place. Before the HTA can approve such cases, the following must be satisfied:

1) no reward has been, or is to be, given.

2) consent to removal for the purpose of transplantation has been given (or removal for that purpose is otherwise lawful).

3) an Independent Assessor has conducted separate interviews with the donor (and if different from the donor, the person giving consent) and the recipient (or the person acting on behalf of the recipient) and submitted a report of their assessment to the HTA.

There are two concerns with regard to living donors. Firstly, the health of the donor maybe adversely affected, with a small risk of death (risk of 1 in 3,000-4,000). Removal of an organ will inevitably cause physical harm, to a lesser or greater extent, to the donor. Hence, living donation may seem difficult to justify, particularly when the risk of harm is considered together with the well-known maxim "first, do no harm". Nevertheless, living donors often gain psychological benefit knowing that their gift has provided an opportunity to dramatically improve the quality of life of another person.

a) Mortality and Morbidity

The most common causes of death after living donation are pulmonary emboli, and cardiac events (myocardial infarction and arrhythmia).

Major short-term morbidity rate after laparoscopic donor nephrectomy is between 4%-5%. Specific complications include DVT/PE; bleeding; bowel injury; wound related problems such as sepsis, hernia and chronic pain; conversion from laparoscopic to open surgery (1%-3%); blood loss and the requirement for blood and blood products (which some donors may find unacceptable e.g. Jehovah's Witnesses); and finally the cosmetic consequences, especially of open surgery.

Studies have shown that long-term survival after donor nephrectomy is at least equal to matched cohorts.

b) Renal Function

A prospective kidney donor should not be considered for donation if the corrected GFR is predicted to fall below a satisfactory level of kidney function within the lifetime of the donor. A predicted GFR of at least 37.5 ml/min/1.73m² at the age of 80 is recommended as a minimum standard.

Compared with a matched cohort of healthy non-donors, kidney donors have an increased risk of end-stage renal disease; however, the absolute incidence of ESRD in donors is very small (<1% at a median follow-up of 8 years).

b) Hypertension

Several large studies with varying duration of follow-up suggest that approximately one third of donors will develop hypertension. Hence, in the pre-operative evaluation of potential donors, careful assessment of blood pressure is important. Evidence of hypertensive end organ damage, poorly controlled hypertension, or hypertension that requires more than two drugs to achieve adequate control are relative contraindications to live donor nephrectomy.

c) Effects of potential malignancy

The presence of a solitary kidney may in certain situations be a major disadvantage, either because it may be affected directly by malignant disease or indirectly by the additional treatment (e.g. chemotherapy) required.

Secondly, although living donation is based on altruism, there is the concern that a 'reward' may be given to the donor, whether it be financial or emotional. For example payment of money can be made without knowledge of the transplant team. Such a reward may only become a factor sometimes later in life e.g. "I gave you my kidney when you were dying now you owe me …".

Transplantation of living donor kidneys from altruistic or stranger donors is on the increase in the UK.

What do you understand by the term 'expanded criteria donor'?

A significant imbalance exists between the number of available organs and candidates awaiting transplantation for end-stage organ failure, and this has led to a reappraisal of donor selection criteria and the utilization of extended criteria allografts. Expanded criteria donors are also known as 'marginal donors' and may provide suboptimal organs that can impact the longevity of the graft function. These donors imply higher risk in comparison with a reference donor. The risk may manifest as increased incidence of poor allograft function, allograft failure leading to death or requiring re-transplantation, or transmission of a donor-derived disease.

For cadaveric kidneys, any deceased donor (DCD or DBD) over the age of 60 years or a deceased donor over the age of 50 years within 2 of the following criteria are classified as marginal:

i)   History of high blood pressure

ii) Serum Cr >1.5mg/dl (>133mmol/l)

iii) Death resulting from a cerebrovascular accident

The long-term survival of such marginal kidneys has been shown to be considerably shorter than that of ideal kidney allografts.

Expanded criteria living kidney donors were defined in one meta-analysis as having any of the following prior to the time of donation:

- age > 60 years old

- hypertension: >140/90 mmHg or on blood pressure medication

- low GFR (either < 80 mL/min or <100 mL/min)

Donors with proteinuria: either $\geq$150 mg/day or $\geq$300 mg/day; microscopic haematuria; or obesity: BMI either >30 kg/m^2 or >35 kg/m^2 were not described in any of the reviewed studies.

An accepted definition of expanded criteria donor livers has not yet been established by the liver transplant community. A donor risk index in liver transplantation has been developed by Feng et al, who analyzed data from deceased donors reported to the Scientific Registry of Transplant Recipients (6). They identified seven donor factors that were significantly associated with graft failure: donor age > 70 years, African-American donors, reduced donor height, cause of death other than cerebral trauma, DCD or split grafts, and prolonged cold ischaemic time. Each additional hour of cold ischaemic time beyond 8 hours was associated with a 1% increase in the risk of graft loss.

Furthermore, the presence of steatosis impacts graft function and survival, with moderately steatotic livers considered as marginal grafts. In addition, livers from other marginal donors may not display graft dysfunction, but can transmit an infection to the recipient: hepatitis C virus-positive (HCV) or hepatitis B core antibody-positive (anti-HBc) donors. HCV$^+$ livers must be transplanted to HCV$^+$ recipients and anti-HBc$^+$ grafts must be initially transplanted to HBV$^+$ patients, but may be transplanted to HBV-negative recipients provided antiviral therapy is used after transplantation.

What percentage of renal dialysis patients are on a transplant list in the UK?

The percentage of dialysis patients on a transplant list varies across the UK from 20%-45%. This would suggest that there is an inequality of access whereby some centres would list a patient whereas others would not. National guidelines and waiting list criteria are available from the NHS Organ Donation and Transplantation website (www.odt.nhs.uk), the British Transplant Society (www.bts.org.uk) and the

UK renal registry (www.renalreg.org). On average the waiting time is around three years, with one in five patients getting a kidney transplant within a year, and about two out of three receiving a transplant by five years. In the UK, diabetes is the most common cause of chronic renal failure.

References

Segev DL, Muzaale AD, Caffo BS, et al. Perioperative mortality and long-term survival following live kidney donation. JAMA. 2010; 303: 959-66.

Muzaale AD, Massie AB, Wang MC, Montgomery RA, McBride MA, Wainright JL, Segev DL. Risk of End-Stage Renal Disease Following Live Kidney Donation. JAMA. 2014;311(6):579-586.

Port FK, Bragg-Gresham JL, Metzger RA, Dykstra DM, Gillespie BW, Young EW, Delmonico FL, Wynn JJ, Merion RM, Wolfe RA, Held PJ. Donor characteristics associated with reduced graft survival: an approach to expanding the pool of kidney donors. Transplantation. 2002 Nov 15;74(9):1281-6.

Lloveras J, Arias M, Puig JM, et al. Long-term follow-up of recipients of cadaver kidney allografts from elderly donors. Transplant Proc 1993;25:3175-6.

Iordanousa Y, Seymoura N, Young A, Johnsona J, Iansavichusa AV, Cuerdena MS, Gillc JS, Poggiod E, Garga AX. Recipient Outcomes for Expanded Criteria Living Kidney Donors: The Disconnect Between Current Evidence and Practice. Am J Transplant 2009; 9: 1558–1573.

Feng S, Goodrich NP, Bragg-Gresham JL, et al. Characteristics associated with liver graft failure: the concept of a donor risk index. Am J Transplant 2006;6:783–90.

Post Liver Transplant Graft Dysfunction

A 63 year old male with hepatitis C disease is listed for liver transplantation. He receives a DCD liver from a 59 year old male, from a CMV positive donor. The operation is performed uneventfully, with the exception of requiring an arterial conduit due to poor recipient vessels, which is placed infrarenally. He makes a good postoperative recovery, and is being managed in the intensive care unit. His ALT peaked immediately postoperatively at 3200, at which point his bilirubin was 78.

Two days postoperatively, his PT has risen from 18 to 22, and his ALT has risen from 2430 to 2890. What is the differential diagnosis and what would be your management plan?

Once a biliary complication is suspected, a Doppler abdominal ultrasound is warranted to evaluate the biliary tree as well as the hepatic vasculature. Hepatic artery thrombosis (HAT) is the most important diagnosis to exclude. Angiographic evidence of more than 50% reduction in caliber of the lumen of the hepatic artery is defined as hepatic artery stenosis. It occurs in approximately 4% of adult liver transplants, with higher rates in paediatric transplantation. Other differentials include preservation injury and initial poor function. An urgent Doppler ultrasound should be performed to exclude a HAT. A low resistive index with increase in focal peak velocity is a suggestive feature of HAT. If there is any doubt regarding arterial flow on ultrasound, a CT angiogram may be required. If there is thrombosis, at this early stage consideration could be given to re-exploration of the arterial anastomosis. Endovascular intervention with thrombolysis or stent insertion may also be considered if there is local expertise. If intervention is not performed, or is unsuccessful, HAT within the first 21 days post transplantation is an indication for urgent re-transplantation.

How do you diagnose primary non-function of the liver graft? What are the risk factors for primary non-function?

Deteriorating lab results may represent either initial poor function (IPF) in the setting of a marginal graft or primary non-function (PNF). Graft dysfunction is common, affecting up to 27% of liver transplants, and published series report PNF rates of up to 8%. PNF is an indication for urgent re-transplantation. It is manifest by a failure to regain consciousness (encephalopathy), sustained elevation of transaminases, increasing coagulopathy and acidosis, and histologic evidence of hepatocyte necrosis in the absence of any vascular complication. It can take more than 72 hours to be certain that the graft will not recover adequate function. One definition of IPF is AST >2000 and PT>16 on postoperative days 2-7. The donor risk factors for PNF include increasing donor age, steatosis, elevated serum sodium level and a DCD donation. Recipient risk factors for PNF include prolonged cold ischaemic and secondary warm ischaemic time and haemodynamic instability.

His Doppler shows a good arterial trace, and his liver function continues to improve. He is transferred to the general ward. On the 10th postoperative day his LFTs show a deterioration (ALT rises from 310 to 510; ALP rises from 209 to 317; bilirubin is static at 33; PT unchanged at 11s). What are the potential causes of these biochemical changes? How would you investigate and manage him?

The current differentials now include hepatic arterial thrombosis, biliary complications (leak/collection), and acute rejection. The initial approach should be to repeat the Doppler ultrasound. If this is normal, then a liver biopsy is indicated to exclude rejection. It is useful to know the trough serum level of the immunosuppression he is receiving. Re-infection with hepatitis C or CMV activation is rare at this stage, with hepatitis usually occurring in the 3rd to 7th weeks, and CMV disease typically occurring around 6 months postoperatively.

The doppler confirms a good arterial trace, and he progresses to undergo a liver biopsy. This shows acute cellular rejection. What are the biopsy characteristics of acute cellular rejection? How would you treat it? How would you monitor response? Does this diagnosis have an impact on the likely longevity of the graft?

Acute cellular rejection occurs in 20%-80% of cases. Typically it occurs between postoperative days 5-30. It has a classic triad of features: portal inflammation, bile duct inflammation and venous inflammation. It is graded according to the Banff criteria, and can be indeterminate, mild, moderate or severe. In the setting of a marginal liver with severe preservation injury, this can be difficult to diagnose, which supports the rationale for an intraoperative protocol biopsy at the time of transplantation. Standard treatment for a first episode of rejection would be 3 doses of intravenous methylprednisolone. In combination with this it is important to optimise the calcineurin inhibitor dose and confirm that the patient is on the correct dose of antiproliferative agent. Response would be monitored by observing the liver function tests for improvement. This may take over 48 hours to become apparent. The role of antibody mediated rejection (AMR) in liver transplantation has only recently been appreciated. Early/mild AMR is characterized by portal oedema, ductular reaction and a neutrophil-rich inflammatory infiltrate. Sinusoidal complement C4d deposition can be a distinguishing feature, and has been found to occur in association with areas of lobular necrosis. Treatment protocols vary between centres, however, high dose steroids remain the standard initial treatment.

A single episode of acute rejection which responds to treatment has no deleterious effect on long-term graft survival (graft survival may actually be better in this patient group). However, recurrent episodes which are steroid refractory do have a negative effect on long-term graft survival and are associated with the onset of chronic rejection.

This scenario is distinct from the context of a follow-up protocol biopsy. Some centres advocate protocol biopsies in the postoperative period, citing a lack of correlation between observed histological changes of rejection with demonstrable biochemical abnormalities. However, less than half of all patients with apparent rejection on protocol biopsies develop biochemical graft dysfunction, hence protocol biopsies are not performed in all centres, as they may be not a good indicator to guide treatment.

If the liver biopsy had not shown rejection, what would your next steps have been?

Biliary complications should be considered. These can occur in up to 30% of cases, and include biliary tract strictures, bile leaks, and bile duct stones. The associated mortality rate with biliary complications is about 10%. The most common biliary complication is bile duct stricture. Strictures are classified as early (within 1 month of transplantation, usually related to technical problems) and late strictures (after 1 month of transplantation, mainly secondary to vascular insufficiency); and as anastomotic (AS) or nonanastomotic (NAS) depending on the stricture site. AS are generally the result of fibrosis, local ischaemia, technical issues, or a bile leak in the post-operative period, whereas NAS can be due to vascular problems and ischaemia, chronic rejection or recurrence of primary sclerosing cholangitis. Whilst a marginal DCD graft is at a higher risk of non-anastomotic strictures, these do not manifest until much later in the postoperative course, typically around 6 months.

MRCP is used to determine the diagnosis, reserving ERCP for those ducts which require intervention, allowing placement of a biliary stent. AS can be successfully treated with endoscopic dilation plus stenting. If the stricture persists, or there is significant disruption of the anastomosis, conversion of a duct-to-duct anastomosis (choledochocholedochostomy) to a choledochojejunostomy with a Roux-en-Y loop should be undertaken. Non-anastomotic strictures require long-term stenting or relisting for transplantation.

Bile leaks are a common complication after liver transplantation with an incidence ranging between 2%-25%. Early bile leaks are either due to a technical problem or biliary ischaemia. It is therefore important to ensure that the hepatic artery is patent (by CT angiogram). If HAT is confirmed, urgent re-transplantation should be considered. Otherwise, either an ERCP with placement of a biliary stent across the leak or surgical repair/biliary reconstruction can be performed.

Further reading:

Moreno R and Bernguer M. Post-liver Transplant Medical Complications. Annals of Hepatology 2006; 5(2): 77-85.

Haydon G. Graft Dysfunction. Graft 2003;6(2):120-128.

Post Transplant Lymphoproliferative Disease

A 65 year old man presents with intermittent right iliac fossa pain associated with weight loss, bloating and occasional vomiting. He has a palpable mass in the RIF. He is 6 years post renal transplant for diabetic nephropathy. A CT scan shows marked thickening of the terminal ileum with proximal distention as well as multiple enlarged mesenteric nodes and stranding.

What is the most likely diagnosis?

He clearly has small bowel pathology and in a transplant recipient one important differential to consider would be post transplant lymphoproliferative disorder (PTLD). However other differential diagnoses to rule out include Crohn's disease as well as other causes of terminal ileitis e.g. infective.

What is PTLD?

PTLD is an increasingly recognised condition as the number of solid organ transplant recipients increases. It affects approximately 8% of solid organ transplant recipients, but is the most common malignancy in solid organ transplant recipients. Certain transplants are more frequently complicated by PTLD than others e.g. small bowel and pancreas.

When do most PTLD cases present following transplant?

The time interval between transplant and development of PTLD is variable, with most occurring within a year. This may correspond to the most aggressive period of immunosuppression. As a general rule patients who present late (>1 year) have more aggressive tumours and a worse prognosis.

What is the pathology of PTLD tumours?

The majority of PTLD tumours demonstrate a polyclonal B-cell Epstein-Barr virus (EBV) positive cell population. Extra-nodal involvement is 3-4 times more common than nodal involvement, and resembles primary lymphoma of those organs. Monoclonal B-cell and T-cell small bowel lymphomas do occur in patients with organ transplants but are less common.

How is a diagnosis of PTLD made?

An accurate diagnosis of PTLD requires a high index of suspicion. Radiologic evidence of a mass in a transplant recipient is suggestive of PTLD. Excisional biopsy is required to ensure an accurate diagnosis.

What is the treatment of PTLD?

Treatment depends on the location and extent of disease. Unlike other malignancies disease regression in response to a reduction in immunosuppression is a unique diagnostic feature of PTLD. Surgical resection of disease may still be required in certain circumstances e.g. bowel obstruction. Other treatment options include radiotherapy and rituximab. If immunosuppression is altered then patients need to be closely monitored for rejection.

What other malignancies are associated with transplant patients?

Human Herpesvirus 8 (HHV8) infection is associated with Kaposi's sarcoma as well as multiple myeloma. Kaposi's sarcoma is an indolent cutaneous disease that rarely disseminates in immunocompetent patients. However under immunosuppression disease is more aggressive, multicentric, and visceral involvement is more common. Initial treatment of Kaposi's sarcoma is a reduction of immunosuppression, which usually prompts regression.

HPV is associated with anogenital cancers including cervical, vaginal, vulval, penile, and anal cancers, head and neck cancer, and is implicated in squamous cell skin cancers.

Merkel cell carcinoma is increased in transplant recipients and is an aggressive, predominantly intradermal, neuroendocrine malignancy, known for local recurrence and lymph node metastases.

Chronic hepatitis B infection is associated with development of hepatocellular carcinoma and risk exacerbated Hep C co-infection.

Renal Vein Thrombosis

You are asked to see a 52 year old female patient (who has been on warfarin) day 3 post renal transplant with pain over the graft, haematuria and hypotension. Describe your assessment of the patient.

Assessment and resuscitation would be by the principles of "ABCD". Particular points of interest would be the patient's observations and the tempo or rate of decline of the patient. Has a sudden drop in the patient's blood pressure and a corresponding rise in heart rate been noted? Examination of the contents of the catheter bag is required and also the documentation of the urine output. If there has been a rapid decline in urine output that could point towards vascular thrombosis. I would examine the patient for signs of graft tenderness/swelling and examine the contents and volume of any drain bag or bottle. An important diagnostic marker is the presence of haematuria. Renal vein thrombosis is often characterised by heavy haematuria and this may differentiate the problem from bleeding from other areas like the vascular anastomoses. Blood in the drain would not be a differentiating factor as this could signify a ruptured kidney secondary to renal vein thrombosis.

Following commencement of immediate resuscitative measures (oxygen, large bore cannulae, intravenous fluids), and guided by the observations, I would request blood tests including full blood count and coagulation. Clearly a drop in haemoglobin would suggest the presence of severe ongoing bleeding. I would also like to know the patient's INR, as she was previously on warfarin. How was the patient's warfarin reversed?

If it was with fresh frozen plasma or concentrated clotting factors and Vitamin K was not included then the warfarin taken by the patient on the day of surgery may still be having an effect and this would need immediate appropriate treatment as well.

You decide that the patient is stable enough for an ultrasound on the ward. The ultrasonographer is unable to demonstrate venous flow and says there is "reverse diastolic" flow. What does this mean and what are you going to do about it?

Lack of venous flow on ultrasonography would suggest renal vein thrombosis. This is further supported by "reverse diastolic flow", where renal arterial flow is reversed in diastole due to vascular outflow obstruction. The diagnosis of renal vein thrombosis is now confirmed, and the patient needs immediate operative intervention. I would therefore ensure there is blood cross-matched, inform the operating theatres and the duty anaesthetist. Consent would be obtained from the patient and/or a discussion with the family if time allowed.

Hyperkalaemia is to be anticipated and would require urgent treatment on the way and in the operating theatre (iv. Calcium gluconate, dextrose/ insulin infusion and haemofiltration).

Describe the operative surgical approach in detail.

Prior to reopening the incision I would ensure that I had appropriate skilled assistants (preferably two) and would have a fixed retraction system set up. I would ask for two pool suction sets to be ready and ensure that the anaesthetic team had blood products ready to be administered. I would also ensure that appropriate vascular clamps were open on the surgical trays. I am anticipating large volume bleeding from a ruptured capsule and reduced working space from a massively swollen graft on opening the deep sutures. If this was to happen I would use finger dissection to develop the planes around the kidney and insert the retractor. The first priority would be to obtain proximal and distal vascular control by applying vascular clamps above and below the arterial and venous anastomosis on the iliac vessels. If this was unsuccessful (or with severe bleeding) a clamp could be placed across the hilum of the kidney and the graft rapidly removed with scissors to obtain access to the deep external iliac vessels. Following vascular control of the pedicle I would pause to allow the anaesthetist to control the blood pressure and obtain formal vascular control of the iliac vessels, identify the ureter and lightly palpate for the presence of thrombus in the renal vein and external iliac vein- a clamp proximal to the thrombus would be applied after clamping the artery. At this stage I would make a decision on the viability of the kidney and in most cases a transplant nephrectomy would be required.

The nephrectomy would be completed by clamping the renal artery and vein and dissecting the ureter free from the bladder. At this stage I would flush the artery and vein to remove any thrombus and ligate them sequentially. I would also make a decision about whether to remove all the donor vascular material and close the arteriotomy and venotomy with native vein patches, although this is not necessary. The bladder should be closed (with ureteric stent removed) primarily in 2 layers with absorbable continuous sutures and washout the wound prior to closure in the standard fashion. A further bladder washout would also be required.

What are the risk factors for renal vein thrombosis?

These can be classified into donor and recipient factors in the immediate perioperative period. Donors after cardiac death (DCD) with long warm ischaemic periods are more susceptible to graft thrombosis (although this is more typically arterial). Right kidneys with short veins and long arteries (kinking) are also predisposed. Multiple veins on the graft (particularly where one has been ligated) and graft position (compression or twisting of the hilum) are also risk factors.

Recipient medical factors include pre-existing (venous) vascular disease and thrombophillia (primary or acquired). Perioperative factors such as dehydration or hypotension leading to hypercoagulability as well as external compression due to haematoma or lymphocoele formation.

Late graft thrombosis (after 1 week) is typically due to graft rejection and is more often arterial.

In what circumstances may you try and salvage a renal graft rather than perform immediate transplant nephrectomy?

The donor and recipient factors need to be evaluated. A live donor graft in a patient with poor vascular access would mandate aggressive attempts at salvage. If the graft looks congested and swollen but viable with only partial occlusion then this may be appropriate. In this situation, prior to nephrectomy, I would ask for a transplant perfusion back table to be set up, explant the graft, cold perfuse with preservation solution to remove all the thrombus from the kidney and then examine the anastomoses for evidence of intimal damage or stenosis prior to re-implantation. Importantly if the graft did not re-perfuse properly I would remove it again and send it for histology prior to finishing the operation.

What are the implications on further transplantation in patients who have a renal arterial thrombosis as opposed to renal vein thrombosis?

In patients who have had a late (>1 month) renal arterial thrombosis the graft may be left in - if there are no signs of graft tenderness or infection. This potentially leads to immunological "sensitisation", but also means that the site of implantation of a re-transplant may need to be the contralateral iliac fossa.

I note that this particular patient has previously been on warfarin. If this is due to previous thrombosis or a primary thrombophillia further investigation may be required prior to listing for re-transplantation. Patients with documented thrombophillia need a perioperative anticoagulation plan at the time of transplantation.

HEPATOBILIARY SURGERY

Jonathon Barnes Tariq Dosani   Rodrigo Figuerido
Jeremy French Bhaskar Kumar   Alexander Phillips
Stuart Robinson   Rehan Saif Avinash Sewpaul
Simon Wemyss-Holden

Contents

Acute Pancreatitis

Scenario 1

A 65 year old man is admitted with severe epigastric pain of sudden onset with a serum amylase of 3500 units. Past medical history includes ischaemic heart disease and type II diabetes. Vital signs are stable and he is passing adequate volumes of urine. His CRP on admission was normal. Modified Glasgow score is 3. He has a bilirubin of 94μmol/l and is icteric. ALP and GGT are raised in an obstructive pattern.

Within 24 hours of admission he is noted to be oliguric with a creatinine of 244μmol/l and a sudden dramatic rise of CRP to 250. He has a metabolic acidosis with pH 7.27 and base excess -11.

What further radiological investigations need to be organised at this stage?

Given the presentation with jaundice and obstructed LFTs this patient is likely to have gallstone pancreatitis. An urgent ultrasound scan of his abdomen should be performed and this can also be done as a portable test if the patient is too unwell to be moved. Should the USS show an obstructed biliary system the patient may require urgent biliary decompression.

What is the role of CT scanning at this stage?

The patient has severe acute pancreatitis, which has rapidly progressed from a mild attack. Although an argument can be made for an urgent CT scan it is justifiable to delay this scan on the basis that necrosis may only be demonstrable from 7 days since the onset of the attack. Also he has acute kidney injury - iodinated contrast media may dramatically worsen his renal function.

The only role of CT at such an early stage is to help exclude other differentials such as mesenteric ischaemia. However in this case the diagnosis is not in any doubt.

An USS shows evidence of gallstones in a thin walled gallbladder with mild intra-hepatic and extra-hepatic dilatation but no definite CBD stone. His bilirubin is now 52μmol/l from 94μmol/l the day before. He is apyrexial and stable but the ICU consultant is pushing you to organise an ERCP.

What is the role of ERCP for this patient?

Although it is possible the patient may have a CBD stone his bilirubin has fallen and he has no sign of cholangitis. In the majority of patients stones/sludge within the CBD pass spontaneously or the jaundice may have been from pancreatic oedema compressing the bile duct. Early ERCP (within 24-72 hours of onset) in gallstone pancreatitis is only indicated when there is evidence of biliary obstruction and clinical signs of cholangitis.

The latest guidelines suggest that early ERCP should only be performed for acute gallstone pancreatitis with evidence of obstruction and cholangitis. Once his general condition improves an MRCP or EUS may be performed to exclude choledocholithiasis.

Would you give antibiotics to this patient?

I would not give antibiotics to this patient as he has no evidence of infected necrosis. Antibiotics are best reserved for patients with infection superimposed on necrosis. There is no evidence to support its use in a prophylactic manner to prevent infection within necrosis. Secondary infection usually occurs in the second or third week following admission.

Although infection of pancreatic necrosis accounts for the majority of late deaths from acute severe pancreatitis, there is no evidence to show a benefit from prophylactic antibiotics. The most recent meta-analysis of 14 RCTs (n=841 patients) concluded that prophylactic antibiotics do not reduce the mortality, infection rates of necrosis or extra-pancreatic infection rates.

A nasogastric tube has drained over 2.5 litres in the past 24 hours. What are the best options for feeding this patient?

Although the evidence would support enteral nutrition this patient has an ileus which limits the ability to feed him enterally. Therefore it would be reasonable to liaise with the nutrition team and insert a PICC line to start peripheral TPN until the ileus resolves.

In acute severe pancreatitis it has been shown by an RCT that enteral nutrition is superior to TPN in terms of reduced morbidity and a trend towards reduced infection. Enteral nutritional support may preserve gut mucosal function and limit the inflammatory response. Enteral feeding options include nasogastric feeding or radiological or endoscopically placed nasojejunal feeding tube, and this depends on local protocols. Recent studies have shown that the NG route is safe and well tolerated in up to 80% of patients. In those who cannot tolerate the NG route after 48 hours then NJ feeding may need to be established.

Ten days into admission an MRCP is performed which shows no evidence of biliary obstruction but gallstones within a thick walled gallbladder. When would you offer this patient cholecystectomy? Would you perform a cholangiogram?

The patient should be offered a laparoscopic cholecystectomy and on table cholangiogram. However I would wait for his general condition to improve significantly and ensure that fluid collections and necrosis stabilise. Given the recent episode of jaundice and obstructed LFTs it would be safer to perform a cholangiogram although the chances of finding a CBD stone are very small since the MRCP did not demonstrate choledocholithiasis.

According to the latest BSG guidelines laparoscopic cholecystectomy should be performed within 2 weeks of hospital discharge for mild acute gallstone pancreatitis. More caution needs to be exercised for severe gallstone pancreatitis though cholecystectomy should ideally be performed once the general condition significantly improves. Given how unstable he was on admission it is best to perform the procedure on the index admission rather than sending the patient home.

Scenario 2

A 75 year old lady presents with vomiting, weight loss and abdominal distention six weeks after a recent admission with idiopathic acute pancreatitis. Clinical examination revealed a distended abdomen with some fullness in the epigastrium. A CT scan was performed and this showed a large (19cm x 10cm) pancreatic pseudocyst causing gastric outlet obstruction (see Figure 1)

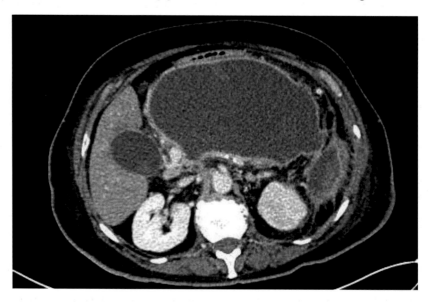

Figure 1: CT pancreas showing large pancreatic pseudocyst causing gastric outlet obstruction.

What is the difference between a pseudocyst and an acute peripancreatic fluid collection (PFC)?

PFCs are seen in the first four weeks after onset of symptoms and are believed to occur due to either ductal rupture or fluid transudation/oedema without the presence of ductal communication. They do not have solid components and result from pancreatic or peripancreatic inflammation without necrosis. PFCs occur in the peripancreatic spaces of the lesser sac and have no defined walls. The majority of PFCs remain sterile and are spontaneously reabsorbed within the first weeks of the acute pancreatitis episode.

What is a pancreatic pseudocyst (PP)?

PPs are seen from about four weeks into the course of acute pancreatitis. They are circumscribed, homogeneous amylase-rich fluid collections with no sign of any solid component/tissue necrosis. They are termed 'pseudo' as they are surrounded by a granulation tissue capsule with no epithelial lining.

How would you manage this lady's pancreatic pseudocyst?

Although asymptomatic pseudocysts do not require intervention this lady's pseudocyst is causing symptoms of gastric outlet obstruction. Symptomatic pseudocysts are managed conservatively for up to 12 weeks from the onset of acute pancreatitis. Up to 50% of these will resolve. Intervention is best performed once a thick wall has formed and the cyst has matured.

The diagnosis of an acute pseudocyst can be made if an acute fluid collection persists for 4–6 weeks and is enveloped by a distinct wall. A pseudocyst is unlikely to resolve spontaneously if: a) it persists for more than 6 weeks, b) chronic pancreatitis is evident, c) there is a pancreatic duct anomaly (except for a communication with the pseudocyst) or d) the pseudocyst is surrounded by a thick wall

What are the treatment options for a pseudocyst?

If available endoscopic ultrasound (EUS) guided transluminal drainage would be the treatment of choice. There have been two RCTs which have conclusively proven that EUS guided drainage is associated with significantly higher rates of technical success than conventional endoscopic drainage. There is also a retrospective study and an RCT that have proven that the clinical outcomes of EUS-guided drainage is comparable to that of surgical cystogastrostomy. Therefore given the high technical success rates, EUS is the endoscopic modality of choice for the drainage of pancreatic pseudocysts, with treatment outcomes comparable to that of surgery.

In some centres metal stents have been popular for the drainage of pancreatic pseudocysts. However despite the enthusiasm for the placement of such stents, current evidence does not support the routine placement of metal stents for drainage of pancreatic pseudocysts. Metal stents do not confer any significant advantage over plastic stents in this context.

Wherever possible percutaneous drainage should be avoided due to the risks of secondary infection and pancreatic fistula. In practice it is probably limited to those patients with infected, fluid-predominant collections with systemic organ dysfunction.

What do you understand by the term 'walled off pancreatic necrosis'?

Pancreatic pseudocysts can occur as a consequence of duct leak or pancreatic inflammation. When the inflammatory process is severe, the liquefied parenchyma matures into a contained collection termed walled-off pancreatic necrosis (WOPN). The distinction between the two has clinical importance, as inadvertent transluminal drainage of a WOPN by using conventional endoscopic cystogastrostomy predisposes the patient to infection, with adverse clinical outcomes.

Characterisation is the first appropriate step in the treatment of fluid collections. Clinical outcomes are directly related to the type of fluid collection being treated, and hence accurate distinction is important before undertaking any intervention. Though used widely contrast-enhanced CT cannot reliably detect necrotic debris within a peripancreatic fluid collection. T2-weighted magnetic resonance imaging (MRI) enables identification of solid debris within a necrotic collection and thereby determines the need for necrosectomy and other interventions.

Although most pseudocysts and WOPN resolve without intervention, those causing pain, gastric outlet, intestinal or biliary obstruction, organ failure, or infection warrant intervention. In a randomized trial that compared a minimally invasive step-up approach to open surgical necrosectomy, one-third of patients managed with percutaneous drainage did not require surgery. There was no difference in mortality between the two groups. There was less organ dysfunction in the step up approach group and overall complications were less in this group.

Although transluminal endoscopic necrosectomy was advocated as a definitive treatment measure in patients with WOPN, the multicenter GEPARD study showed that the procedure is associated with high morbidity and mortality.

Superior outcomes can be achieved by tailoring the endoscopic approach to the specific characteristics of each collection.

What is the difference between a pancreatic pseudocyst and WOPN?

The two entities differ by the fact that WOPN replaces part of the pancreatic parenchyma and contains pancreatic necrotic debris, while pseudocysts do not contain necrotic debris and most commonly develop in the peripancreatic spaces. It is not uncommon that the presence of areas of walled off pancreatic necrosis are still reported as pseudocysts.

Pseudocysts have a better prognosis than WOPN as they can be more easily drained.

How is minimally invasive necrosectomy performed?

This is a technique developed by the Glasgow group in which first a radiological drain tract is dilated and a nephroscope inserted. Debridement can be performed through this system. Several sessions may be required for complete debridement. An alternative is Video Assisted Retroperitoneal Dissection (VARD) in which a small 5cm incision is made in the left flank allowing video assisted removal of necrotic material.

Are you aware of any trials which have compared minimally invasive techniques for necrosectomy?

Minimally invasive necrosectomy strategies have never been compared in a randomised controlled trial. The PANTER study (PAncreatitis, Necrosectomy versus sTEp up appRoach) is an RCT comparing:

Group A: minimally invasive 'step-up approach' starting with drainage followed, if necessary, by videoscopic assisted retroperitoneal debridement (VARD)

Group B: maximal necrosectomy by laparotomy.

- Both procedures are followed by CPL.

- Patients will be recruited from 20 hospitals, including all Dutch university medical centers, over a 3-year period. The primary endpoint is the proportion of patients suffering from post-operative major morbidity and mortality. Secondary endpoints are complications, new onset sepsis, length of hospital and intensive care stay, quality of life and total (direct and indirect) costs.

Are you aware of any trials looking at the role of early enteral nutrition in acute pancreatitis?

The PYTHON trial is a multicentre RCT set up by the Dutch Pancreatitis study group. They conducted a multicenter, randomized trial comparing early nasoenteric tube feeding with an oral diet at 72 hours after presentation to the emergency department in patients with acute pancreatitis. This trial did not show any difference in reducing the rate of infection or mortality.

References

UK guidelines for the management of acute pancreatitis. Working Party of the British Society of Gastroenterology; Association of Surgeons of Great Britain and Ireland; Pancreatic Society of Great Britain and Ireland; Association of Upper GI Surgeons of Great Britain and Ireland. Gut. 2005 May;54 Suppl 3:iii1-9.

van Santvoort HC, Besselink MG, Bakker OJ, et al. A step-up approach or open necrosectomy for necrotizing pancreatitis. N Engl J Med. 2010;362:1491–1502.

Besselink MG, van Santvoort HC, Nieuwenhuijs VB, et al of the Dutch Acute Pancreatitis Study Group. Minimally invasive 'step-up approach' versus maximal necrosectomy in patients with acute necrotising pancreatitis (PANTER trial): design and rationale of a randomised controlled multicenter trial BMC Surg. 2006 Apr 11;6:6.

Bakker OJ, van Brunschot S, van Santvoort HC, Besselink MG et al. Early versus on-demand nasoenteric tube feeding in acute pancreatitis. N Engl J Med. 2014 Nov 20;371(21):1983-93.

Wittau M, Mayer B, Scheele J, Henne-Bruns D, Dellinger EP, Isenmann R. Systematic review and meta-analysis of antibiotic prophylaxis in severe acute pancreatitis. Scand J Gastroenterol. 2011 Mar;46(3):261-70. Epub 2010 Nov 10.

Varadarajulu S, Christein JD, Tamhane A, Drelichman ER, Wilcox CM. Prospective randomized trial comparing EUS and EGD for transmural drainage of pancreatic pseudocysts (with videos) Gastrointest Endosc. 2008;68:1102–1111.

Park DH, Lee SS, Moon SH, et al. Endoscopic ultrasound-guided versus conventional transmural drainage for pancreatic pseudocysts: a prospective randomized trial. Endoscopy. 2009;41:842–848.

Varadarajulu S, Lopes TL, Wilcox CM, Drelichman ER, Kilgore ML, Christein JD. EUS versus surgical cyst-gastrostomy for management of pancreatic pseudocysts. Gastrointest Endosc. 2008;68:649–655.

Varadarajulu S, Bang JY, Sutton BS, Trevino JM, Christein JD, Wilcox CM. Equal efficacy of endoscopic and surgical cystogastrostomy for pancreatic pseudocyst drainage in a randomized trial. Gastroenterology. 2013;145:583–590.

Benign Liver Lesions

A 52 year old woman complained of vague upper abdominal pain. No other signs or symptoms were discovered on clinical examination apart from hepatomegaly. Liver function tests and full blood count were normal. She has an elevated level of carbohydrate antigen 19-9 (CA 19-9) 123ng/ml (normal value: <37). The remaining tumour markers including carcinoembryonic antigen (CEA), carbohydrate antigen 125 (CA 125) and alpha-fetoprotein (AFP) were normal. Anti-echinococcal IgM and IgG antibodies and viral markers for hepatitis B and C were negative. Ultrasound examination of the liver shows a cystic, well-defined lesion of maximum diameter 14 cm occupying liver segments 4 and 8.

List the types of benign liver lesions. Which are the most common?

- hepatic cyst
- haemangioma
- focal nodular hyperplasia
- hepatic adenoma
- biliary cystadenoma
- nodular regenerative hyperplasia
- angiomyolipoma
- endothelioid haemangioendothelioma
- bile duct hamartoma
- peliosis

It is noted that most benign liver lesions are asymptomatic incidental findings on cross-sectional imaging.

What is the first step in radiological assessment of a benign liver lesion?

- characterisation of the lesion as cystic or solid
- simple hepatic cysts have characteristic appearances on imaging, such as anechogenicity on ultrasound, water density on CT scan and homogenous bright signal intensity on T2 weighted MRI

What features on imaging of a cyst would cause concern and why?

- internal septa, wall enhancement and mural nodularity raise suspicion of a biliary cystadenoma or biliary cystadenocarcinoma

- other findings such as thickening of the wall, proteinaceous debris within the lesion or loculation, in the correct clinical context, may be suggestive of liver abscess

- identification of an endocyst/pericyst interface, calcification, and daughter cysts in the periphery of the main lesion are suggestive of a hydatid cyst

What are the indications for surgery for benign liver lesions?

- symptoms

- inability to rule out malignancy

- prevention of malignancy or other complications

What is the most common benign neoplasm of the liver, and how can it be definitively diagnosed?

Haemangioma:

- definitive diagnosis can be established using contrast CT or multiphasic MRI scan

- typical characteristics include peripheral "puddling" of early phase contrast within the lesion, followed by centripetal enhancement on portal venous phase images

- they are universally benign, and carry an exceedingly low risk of rupture or bleeding

- there is usually NO indication for resection

What is Kasabach-Merritt syndrome?

A syndrome of giant cavernous haemangiomas characterised by consumptive coagulopathy mimicking DIC, plus high output cardiac failure due to AV shunting, usually observed in children. It is extremely rare.

Describe the clinical features and management of Focal Nodular Hyperplasia.

Focal nodular hyperplasia is a nodular polyclonal proliferation within the liver containing all cellular elements of liver parenchyma and is usually completely asymptomatic.

- it has no potential for malignancy, spontaneous rupture or haemorrhage

- management is almost universally conservative

- the only indications for surgery are to control symptoms (e.g. pain, early satiety or weight loss associated with larger lesions) or the inability to rule out malignancy. Operations for FNH are rare

- they can usually be identified on imaging as well circumscribed and with a central scar

What are management considerations for patients with hepatic adenomas?

- Specialised MRI with contrast agents can differentiate adenomas from FNH. It is more difficult to differentiate adenomas from regenerative nodules or HCC.

- Surgical resection should be considered in lesions above 5cm. (There is a small risk of malignancy). Biopsy of lesions is to be considered as tumours expressing a beta-catenin activating mutation are at a higher malignancy risk. Inflammatory lesions can be safely monitored. If growth occurs during monitoring, surgical resection should be considered.

- Patients should be advised not to take an oestrogen-containing contraceptive pill

- If patients with adenomas become pregnant, frequent USS monitoring (every three weeks) is necessary to monitor lesional volume

- Patients with adenomas from exogenous steroid use have a very high malignancy risk and should be counselled for surgery

The patient undergoes cross-sectional imaging and CT shows a large 14cm x 12cm well encapsulated cystic formation with internal septa and other cystic lesions of different density within it. The lesion occupied liver segments II, III and IV and appeared to exceed the limits of the liver causing mild compression of surrounding structures. What is the likely diagnosis?

Biliary cystadenomas are rare (benign but potentially malignant) multi-locular cystic neoplasms of the biliary ductal system, accounting for less than 5% of cystic neoplasms of the liver. Hepatobiliary cystadenomas can occur at any age, but they are usually seen in middle-aged women. They usually arise in the liver (80%-85%), less frequently in the extra-hepatic bile ducts and rarely in the gallbladder.

The typical patient is a Caucasian female presenting with abdominal discomfort, swelling, gradual increase in abdominal girth and/or pain and a palpable mass. Less frequently the patients have gastrointestinal obstruction leading to nausea and vomiting, dyspepsia, anorexia, weight loss or ascites. Other less common symptoms include painful intracystic haemorrhage, rupture and fever from secondary infection. Vena cava obstruction and thrombosis have also been reported. Any patient suspected of having a cystadenoma should be considered for surgical resection.

Serum level of CA 19-9 may be elevated and is a valuable marker in the diagnoses and monitoring of postoperative follow up since it has been reported by several authors to return to normal after complete resection.

Bile Leak after Cholecystectomy

A 36 year old female undergoes a laparoscopic cholecystectomy for biliary colic as a day case procedure in a DGH. The procedure is uneventful and the patient is discharged the same day. The patient gets readmitted 48 hours later with a history of severe abdominal pain.

Outline the initial management of this patient. What initial investigations would you perform? What is the likely diagnosis?

After initial resuscitation and exclusion of generalized peritonitis, an ultrasound scan should be performed to look for a collection in the right upper quadrant. The ultrasound scan may also demonstrate biliary dilatation, which in the presence of deranged liver function tests may indicate retained ductal calculi. The most likely diagnosis here is a bile leak post cholecystectomy. The differential diagnosis includes: intra-abdominal haematoma, bowel/duodenal perforation/coincidental unrelated pathology. If the ultrasound is inconclusive a CT scan should be performed. If a discrete localised collection is identified a percutaneous drain may be inserted. Successful drainage of a bile leak is critical to management. If there is free intra-abdominal fluid a repeat laparoscopy and washout with placement of a large drain in the RUQ is indicated.

What is the incidence of bile leak post cholecystectomy?

A bile leak post laparoscopic cholecystectomy is uncommon. The incidence is between 0.3-2.7%.

Bile leaks can arise as a result of injury to the common bile duct but the vast majority arise from the cystic duct stump or a sub-vesical duct of Luschka. If not identified and treated early, bile leaks can cause significant morbidity and mortality. Bile leaks less commonly can occur from the gallbladder fossa. The fossa should always be meticulously inspected after removing the gallbladder. A further possibility is unrecognized damage to a segment 6 bile duct that inserts separately into the CBD.

What is the role of laparoscopy?

The presence of sepsis and biliary peritonitis implies that simple percutaneous drainage is inadequate to control the bile leak. An urgent laparoscopy and washout of abdominal cavity with adequate drainage should be performed. The peritoneal cavity should be irrigated with copious lavage until the effluent is clear. The role of laparoscopy is to washout the bile and achieve adequate external drainage in order to prevent re-accumulation.

How would you manage a bile leak? What is the role of ERCP?

With adequate percutaneous drainage biliary sepsis is unlikely to develop. In this situation conservative management with antibiotics and daily drain output measurement is all that is necessary. It is likely that the bile drainage will subside over the course of a few days. However in the presence of a large volume bile leak (>200 ml/day) or if the output does not decrease further intervention is necessary. An ERCP should be performed. This has both a diagnostic and therapeutic role. It will demonstrate the site of the bile leak and also any CBD stones or sludge can be identified and removed. A biliary stent can be placed across the ampulla, which will decrease the pressure gradient between the bile duct and duodenum. This will help in attenuating the bile leak and allows the site to heal. It is unusual for a sphincterotomy to be necessary unless stone extraction is planned.

In the presence of significant sepsis an urgent ERCP and biliary stent should be performed urgently to help reduce the bile leak. Following successful resolution of the bile leak, the biliary stent should be removed after 6 weeks.

When would you refer to the regional HPB unit?

Referral should be made if a bile duct injury is suspected or in the presence of severe biliary sepsis. Advice from the regional tertiary HPB unit should be taken early in the course of management.

Chronic Pancreatitis

A 45-year-old woman with a long history of smoking and alcohol abuse presents to the Emergency Department with constant severe upper abdominal pain radiating to her back. Serum amylase is normal. Chest X-ray is normal. A plain abdominal X-ray shows multiple calcifications in the upper abdomen but little else of note.

What is the diagnosis?

Chronic pancreatitis is the most likely diagnosis.

What causes chronic pancreatitis?

Several theories have been described to explain the pathogenesis of chronic pancreatitis. Recently research in the immunology of pancreatitis has demonstrated the primary role of pancreatic stellate cells. The sentinel acute pancreatitis event (SAPE) hypothesis encompasses past theories and the new knowledge about pancreatic stellate cells. This model includes 3 sequential phases on a continuum – a) pre acute pancreatitis, b) the sentinel attack of acute pancreatitis and c) the progression phase. It presupposes that CP occurs in patients who are genetically or environmentally at risk of pancreatitis (pre-acute pancreatitis stage). The sentinel event of pancreatitis (second stage) in a predisposed patient leads to triggering of chronic inflammation in the pancreas and importantly, activation and recruitment of stellate cells. Factors are listed here:

- Up to 30% of cases are idiopathic

- Alcohol abuse – 60%-70%

- Obstruction of pancreatic ducts – ductal strictures, pseudocysts, gallstones, periampullary tumours, abnormalities of sphincter function

- Congenital anatomical abnormalities – pancreas divisum

- Genetic – CFTR mutations, SPINK1, PRSS-1

- Autoimmune pancreatitis – usually associated with raised levels of IgG4

- Tropical pancreatitis

How does chronic pancreatitis typically present?

- **abdominal pain** – recurrent or persistent episodes of epigastric abdominal pain radiating through to the back is the predominant symptom of chronic pancreatitis, but 5-10% of patients will remain pain-free. Patients will usually also complain of varying degrees of nausea, anorexia and weight loss. Aetiological mechanisms contributing to pain include ductal obstruction, parenchymal hypertension, acute inflammation and perineural inflammation.

- **endocrine dysfunction** – type 1 diabetes mellitus. About two-thirds of patients will have abnormal glucose tolerance tests. Overt diabetes is present in only 30-50% of cases.

- **exocrine dysfunction** – fat malabsorption and steatorrhoea. Frank steatorrhoea is only present in 10-15% of cases. Gross steatorrhoea tends to manifest itself when the patient's pancreatic exocrine function is <10% of the normal level.

- there may be an incidental finding of pancreatic calcifications on X-ray/CT.

- Note - serum amylase is not typically elevated.

What tests would you perform next to confirm the diagnosis in the patient?

- diagnosis is made based upon the clinical history and the presence of morphological features

- our patient has visible calculi on a plain abdominal film, which is indicative of large duct disease

- A triple phase pancreatic protocol CT may show pancreatic calcification, gland atrophy, duct dilatation/structuring, and pseudocysts

- MRCP is a sensitive method for looking at pancreatic ductal strictures and will also help localise calculi

- Endoscopic ultrasound is the most sensitive modality. Additional features are loss of lobularity, subtle parenchymal calcification and a firm gland using elastography

A 48-year old gentleman with idiopathic chronic pancreatitis suffering with severe symptoms has been extensively investigated by the HBP team. He has proven endocrine and exocrine insufficiency. MRCP has revealed a dilated pancreatic duct with multiple strictures and stones. Subsequent EUS showed a dilated pancreatic duct with a diameter of 9mm, with significant calcifications and fibrosis concentrated mainly in the head of the pancreas.

What are the available non-surgical options in the management of this patient?

- cessation of toxic habits (smoking and alcohol)

- medical pain control

- control and monitoring of diabetes mellitus

- administration of exogenous pancreatic enzyme preparations with meals

- Nutritional assessment and dietary advice

- ERCP to remove pancreatic duct stones. Dilatation and stenting strictures in the pancreatic duct

What surgical options are available and what is the rationale for using them?

- The main aim of surgery is to relieve pain and prevent further pancreatic parenchymal damage. The pain of chronic pancreatitis is multifactorial, but there are two main aetiological theories which form the rationale for surgical therapies:

1) increased pressure within the pancreatic ducts and parenchyma leads to a "compartment syndrome" effect with ischaemia and tissue death

2) an inflammatory mass – usually in the head of the pancreas – releases neurotransmitters which lead to the generation of painful stimuli

- **drainage procedures** aim to relieve pressure within the pancreatic duct system. Drainage via lateral pancreaticojejunostomy (Puestow procedure). At the same time it is common to perform pancreatic head parenchyma 'coring' out (Frey's procedure).

- **resections** of pancreatic head aim to remove the inflammatory mass (The Whipple's Procedure or its pylorus preserving variant). This is generally indicated if the pancreatic head exceeds 4 cm in its anterior-posterior diameter.

- total pancreatectomy is usually reserved for those in whom multiple less radical procedures have failed to provide symptomatic relief, as it guarantees exocrine and endocrine insufficiency with brittle diabetes.

- auto-islet transplantation in non-diabetic patients is an alternative in selected patients.

Which option do you think would be most appropriate in this patient and why?

- medical management is unlikely to be effective in isolation here, as this patient has advanced disease and severe symptoms.

- ERCP is unlikely to prove effective in relieving the pancreatic duct pressure, as he has multiple strictures and stones.

- the finding of a severely diseased pancreatic head would indicate the need for surgery to remove the inflammatory mass, alongside surgical pancreatic duct decompression and drainage. Therefore a Frey's procedure is likely to be the best option in controlling his symptoms and relieving the disease burden.

- total pancreatectomy is an option if symptoms persist following a Frey's procedure.

Is there any evidence comparing endoscopic and surgical methods of pancreatic duct drainage?

A randomised control trial of endoscopic versus surgical therapy for patients with chronic pancreatitis and main duct dilation showed 95% of patients who underwent surgery did not require further treatment versus only 32% who had endoscopic procedure (Gouma et al).

Can you name a few complications of chronic pancreatitis?

- Pseudocyst formation

- Pancreatic cancer – 4% lifetime risk in patients with chronic pancreatitis, likely due to combination of oncogenic KRAS mutations and presence of ongoing inflammation

- GI bleed - either due to pseudoaneurysm formation or to variceal bleeding (gastric due to splenic vein thrombosis and segmental portal hypertension)

- Biliary duct obstruction

- Duodenal obstruction

Reference

Gouma DJ, Laramee P: Long-term outcomes of endoscopic versus surgical drainage of the pancreatic duct in patients with chronic pancreatitis, Gastroenterology 141:1690-1695,2011

Common Bile Duct Stones

You are performing an elective laparoscopic cholecystectomy for gallstones. The patient has mildly deranged preoperative LFTs. A routine intraoperative cholangiogram is performed.

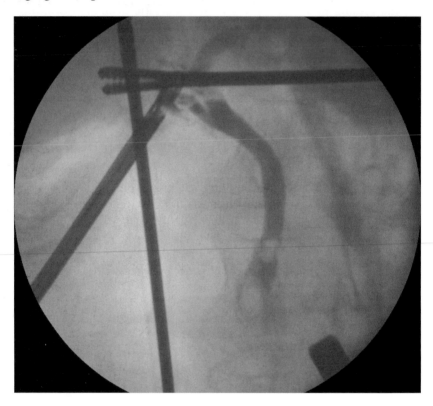

Please describe the findings of the cholangiogram.

The cholangiogram shows the presence of two filling defects within a dilated CBD and absence of filling of the duodenum. There is inadequate visualisation of the proximal ducts, and these need to be reimaged more proximally. These findings would be consistent with obstructing CBD stones.

What would you do in this scenario?

Given the finding of multiple stones, my preferred option, as a non-upper GI trainee, would be to secure the cystic duct with an endoloop and leave a drain in situ pending a post-op ERCP. I realise that there is the option of performing an intraoperative ERCP, but this approach is usually limited by logistical problems. However I am also aware that those who are trained in bile duct exploration may wish to do this.

Your answer here will be guided by your experience of bile duct exploration and stone extraction. An awareness of the different available options is important even if you are not trained at doing them.

If you were to explore the CBD to remove the stones what are your options?

There are two approaches available in this scenario. One is to consider a laparoscopic transcystic exploration. For a transcystic approach the following criteria need to be satisfied:

- patients with stones smaller than 10 mm

- stones below the CBD/cystic duct junction, as the equipment cannot retroflex into the Common Hepatic Duct (CHD)

Stone retrieval may be performed with a fluoroscopically-guided wire basket (e.g. Dormia basket) or biliary Fogarty catheter, although the latter approach carries the risk of stone displacement into the common hepatic duct as the stones are not grasped directly. Transcystic choledochoscopy may be performed via a 5mm port if the necessary equipment is available.

Choledochotomy should be reserved for patients with large occluding stones or those in whom the duct cannot be cleared using a transcystic approach.

What are the pre-requisites for successful trans-ductal laparoscopic CBD exploration?

CBDE through this route requires a dilated duct of at least 8 to 10 mm, because smaller ducts have increased risk of iatrogenic injury and are more likely to stricture at the choledochotomy site. Severely inflamed ducts may predispose to greater likelihood of bile leak.

What are the essential steps of performing a trans-choledochal CBD exploration?

- An anterior longitudinal choledochotomy approximately 10 to 15 mm in length. Care is taken to avoid injury to the vascular supply of the CBD, which parallels the duct at the 3 and 9 o'clock positions.

- Stay sutures may be placed at both sides of the opening using 4-0 vicryl which may assist in duct exposure and allow easier instrumentation.

- The intra and extra-hepatic biliary tree is then visualized endoscopically. Either a choledochoscope or a flexible cystoscope can be used. The use of a cystoscope has the advantage that balloon catheters, wires and baskets can be passed down the scope and used under direct vision.

- Small stones can often be flushed or 'pushed' through to the duodenum.

- Larger stones can be retrieved using a combination of a Dormia basket or 'biliary' Fogarty catheters.

- Stones which are impacted at the ampulla can often be displaced using a stiff guidewire.

- After successful stone retrieval the intra and extra-hepatic ducts should be clearly visualized to ensure there are no residual stones.

- Post-operative biliary drainage can be achieved either by inserting a traditional T-tube through the choledochotomy or inserting a 10cm 10F 'straight' ERCP stent through the ampulla. (The author prefers the latter approach as it achieves good drainage and reduces the morbidity associated with a T tube.)

- The choledochotomy is closed using 4.0 vicryl using interrupted sutures.

- A non-suction tube drain is left adjacent to the choledochotomy.

Following choledochotomy what are the options for CBD closure?

After choledochotomy the CBD is closed with either a T tube or primarily.

T tube advocates would argue that it allows spasm or oedema of sphincter to settle. The T-tube may also provide an easy percutaneous access for cholangiography and extraction of retained stones.

A second option is primary closure of the choledochotomy with placement of a biliary stent. The stent would also allow biliary decompression. The presence of the stent in the duodenal lumen makes ERCP easier in the presence of residual CBD stones. There is evidence that such an approach leads to lower morbidity, shorter post-operative hospital stay, less post-operative discomfort, and earlier return to full activities, compared to T-tube placement.

A third option for choledochotomy closure is primary closure without the use of T-tube or biliary stent.

Do you routinely perform an intraoperative cholangiogram (IOC) for laparoscopic cholecystectomy?

It is my practice to perform IOC on a selective basis. I reserve an IOC for cases where the likelihood of a CBD stone is high e.g. gallstone pancreatitis or deranged LFTs or if I am uncertain of anatomy during the operation. I am aware of the advantages of performing it routinely such as maintaining the technical skill of cannulation as well as image interpretation, but in my experience the benefits on a routine basis are not significant.

Or

It is my practice to perform a routine IOC as it not only helps me to clarify the anatomy before making an irreversible step, but it also may detect CBD stones as well as maintaining my technical skills and familiarity with image interpretation. However I am aware of the need to be flexible and omit the procedure when cannulation may be hazardous e.g. short cystic duct.

There is no right or wrong answer here but whichever option you choose you must be able to speak from experience. In a recent large retrospective cohort study over a 9 year period there was no statistically significant association between IOC use and CBD injury. They concluded that IOC is not an effective preventive strategy against common duct injury during cholecystectomy.

References

ElGeidie AA. Single-session minimally invasive management of common bile duct stones. World J Gastroenterol. 2014 Nov 7;20(41):15144-15152.

Orenstein SB, Marks JM, Hardacre JM. Technical aspects of bile duct evaluation and exploration.Surg Clin North Am. 2014 Apr;94(2):281-96.

Sheffield KM, Riall TS, Han Y, et al. Association between cholecystectomy with vs without intraoperative cholangiography and risk of common duct injury. JAMA 2013;310(8):812–20.

Colorectal Liver Metastases

A fit 55 year old man has had an elective laparoscopic right hemicolectomy 6 months ago for an adenocarcinoma of the colon pT3 N1 (2/23) nodes. He made a good post-operative recovery. He has completed a course of adjuvant chemotherapy (5-FU/Oxaliplatin). He is attending your clinic for on-going surveillance.

How would you perform surveillance?

Surveillance should be two-fold. Colonoscopic surveillance should commence one year after surgery. Provided this is satisfactory then colonic surveillance should be every three years. Metastatic surveillance should be via a thorough history, clinical examination and serum CEA every six months up to 10 years post resection. There is no robust evidence for routine cross-sectional imaging. Even if patients had a normal CEA prior to colonic resection (i.e. a non-secretor) the majority of patients with liver metastases will have a raised CEA.

What investigations/imaging would you do if the CEA was raised?

I would first see the patient urgently in clinic and explain that I am concerned they may have recurrence. Note the reference range for CEA is different in people who smoke (higher normal range). Consider colonoscopy, but the local recurrence is usually extra-luminal. Cross–sectional imaging with a triple phase CT chest abdomen and pelvis should be urgently performed.

What are the potential sites of recurrence?

- Local recurrence – more likely if resection margins were close after the primary operation

- Liver – the most common site of recurrence. About 50% of patients that have colorectal cancer will get liver metastases

- Lungs – the site of occurrence after the liver, however in about 10% of cases the liver is skipped and there are isolated lung lesions

- Lymph nodes – typical places would be inguinal, para-aortic, portocaval, and/or mediastinal lymph node stations

Liver MRI and CT-PET should be performed if liver surgery is to be considered, as additional lesions are often detected that are not seen on CT. CT-PET is useful to exclude extra-hepatic disease.

Following CT, MRI and CT-PET there are 3 lesions detected in the right liver lobe plus another lesion in segment IVa. There is no extra-hepatic disease. The left lobe represents 40% of the liver volume. The patient is fit for surgery. What are your management options?

- Primary liver resection – there is adequate FLR (future liver remnant). 25% is required in patients with a normal liver; 30% in patients who have chemotherapy; 40% in patients with fibrosis. Primary resection is a reasonable approach and many centres would do this.

- Neo-adjuvant chemotherapy, followed by liver resection – this is another approach with many attractive aspects. Chemotherapy can theoretically sterilise 'in-transit' disease. It can also provide disease stabilisation within the liver. There is also a 'test of time' in that if patients progress while on chemotherapy then it is highly likely they will have had a poor outcome following surgery. Remember that major surgery produces a profound immunosuppressive effect resulting in rapid proliferation of residual disease. The negative aspects of this approach are that chemotherapy agents can cause Chemotherapy Associated Liver Injury (CALI).

What chemotherapy agents are used to treat colorectal liver metastases?

Chemotherapy agents that are used in this context (and combinations) are Capecitabine, Oxaliplatin (FOLFOX) or Capecitabine and Irinotecan (FOLFIRI). Biologicals (antibodies) – Cetuximab (Platelet derived growth factor antagonist) – is only given if patients are *K-ras* wild-type positive (patients with mutant *K-ras* have a lower response rate) or Bevacizumab (Vascular endothelial growth factor inhibitor). Usually FOLFOX or FOLFIRI is given with one of the biological agents.

What is Chemotherapy Assisted Liver Injury - CALI?

CALI refers to a spectrum of liver injury particularly from the use of oxaliplatin which can cause sinusoidal obstruction (blue-liver) which is not reversible. Irinotecan can cause steatohepatitis (red-liver) which is partially reversible. Bevacizumab can be problematic in patients with coronary artery disease and peripheral vascular disease. It can cause hypertension and promote bleeding. It needs to be stopped at least 6 weeks before surgery.

The patient has had 6 cycles of FOLFIRI and Bevacizumab. The patient has been restaged 4 weeks after chemotherapy has been stopped, and has stable disease. How would you consent the patient for an open right hepatectomy?

The operation proposed to achieve disease clearance is an extended right hemi-hepatectomy. This is a major procedure. It involves a general anaesthetic with multiple in dwelling catheters including frequently an epidural, a large incision, 3-6 hours operating, HDU care post-operatively for at least 1 day, and in hospital stay of 7-10 days. Benefit for the patient is potential cure in about 40%-50% of cases and a survival benefit. Undetected liver metastases can result in patient death in approximately 1 year. Mortality rate is approximately 1%-2%. Morbidity may occur in up to 20% of cases (Infection, bleeding, bile leak, cardiovascular, thromboembolic, hernia).

Ablative therapies including radiofrequency ablation (RFA) and microwave ablation (MA) have shown promising results. RFA though safe is limited by an increased risk of local recurrence with lesions greater than 2cm. MA can achieve effective ablation of much larger tumours (up to 6cm-8cm) through higher intra-tumoural temperatures and faster ablation times.

When would you use portal vein embolization (PVE)?

PVE is a technique that is used to increase the Functional Residual Volume (FRV). The volume of segments I, II and III (the segments remaining after such a resection) may be too small and if the operation was performed the patient would be in danger of dying from liver failure and experiencing small-for-size syndrome. PVE is performed via a percutaneous approach. The right portal vein (and sometimes segment IV vein) is occluded with coils. Within 6 weeks this normally causes hypertrophy of segments I, II and III. A safe resection can then be performed.

What are the potential benefits of laparoscopic liver resection?

Many reports now state numerous advantages including: less blood loss, less blood transfused, shorter hospital stay, no epidural, earlier ambulation, less post-operative pain, less wound infection, earlier return to work. There is no compromise in terms of resection margin. It is noted however that there are no randomised controlled trials versus open resection. Furthermore it is widely thought that the anterior liver segments are more amenable to laparoscopic surgery although many centres now are performing major and complex resections using this technique.

When would you consider a synchronous liver (for metastases) and bowel (for the primary tumour) resection?

A general principle is that a major colorectal procedure (e.g. anterior resection, APR) should not be performed with a major liver resection (e.g. Hemi-hepatectomy). The main risk is sepsis from anastomotic dehiscence. However if a stoma is planned e.g. APR, then synchronous major liver resection can be considered. If one of the procedures is 'lesser', then the other can be major e.g. a right hemi-colectomy and right hepatectomy. APR and left lateral segmentectomy.

For inpatients with non-operable disease - what other liver targeted therapy do you know?

- Chemotherapy as described above. There are also a large number of other agents that can be used (e.g. panitumumab, regorafinib).

- Thermal ablation using radiofrequency or microwave. Sometimes these techniques are used in combination with liver resection.

- Ablation using irreversible electroporation (IRE) (Nanoknife®).

- Selective intrahepatic radiation therapy (SIRT). Yttrium ^{90} labelled resin or glass spheres that are delivered to the liver via the hepatic artery. They lodge in the small vessels in and close to metastases where they have an embolic effect and also deliver targeted radiation to the cancer.

Hepatocellular Carcinoma

A 54-year-old man with known hepatitis B is seen in the hepatology clinic with worsening right upper quadrant pain over the last few months. A serum Alpha Fetoprotein (AFP) is 422 ng/ml and an USS reveals a grossly cirrhotic liver with at least one hyperechoic lesion, measuring approximately 4cm x 4cm, in the right liver lobe. Doppler assessment reveals significant arterial blood flow to this lesion.

What is the likely underlying pathology and diagnosis?

This patient has hepatitis-induced cirrhosis with a hepatocellular carcinoma (HCC) as the most likely diagnosis of the liver mass. The differential diagnosis of this mass is a hepatic adenoma, a hypervascular metastasis (e.g. renal cell cancer, neuroendocrine tumour), focal nodular hyperplasia, a liver abscess, liver cyst or a haemangioma.

The raised AFP is suggestive of HCC. A level over 400ng/ml is considered diagnostic in the presence of concordant imaging (e.g. EUS, CT or MRI). AFP is also an important prognostic factor. Although not a strong marker a high AFP (>400) is associated with a poorer prognosis. AFP is, however, not specific for HCC. It has sensitivity for HCC from 39% to 97% and specificity of 76% to 95%. Other causes of a raised AFP are: metastatic liver tumours, germ cell tumours, neural tube defects and ataxia telangiectasia.

What is the aetiology and epidemiology of this condition?

Chronic inflammation, with necrosis and fibrosis and then cellular regeneration, from any cause underlies the development of HCC in most patients. The commonest underlying conditions that lead to HCC are blood borne viral hepatitis infections (B and C) with or without cirrhosis, and cirrhosis, of which the causes include alcohol (commonest), non-alcoholic fatty liver disease, haemachromatosis (iron deposition) and Wilson's disease (copper deposition). Environmental exposure to aflatoxins (from Aspergillus) may also lead to HCC development.

HCC is the third leading cause of cancer deaths worldwide and is the fastest growing cause of cancer mortality in the US. It is twice as common in less economically developed countries as it is in more economically developed countries.

What further investigations would you like to arrange at the clinic?

A definitive diagnosis and staging is now needed. For diagnosis, he should have cross sectional imaging to characterise the lesion and assess the liver for any other lesions or evidence of structural liver disease. A triple phase CT scan would be the most appropriate investigation (extra-hepatic and hepatic disease). An MRI liver would be an alternative (showing hepatic disease). CT is more readily available so is often first line. However, MRI is more sensitive and specific for the diagnosis of HCC. MRI also better characterises the primary lesion as well as the tumour relationship to surrounding structures.

What is the typical appearance of an HCC on CT scanning?

On CT scan HCCs are hypervascular lesions exhibiting arterial enhancement and rapid washout in the portal phase. There may also be a visible tumour capsule and/or a visible portal venous thrombus. If tumour was confirmed on initial imaging a full staging CT (chest/abdomen/pelvis) would also need to be arranged for completion.

What blood tests should be performed?

He also needs further blood tests to fully assess the synthetic liver function. These should include:

- FBC – to look for signs of infection and thrombocytopenia, which may indicate splenomegaly
- Coagulation profile – the pro-thrombin time (PT) is a sensitive marker of synthetic liver dysfunction
- Albumin
- Urea and electrolytes to assess renal function and degree of fluid retention, liver function tests to look for liver tissue damage and obstruction, a CRP to assess inflammation (although this may be normal in liver failure) and a serum glucose (hypoglycaemia can indicate liver failure) are all needed
- Bone profile (HCC can lead to para-neoplastic parathyroid hormone release and hypercalcaemia)
- Hepatitis B and C serology, iron and copper studies

How do you stage the liver disease and HCC? What are the systems you know?

Several staging systems exist. The TNM staging does not incorporate liver function whilst the Child-Pugh score is based solely on liver function and not tumour characteristics. These scores are therefore useful for prognostication but not as useful as scores that incorporate both tumour characteristics and markers of liver function. This is because in HCC there are two pathologies to consider, the tumour burden, but also the associated/underlying liver dysfunction. Examples of integrated scores include the Barcelona Cancer Liver Clinic (BCLC) score, the Japan Integrated Staging System and the Cancer of the Liver Italian Programme (CLIP) score.

What do you need to do now?

You would need to explain to the patient your concerns (that he may have a liver tumour) and outline for him the next steps – these would include further imaging, tissue diagnosis and then treatment. He should be discussed at the multidisciplinary team meeting and a management plan created. Tissue biopsy is not mandatory. In patients with lesion(s) who are not candidates for therapy, it is not needed. In patients (such as this patient) with clear radiological and biochemical findings, it is also unnecessary.

What are the management options for this patient?

Patients should be under the joint care of hepatology, hepatobiliary surgery and oncology. They should also be referred to local specialist nursing teams and a local cancer support network. Management options include medical, radiological and surgical.

Medical options are limited. Multiple chemotherapy agents have been trialled with no real success. More recently Sorafenib, a tyrosine protein kinase inhibitor, has been shown to be potentially beneficial in advanced disease (Llovet et al.) Although it has not been shown to cure HCC, it has been shown to increase the time to disease progression, from less than three, to almost six months. It is not currently recommended for use by NICE (TA189).

Symptom control may also be difficult as analgesia may precipitate worsening encephalopathy in patients with end stage liver failure. Fluid overload associated with liver failure is best managed with furosemide and spironolactone and paracentesis. HCC is relatively insensitive to external beam radiotherapy. Symptomatic bone metastases however respond extremely well to this modality.

The most commonly used radiological option is TACE (trans-arterial chemoembolisation) in which large doses of chemotherapy are injected into the arteries supplying the tumour, to cause tumour cell death. To prevent backflow and encourage necrosis the supplying artery is then embolised with foam and/or coils. TACE can be given multiple times, however it is contraindicated in some patients (e.g. decompensated liver disease, reduced portal flow, renal failure) (Lencioni et al.)

SIRT (selective internal radiotherapy) is a form of brachytherapy in which small glass beads (30μm) coated in radioactive yttrium are injected into the tumour angiographically via the hepatic artery. HCCs receive most of their blood supply from the hepatic artery thus targeting the tumour whilst minimising injury to healthy liver tissue. Initial experiences have suggested that SIRT may be an appropriate therapy both with palliative intent and as a bridge to surgery and may be more effective than TACE (NICE IPG490). Nice currently recommends that patients may be offered SIRT after careful MDT consideration and all patients should be entered into local or national trials/audit to monitor results.

Ablation can be done as a percutaneous procedure using ultrasound/CT guidance or via laparoscopy, and can be curative in small tumours (<3cm), Traditionally ethanol injection (PEI) was used to kill tumour cells but radiofrequency ablation (RFA) is now the standard ablative method. One drawback with RFA however is that blood can act as a heat sink, meaning tumours near vascular structures can be more difficult to treat. A third effective ablative option is microwave ablation. With modern microwave systems it is possible to produce larger ablation zones than with RFA, whilst avoiding the heat sink effect.

A final radiological treatment option is irreversible electroporation (IRE) using the Nanoknife®. Unlike RFA, IRE is effective when tumours are near major vascular structures. In IRE electrodes are positioned around the tumour under radiological guidance. A potential difference is then generated between the two electrodes and an electrical field created. The flow of electrons causes nanopores to be produced in the cell membrane leading to cellular apoptosis. One main advantage of this method is that it is highly tissue selective, minimising damage to surrounding structures. Further data is needed using the technique to fully assess its effectiveness but initial results are promising (Narayanan et al.)

Surgical management consists of resection or transplantation.

Outline the indications for surgical resection.

Liver resection is the treatment modality of choice for appropriately selected patients. The indications are localised disease fully resectable tumours and a non-cirrhotic or Child-Pugh Score A liver. In non-cirrhotic patients up to 50% of the liver can be removed with good liver function preserved. In those with mild liver disease (i.e. Child-Pugh A) only minimal resection is advised (two segments or less). In advanced liver disease (Child-Pugh B or C) and cirrhosis, resection is inappropriate.

Which patients are eligible to be considered for liver transplantation?

Indications for liver transplantation in patients with HCC are based on the Milan Criteria (Mazzaferro et al). These state that:

- The patient must have only one lesion under 5cm, or less than three lesions each under 3cm
- There must be no extra hepatic disease
- There must be no vascular invasion (portal vein/hepatic vein/hepatic artery)
- Extended criteria have been described. The University of California San Francisco (UCSF) criteria are (Yao et al):
  - Single tumour less than 6.5cm, or 2-3 tumours > 4.5cm or total tumour diameter < 8cm
  - There must be no vascular invasion

5-year survival rate is thought to be over 70% based on the Milan criteria and over 60% based on the UCSF criteria (Decaens et al.) As well as being physiologically fit for the procedure, patients in the UK must be 70 years or younger.

How do you interpret hepatitis B antibody/antigen results?

- HBsAb – This will be present in anyone who has ever had contact with hepatitis B – either by vaccination or by infection
- HBsAg – Surface antigen indicates active infection
- HBcAb – Core antibody will only be present in someone who has been infected

- IgM indicates current infection whilst IgG indicates a resolved infection
- HBeAg – Indicates infectivity
- HBeAb – Indicates a resolved infection

Therefore:

An immunised patient will just have HBsAb.

An acutely infected patient will have antigens (HBsAg and HBeAg) and antibodies (HBsAb and IgM HBcAb). The infected patient will then go on to recover or to develop chronic active infection.

A patient who has recovered from infection will have no antigens but will have HBsAb, HBeAb and HBcAb (IgG).

A patient who is chronically infected will have HBsAb and HBcAb (IgG) but will also have on-going HBsAg and/or HBeAg. These are the patient sub-groups who are at risk of developing structural liver disease, including HCC.

References:

Llovet et al., 2008, Sorafenib in advanced hepatocellular carcinoma, *N Engl J Med*, 359(4), 378-390

National Institute for Health and Care Excellence, 2010, Sorafeinb for advanced hepatocellular (liver) cancer (TA189), London; National Institute for Health and Care Excellence.

Lencioni et al., 2013, Chemoembolization for Hepatocellular Carcinoma, *Semin Intervent Radiol*, 30(1), 3-11

National Institute for Health and Care Excellence, 2013, Selective Internal Radiation Therapy for Primary Hepatocellular Carcinoma: guidance (IPG460), London: National Institute for Health and Care Excellence.

Lin, SM., 2013, Local Ablation for Hepatocellular Carcinoma in Taiwan, *Liver Cancer*, 2(2), 73-83.

Narayanan et al., 2013, Irreversible Electroporation of Hepatic Malignancy, *Semin Intervent Radiol*, 30(1), 67-73.

Mazzaferro et al., 1996, Liver transplantation for the treatment of small hepatocellular carcinomas in patients with cirrhosis, *N Engl J Med*, 334(11), 693-9.

Yao et al., 2002, Liver transplantation for hepatocellular carcinoma: comparison of the proposed UCSF criteria with the Milan Criteria and the Pittsburgh modified TNM criteria, *Liver Transpl*, 8(9), 765-74.

Decaens et al., 2006, Impact of UCSF criteria according to pre- and post-OLT tumour features: analysis of 479 patients listed for HCC with a short waiting time, *Liver Transpl*, 12(12), 1761-9.

Neuroendocrine Cancer

A 52 year old lady presents. She gives a history of intermittent abdominal pain, nausea and vomiting. She also gives a history of intermittent flushing episodes and diarrhoea. There is no significant past medical history. Clinical examination is otherwise unremarkable. You suspect she has a neuroendocrine tumour (NET).

How would you fully diagnose and stage a patient with a suspicion of a NET?

Diagnosis of NET is based on clinical manifestation, biochemistry, specialized radiological and nuclear imaging. Biochemistry includes fasting gut hormones and urinary 5HIAA. Serum Chromogranin A (CgA) is usually found in high concentration. This helps in initial diagnosis and to assess the efficacy of treatment and changing prognosis. Pancreatic polypeptide (PP) is a useful additional marker.

Imaging involves a multi-modality approach to identify the primary tumour and secondary deposits. CT, MRI and Octreoscan are used. Additional imaging modalities may include EUS, endoscopy, DSA, venous sampling and PET.

How common are NETs?

NETs are rare with an incidence of 1-2 per 100,000. They are characteristically slow growing and metastasise primarily to the liver. The majority are non-functioning and found incidentally. Functioning tumours present with symptoms due to excess hormone production and many will have metastatic disease at presentation.

What is the aetiology of NETs?

The aetiology of NETs is poorly understood. The majority of NETs are sporadic but there is a small familial risk. They are a heterogenous group of neoplasms that share characteristic biological features and arise from pluri-potential progenitor cells that develop neuroendocrine characteristics. They may also occur as part of familial endocrine cancer syndromes such as MEN.

How are NETs classified?

Historically gut NETs were classified into tumours of the foregut, midgut and hindgut. The current WHO classification is based on histopathological characteristics.

These characteristics are related to grade (G1-high grade Ki67 >20%, G2-intermediate grade Ki67 3-20%, G3-low grade Ki67 <3%). Well differentiated are low and intermediate grade. Poorly differentiated are high grade tumours.

What are the clinical features of NETs?

A high index of suspicion is necessary for the diagnosis of gastroenteropancreatic NETs. Most NETs are non-functioning and may present with non-specific symptoms such as abdominal pain, anaemia, nausea and vomiting. They may also present with bowel obstruction or mesenteric ischaemia. They usually present with liver metastases.

Functioning NETs present with symptoms due to peptide and hormone release. Examples of these hormones are serotonin, gastrin, secretin, insulin.

What is carcinoid syndrome and crisis?

Carcinoid syndrome occurs in approximately 20% of well-differentiated mid-gut NETs. It occurs less commonly with NETs of other origin. Patients usually present with symptoms of abdominal pain, flushing, palpitations and diarrhoea. There may also be symptoms of wheezing, lacrimation and rhinorrhea. It is usually due to metastasis to the liver with the release of vasoactive compounds, serotonin and tachykinins.

Carcinoid crisis is characterized by profound flushing, bronchospasm, tachycardia and fluctuating blood pressure. It is precipitated by anaesthesia, intraoperative handling of tumour or any invasive therapeutic procedure.

All patients with NETs should have prophylactic administration of somatostatin analogues when an intervention is planned in order to prevent a carcinoid crisis.

What are the principles of treatment?

The aim of treatment should be curative if possible although in the majority of cases treatment is palliative. The aim of treatment is to keep the patient free of symptoms and disease for as long as possible and to maintain a good quality of life.

Surgery is offered when NETs are resectable (curative intent) or for debulking (palliative intent). Surgery is also offered in the presence of liver metastases. Resection of the primary tumour and associated mesenteric lymphadenopathy is appropriate to delay progression of disease. Resection of mesenteric metastases alleviates symptoms (e.g. intestinal obstruction) and is associated with prolonged survival. There is no clear guidance on the resection of asymptomatic primary NETs. In the presence of liver metastases, if a curative liver resection is not possible, a debulking operation is performed for palliation with better outcomes and where there is resistance to medical therapy.

For patients who are not fit for surgery, treatment is aimed to improve symptoms and quality of life and prolong survival. This includes somatostatin analogues, biotherapy (interferon), targeted radionuclide therapy, loco-regional treatments (ablation, chemoembolization, radioembolisation / cytoreductive approach) and chemotherapy. Sunitinib or Everolimus are licensed for use in pancreatic NETs.

What is the prognosis of NETs?

NETs are slow growing tumours and survival depends on a number of factors. 5 year survival varies from 27%-95%. Survival depends on the histopathological type of tumour, Ki-67 proliferation index, size, location and age of the patient and response to treatment.

Pancreatic Cancer

A 73 year old gentleman is referred by his GP with progressively worsening painless jaundice over the last month. Abdominal ultrasound has already been performed which demonstrated intra- and extra-hepatic biliary dilatation. His gallbladder is normal with no evidence of gallstones. How would you investigate this gentleman further?

The most important differential diagnosis here is malignant process of the distal CBD, pancreatic head or ampulla. The investigation of choice would be a pancreatic protocol CT which is a three phase scan consisting of non-contrast, arterial and venous phases.

Gadolinium enhanced MRI/MRCP is an alternative investigation but has a lower sensitivity/specificity than triple phase CT and is best reserved for those patients where CT is contraindicated.

Endoscopic Ultrasound (EUS) and FNAC for tissue diagnosis are now routinely performed in many centres and should be considered depending on local protocols.

Imaging demonstrates dilatation of both the extra-hepatic biliary tree down to the level of the pancreatic head along with dilatation of the main pancreatic duct with a small mass in the head of the pancreas, in keeping with a diagnosis of pancreatic ductal adenocarcinoma. What are the key imaging features to consider when assessing if this lesion is resectable?

The presence of extra-pancreatic disease should be considered an absolute contraindication to surgery.

The relationship of the tumour to local vascular structures is key in determining resectability. Encasement of major arterial structures (e.g. SMA, common hepatic artery) should be considered a contraindication to surgery – arterial resection is associated with increased perioperative morbidity and mortality as well as poor long term outcomes. By contrast involvement of the superior mesenteric vein/portal vein confluence is not necessarily a contraindication to resection - outcomes following venous resection are comparable to those patients in whom this is not necessary.

How would you manage this patient's jaundice prior to surgery?

This would depend on the bilirubin level. Recent evidence has demonstrated that in patients with a bilirubin of less than 250mµ/l (with no renal dysfunction or biliary sepsis) early surgery without biliary drainage is associated with a significant reduction in the incidence of serious perioperative complications.

In more jaundiced patients or in those in whom there is going to be a significant delay prior to surgery, biliary drainage is appropriate. In the majority of cases this can be achieved by ERCP and stent insertion. Conventional management advocates the use of plastic stents in this context. More recent evidence has suggested that short self-expanding covered metal stents are associated with improved biliary drainage without compromising surgical outcomes. Percutaneous transhepatic cholangiography (PTC) with external drainage is an alternative in reducing the risk of septic complications if ERCP could not be successfully performed.

If the patient is found to have inoperable disease how would you proceed?

Patients with metastatic disease should be considered for palliative chemotherapy ideally with the combination of gemcitabine/capecitabine, which has been shown to increase survival in comparison to either single agent treatment or best supportive care.

For those patients with locally advanced disease who are otherwise fit for surgery then the triplet regimen of 5-FU/Folinic acid, Oxaliplatin and Irinotecan (FOLFIRINOX) should be considered. This regimen is associated with an improved objective response rate as compared to conventional chemotherapy and may facilitate resection in a proportion of patients. However its use is associated with significant toxicity and unfortunately is often poorly tolerated.

Prior to palliative chemotherapy a tissue diagnosis is essential and, if this has not been achieved with brushings taken at ERCP, then EUS/FNA should be performed.

What is the evidence for adjuvant chemotherapy following resection of pancreatic ductal adenocarcinoma?

The ESPAC-1 study randomized patients following resection of pancreatic adenocarcinoma to receive either chemoradiation (20 gray over 2 weeks and 5-FU) or chemotherapy alone (6 cycles of 5-FU/Folinic acid). Whilst there was no advantage in chemoradiation treatment, the use of 5-FU chemotherapy was associated with a 6 month improvement in median survival as compared to observation.

The ESPAC-3 study randomised patients to receive treatment with either 5-FU/folinic acid or gemcitabine. There was no difference in median survival between the two groups.

As a consequence of these trials either regimen is considered appropriate for use as adjuvant chemotherapy following resection of pancreatic cancer.

The ESPAC-4 trial is currently running and aims to compare single agent gemcitabine to the combination regimen gemcitabine/capecitabine.

Do you know of any environmental or genetic risk factors for the development of pancreatic cancer?

Cigarette smoking is strongly linked to the development of pancreatic cancer with smokers having an approximately 3 fold increased risk of developing the disease as compared to the general population.

Several genetic syndromes have been linked with an increased incidence of pancreatic cancer:

- Peutz-Jeghers Syndrome, an autosomal dominant condition linked to mutations in the STK11 gene. It is associated with a life time cumulative risk of developing cancer of up to 36%

- BRCA2 mutation is associated with a 3.5 fold increased risk of developing pancreatic cancer as compared to the general population

- Lynch syndrome (i.e. mutation in one of the DNA mismatch repair genes MLH1, MSH2, MSH6, PMS2) is associated with a 8.6 fold increased risk of developing pancreatic cancer

- Mutations in the p16 tumour suppressor gene are associated with an up to 22 fold increased risk of developing pancreatic cancer

References

Riediger H, Makowiec F, Fischer E, Adam U, Hopt UT, Riediger H, et al. Postoperative morbidity and long-term survival after pancreaticoduodenectomy with superior mesenterico-portal vein resection. Journal of Gastrointestinal Surgery. 2006;10:1106-15.

van der Gaag NA, Rauws EA, van Eijck CH, Bruno MJ, van der Harst E, Kubben FJ, et al. Preoperative biliary drainage for cancer of the head of the pancreas. N Engl J Med. 2010;362:129-37.

Cavell LK, Allen PJ, Vinoya C, Eaton AA, Gonen M, Gerdes H, et al. Biliary self-expandable metal stents do not adversely affect pancreaticoduodenectomy. Am J Gastroenterol. 2013;108:1168-73.

Cunningham D, Chau I, Stocken DD, Valle JW, Smith D, Steward W, et al. Phase III randomized comparison of gemcitabine versus gemcitabine plus capecitabine in patients with advanced pancreatic cancer. J Clin Oncol. 2009;27:5513-8.

Conroy T, Desseigne F, Ychou M, Bouche O, Guimbaud R, Becouarn Y, et al. FOLFIRINOX versus gemcitabine for metastatic pancreatic cancer. N Engl J Med. 2011;364:1817-25.

Neoptolemos JP, Dunn JA, Stocken DD, Almond J, Link K, Beger H, et al. Adjuvant chemoradiotherapy and chemotherapy in resectable pancreatic cancer: a randomised controlled trial. Lancet. 2001;358:1576-85.

Neoptolemos JP, Stocken DD, Bassi C, Ghaneh P, Cunningham D, Goldstein D, et al. Adjuvant chemotherapy with fluorouracil plus folinic acid vs gemcitabine following pancreatic cancer resection: a randomized controlled trial. JAMA. 2010;304:1073-81.

Pancreatic Cysts

A 70 year old lady undergoes a routine CT KUB to investigate renal stone disease. An incidental finding on this scan is of a 6cm cystic lesion located in the tail of the pancreas. What is the differential diagnosis and how would you begin to investigate this patient?

The differential diagnoses here include:

- Pancreatic pseudocyst

- Serous cystadenoma

- Mucinous cystic neoplasm

- Intraductal papillary mucinous neoplasm (IPMN)

- Cystic variant of a solid tumour (e.g. NET, ductal carcinoma etc)

An appropriate initial investigation would be with cross sectional imaging of the pancreas using either pancreas protocol CT (i.e. non-contrast, arterial and portal venous phases) or, in patients unsuitable for CT, MRI which should consist of MRCP as well as contrast enhanced MR of the pancreas.

What is the role of EUS and cyst sampling in the assessment of pancreatic cystic lesions?

EUS alone as an imaging modality probably adds little to the assessment of pancreatic cystic lesions in terms of either cyst size or cyst features as compared to conventional cross sectional imaging. EUS is however more accurate in determining multi-focality.

The real strength of EUS is in the ability to obtain samples of cyst fluid for biochemical and cytological analysis. Measurement of cyst fluid CEA is useful in differentiating mucinous cysts from other lesions (typically elevated >192ng/ml). A low cyst fluid amylase (<250u/l) has a good exclusion value for pancreatic pseudocysts.

Cyst fluid cytology can also be of value in determining the aetiology of these lesions. Mucin producing cells will typically be present on aspirates from either mucinous cystic tumours or IPMNs. Glycogen producing cells may be demonstrated in aspirates from a serous cystadenoma. Cytology from a pseudocyst will typically demonstrate inflammatory cells. In addition dysplastic cells may be demonstrated on FNA aspirates, which may aid in decision making in regard to further treatment.

What are the typical imaging features of a serous cystadenoma? What is the natural history of this lesion and how would you manage it?

Serous cystadenomas are benign cystic pancreatic neoplasms. They can be classified as either microcystic or macrocystic lesions. The majority however are microcystic, consisting of multiple small cysts (<2cm in diameter) surrounding a fibrotic calcified central scar. Macrocystic lesions are unilocular or bilocular cysts that can be much more difficult to differentiate from mucinous neoplasms.

Serous cystadenomas typically occur in female patients with a peak incidence over the age of 70. Malignant transformation is exceedingly rare with approximately 30 reported cases in the literature. As such surgical treatment is generally not required unless the patient is symptomatic.

Serous cystadenomas may be associated with mutations of the von Hippel-Lindau gene (a tumour suppressor gene). In this situation other associated lesions may be demonstrated on abdominal CT e.g. renal tumours, phaeochromocytoma etc.

How would you sub-categorize IPMNs? How does this categorization affect management?

In contrast to mucinous cystic neoplasms, IPMNs do communicate with the pancreatic duct. They can be categorized according to whether they communicate with either the main pancreatic duct (main duct IPMN) or a side branch of it (branch duct IPMN) which is typically dilated on imaging.

The incidence of either high grade dysplasia or invasive carcinoma is much higher in main duct IPMNs (up to 50%) as compared to branch duct IPMNs (approximately 10%). For this reason current guidelines suggest resection should be offered to all medically fit patients presenting with main duct IPMNs. By contrast resection is only recommended for branch duct IPMNs in the presence of positive cytology, high risk radiological features (size > 3cm, presence of mural nodules or main duct dilatation >6mm).

How would you manage a patient with a mucinous cystic neoplasm?

Mucinous cystic neoplasms occur predominantly in young female patients. There is a real risk of malignant transformation in these lesions with either high grade dysplasia or invasive carcinoma being present in up to 17% of patients at diagnosis. For this reason surgical resection is generally advocated, provided the patient is otherwise fit. These lesions primarily occur in the left pancreas and can be treated with distal pancreatectomy in the majority of patients utilizing a laparoscopic approach.

If post resection histology does not reveal evidence of invasive carcinoma then follow up imaging is not required as multi-focality is not a characteristic feature of these lesions. In the presence of invasive carcinoma then follow up should be as for invasive ductal carcinoma – the reported recurrence rate is between 40% and 80% at 5 years.

References

Del Chiaro M, Verbeke C, Salvia R, Kloppel G, Werner J, McKay C, et al. European experts consensus statement on cystic tumours of the pancreas. Dig Liver Dis. 2013.

Brugge WR. The incidental pancreatic cyst on abdominal computerized tomography imaging: diagnosis and management. Clin Gastroenterol Hepatol. 2008;6:140-4.

Tanaka M, Fernandez-del Castillo C, Adsay V, Chari S, Falconi M, Jang JY, et al. International consensus guidelines 2012 for the management of IPMN and MCN of the pancreas. Pancreatology. 2012;12:183-97.

OESOPHAGOGASTRIC SURGERY

Edward Cheong Bhaskar Kumar
Alexander Phillips Dimitri Pournaras

Contents

Achalasia

A 45 year old man presents to your outpatient clinic with a 6 month history of dysphagia to solids and liquids, and post-prandial chest pain which has progressively got worse. He also states that he has lost 5kg weight over this time period.

What primary investigations are you going to carry out?

My main concern with this patient is whether he has an underlying malignancy. I would organise an urgent gastroscopy to exclude this diagnosis. There are also benign differentials that might become apparent at gastroscopy and include complications of GORD such as a peptic stricture, though this is unlikely to be the cause of his chest pain. Though rare, achalasia is another possibility as the symptoms he describes are consistent with this.

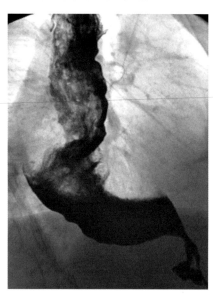

What endoscopic abnormalities might you expect to find in achalasia?

In the early stages of achalasia there may not be too many abnormalities other than a distinctive 'pop' as the scope traverses the lower oesophageal sphincter. In the later stages there may be gross evidence of fluid/food residue and a dilated atonic oesophagus. Upon clearing some of the residue there may be underlying oesophagitis. Achalasia is associated with squamous cell carcinoma of the oesophagus, but this is not a common finding.

Having suspected achalasia on history and endoscopy how would you investigate this further?

I would then wish to carry out a barium swallow which may demonstrate a characteristic "bird's beak" appearance. However, to confirm the diagnosis I would like to carry out oesophageal manometry, which would demonstrate a hypertensive lower oesophageal sphincter and lack of oesophageal peristalsis.

What does the earlier barium swallow image show?

The barium swallow shows a grossly distended oesophagus, which demonstrates aperistalsis and contains food residue. The GOJ or lower oesophageal sphincter is contracted with a typical 'rat tail appearance', supporting a significant barium column in the erect position. I would expect to see aperistalsis of the oesophagus on the dynamic imaging.

What is the definition of achalasia?

Achalasia is defined as a primary motility disorder of the oesophagus of unknown aetiology characterised by absence of oesophageal peristalsis, high resting lower oesophageal sphincter tone and failure of relaxation of the lower oesophageal sphincter. Achalasia is due to progressive loss of ganglion cells in the myenteric plexus.

Can you draw and describe the manometric tracing seen in a patient with achalasia?

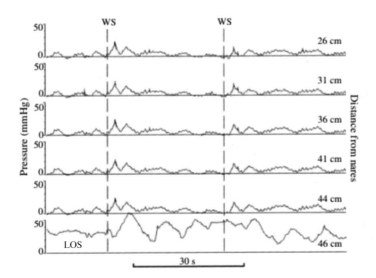

The manometry tracing has pressure on the Y axis and time on the x-axis. The distance from the nares is indicated on the right. The LOS (lower oesophageal sphincter) corresponds to the most distant sensor. The most striking feature of the tracing is the absence of relaxation of the LOS with wet swallows (WS) as well as the simultaneous low amplitude contractions seen in the whole oesophagus.

What are the treatment options once the diagnosis of achalasia has been confirmed?

Treatment options for achalasia can be classified as interventional (pneumatic dilatation/cardiomyotomy/POEM/oesophagectomy) or medical (calcium channel blockers/endoscopic botox injection). The most effective treatment options are pneumatic dilatation or laparoscopic Heller's cardiomyotomy. The latter may or may not be carried out with a fundoplication procedure to reduce reflux symptoms. Pneumatic dilation may be carried out as required and repeatedly in order to give symptomatic relief. It is important for the patient to understand that these treatments are not curative and are performed to control symptoms of achalasia. Oesophagectomy is reserved for end stage achalasia or cases associated with cancer.

Endoscopic botox injection decreases the LOS pressure by blocking the release of acetylcholine. Although it is a safe treatment and has a good initial relief rate (85%), its effects decline over time with nearly two-thirds having recurrence of symptoms at one year. The transmural inflammation it produces makes subsequent attempts at cardiomyotomy much more difficult and less effective. Therefore botox is best reserved for candidates unsuitable for other treatments.

Heller performed the first myotomy on April 14, 1913 and described "A longitudinal cut of approximately 8cm on the anterior oesophageal wall which includes about 2cm cut on the dilated part (oesophagus) and a short cut over the cardia into the fundus".

What do you understand by a POEM procedure?

POEM stands for Per Oral Endoscopic Myotomy. It is usually performed under general anaesthetic whereby a 2-cm longitudinal mucosal incision is made on the mucosal surface to create a mucosal entry to the submucosal space. Thereafter a submucosal tunnel is created in a similar manner to ESD (endoscopic submucosal dissection) passing over the OGJ and entering the proximal 3cm of stomach. Myotomy of the circular muscle is performed using spray coagulation current keeping the longitudinal layer intact and extending for approximately 3cm into the cardia. The mucosal defect is closed with endoclips.

This procedure was first described in 2007 and is in its relative infancy. Experienced operators report results as good as laparoscopic myotomy but more substantive short and long term data is awaited.

Tell me about the evidence base for the management of achalasia.

Due to the rarity of achalasia there are very few high quality studies with good numbers of patients. There has been only one RCT comparing pneumatic dilatation (PD) with laparoscopic Heller's cardiomyotomy (LHM) and Dor fundoplication. The European Achalasia Trial randomised a total of 201 patients between the groups and demonstrated no advantage with LHM over pneumatic dilatation at two years (Boeckxstaens et al). The primary outcome measure was therapeutic success (defined as a drop in Eckardt score </-3). There was no difference in the primary outcome measure in the two groups. One of the secondary outcome measures was need for re-treatment. This was significantly lower for the surgery group than balloon dilatation. Although this study remains the best comparison of the two treatments there were significant flaws in the design.

Surgical group - On average only one myotomy was performed per centre each year. The length of the gastric myotomy was 1 to 1.5cm in the surgical group while there is evidence that a 2.5cm myotomy has a better outcome. There was no description of how the Dor fundoplication was performed.

Dilatation group: The dilatation protocol changed after an initial 31% perforation rate using a 35mm balloon. The follow up period was short – this is significant as the effects of pneumatic dilatation may not be durable.

Are you aware of any meta-analyses on the treatment of achalasia?

The most contemporary meta-analysis compared PD and LH in 346 patients with new diagnoses of achalasia (Yaghoobi). This meta-analysis showed that LHM is more effective than PD, with fewer immediate adverse events. LHM provided a 14% higher response rate (86% vs 75.6%), with a rate of significant adverse events 8 times less than that of PD (0.6% vs 4.8%) for as long as 1 year after treatment. The rates of major mucosal tears requiring subsequent intervention with LHM were also significantly lower than those of oesophageal perforation with PD. The rates of gastroesophageal reflux, lower oesophageal sphincter pressures, and quality-of-life scores were not different. Therefore LHM may be more promising in providing long-term remission.

What are the principles of performing a laparoscopic cardiomyotomy?

This is usually a five port laparoscopic technique. The gastro-oesophageal junction is identified by the fat pad, which is lifted away to expose it, and the oesophagus is mobilised anteriorly at the hiatus. A myotomy is performed for 2.5 to 3.0 cm on the gastric side and 6cm on the oesophageal side. Myotomy can be done in a variety of ways including use of hook diathermy to split the muscle. Some surgeons use an adrenaline soaked gauze for haemostasis with blunt dissection to ensure no heat is placed near the mucosa, eliminating the risk of a delayed perforation from ischaemia due to cautery. An endoscopy can be performed at the end to ensure adequate myotomy and no oesophageal perforation. A DOR fundoplication without any tension may be performed at the end to help minimise reflux and provide coverage for any oesophageal leak.

What are the long term concerns of achalasia?

Achalasia is associated with an increased risk of developing squamous cell carcinoma of the oesophagus. The increased lifetime risk is thought to be around thirty times the rest of the population.

What is pseudoachalasia?

Pseudoachalasia is defined as signs and symptoms consistent with achalasia but due to invasion of the distal oesophagus by tumour.

What is vigorous achalasia?

This term was first coined to describe patients whose clinical features and manometry findings were of both achalasia and diffuse oesophageal spasm. Dysphagia, regurgitation, and pain are the most common symptoms, with pain occurring in approximately two thirds of patients. This is usually described as a sharp crampy spasmodic pain in the epigastric region and referred to the back or into the neck. Manometry will confirm the diagnosis, which shows high amplitude contractions (>37mmHg) on swallowing as opposed to low amplitude contractions seen in classic achalasia. There is also minimal oesophageal dilatation and prominent tertiary contraction.

References

Boeckxstaens GE, Annese V, des Varannes SB, Chaussade S, Costantini M, Cuttitta A, Elizalde JI, Fumagalli U, Gaudric M, Rohof WO, Smout AJ, Tack J, Zwinderman AH, Zaninotto G, Busch OR, European Achalasia Trial Investigators Pneumatic dilation versus laparoscopic Heller's myotomy for idiopathic achalasia N Engl J Med. 2011;364(19):1807

Wang YM, Li L. Meta-analysis of randomized and controlled treatment trials for achalasia. Dig Dis Science 2009;54:2303-11.

Yaghoobi M, Mayrand S, Martel M, et al. Laparoscopic Heller's myotomy versus pneumatic dilation in the treatment of idiopathic achalasia: a meta-analysis of randomized, controlled trials. Gastrointest Endosc 2013;78:468-75.

Bariatric Complications

A 45 year old lady who underwent a gastric band procedure privately in Europe two years previously has attended A & E with worsening dysphagia. What are the complications of a gastric band, and how would you manage this lady?

There are a number of complications associated with these procedures including:

Slippage

- The stomach prolapses through the band and may become strangulated
- With the pars flaccida approach instead of perigastric placement this complication is now less common

Erosion of the gastric band into the stomach

History may reveal the underlying cause, and this lady may have had a recent adjustment which may explain the symptoms.

A plain x-ray (chest/abdomen) will allow visualization of the band which may appear more horizontal if slippage has occurred. Other investigations that would assist diagnosis are a contrast swallow, and OGD.

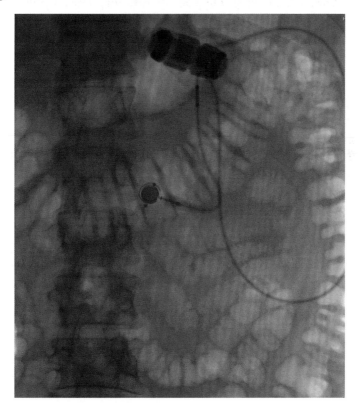

The superior angle formed by the longitudinal axis of the gastric band and the spine, the φ (phi) angle, should be between 4° and 58°. In the preceding picture the gastric band lies in a position with a larger angle, therefore representing a band slippage.

Initial management involves resuscitating as appropriate and immediate deflation of the balloon to completeness, which can be done with any needle but ideally requires a non-coring needle (such as a Huber needle).

She may subsequently require removal of the band if the deflation did not alleviate the symptoms. This can be done laparoscopically, and requires the band to be freed from the fibrous capsule that forms around it. The buckle of the band can then be cut behind the locking head, or the locking head undone, and the band pulled through.

The access port will also need to be removed with an incision over where it can be palpated.

Another 45 year old lady attends A & E who has been complaining of diffuse abdominal pain for two weeks, with intermittent episodes of vomiting. She has had a previous laparoscopic bypass operation two years previously, again privately overseas, and has had a significant (10stone/64kg) weight loss. What are your concerns and how would you manage this lady?

This lady needs a full history and examination to be taken, as well as plain x-rays. She has had previous obesity surgery, but a full assessment must be made and it cannot be assumed that the problem is related to this surgery - a new intrabdominal pathology may be responsible. She also needs assessing regarding the level of resuscitation required, she has been unwell for some time, and may be dehydrated. Further, she has lost a significant amount of weight, which might be appropriate for her, but she may have lost so much that she has become malnourished. Given that she had her surgery abroad she may have had no follow up in terms of vitamin supplementation and regular blood tests.

Given her symptoms (which are generally vague, and sound as if there is an obstructive feature) and that she is two years post obesity surgery with significant weight loss, my specific concern would be of an internal hernia (eg Petersen's hernia). Adhesions causing obstructive symptoms would be a further possibility.

How would you further investigate this lady?

Further to routine blood tests and plain x-rays, probably the most useful investigation to carry out would be a CT scan with contrast. This may demonstrate an internal hernia or confirm whether there is another explanation for this lady's symptoms. However, the CT may not reveal an underlying cause and a diagnostic laparoscopy may be required.

What is a Petersen's hernia?

This is herniation of loops of small bowel into Petersen's space: the area between the gastrojejunostomy and the transverse colon. The incidence is reported as <3%, and some surgeons routinely try to close this space when doing the initial procedure.

Further potential spaces exist behind the biliopancreatic limb and roux limb at the jej—jej anastomosis and, if a retrocolic anastomosis is made, the defect in the transverse mesocolon can also allow herniation.

CT confirms the diagnosis of an internal hernia. How would you proceed?

I would explain the findings to the patient and the nature of the problem. This needs to be repaired. There is a risk of strangulation to the bowel and a possible need for resection which I would explain to the patient. I would aim to carry out a laparoscopy to confirm the diagnosis and hopefully treat the problem by reducing any herniated bowel before closing the space.

Further Reading

Higa KD, Ho T, Boone KB. Internal hernias after laparoscopic Roux-en-Y gastric bypass: Incidence, treatment and prevention. Obes Surg2003;13(3):350–4.

Geubbels N1, Lijftogt N, Fiocco M, van Leersum NJ, Wouters MW, de Brauw LM. Meta-analysis of internal herniation after gastric bypass surgery.Br J Surg. 2015 Apr;102(5):451-60. doi: 10.1002/bjs.9738. Epub 2015 Feb 24.

Barrett's Oesophagus

You endoscope a 46 year old female as part of a Barrett's surveillance programme. Over the years she has not been compliant with PPI or surveillance endoscopies. At endoscopy you find a circumferential highly inflamed segment of Barrett's starting at 28cm extending for 10cm (see figure below).

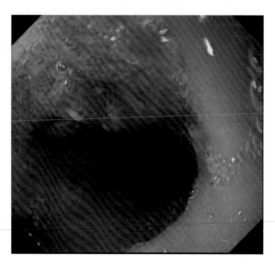

Figure 1. Endoscopic image from 28cm.

Can you describe the endoscopic findings above? What are your concerns with these findings?

The endoscopy image demonstrates a visible abnormality in the form of nodularity on a background segment of columnar epithelium, which would be consistent with Barrett's oesophagus. My main concern is the finding of marked nodularity, as this represents a visible lesion and may be consistent with an underlying neoplastic lesion.

Visible lesions should be considered malignant until proven otherwise.

The biopsies confirm the diagnosis as Barrett's oesophagus (BE) – what is Barrett's oesophagus?

Barrett's oesophagus (BE) is defined as an acquired metaplastic condition of the oesophagus in which any portion of the normal squamous epithelium has been replaced by macroscopically visible columnar epithelium which is confirmed histologically. The development of the metaplastic Barrett's mucosa occurs when there is a switch in differentiation from one cell type to another – specifically the normal stratified squamous mucosa is replaced by columnar mucosa.

How would you manage this patient?

I would extensively biopsy the nodular segment and perform four quadrant biopsies for the remaining segment as per the Seattle protocol. These need to be sent for urgent histology. In the meantime I would strongly advise the patient to be compliant with a high dose PPI which needs to be taken twice a day. Depending on the histology from biopsies a repeat endoscopy may need to be performed in 4 to 6 weeks once the inflammation has subsided.

Visible abnormalities can be very subtle and easily overlooked at endoscopy. Abnormal surface patterns may correspond with dysplastic epithelium. These features can be missed and so 'freeze frame' analysis should be performed at the time of endoscopy. A high quality endoscopy is essential in the management of BE to map out any visible lesions and extent of dysplasia. If a patient has biopsy-proven HGD then an expert high resolution endoscopy is essential.

The histology from the nodular area at 28cm confirms the presence of high grade dysplasia (HGD). The remaining biopsies confirm non dysplastic Barrett's oesophagus. How will you proceed?

The histology needs to be discussed in an oesophagogastric cancer MDM following review by two expert GI pathologists. If a consensus opinion is reached to confirm HGD and no evidence of cancer then the nodular area should be considered for an Endoscopic Mucosal Resection (EMR) which would effectively provide a 'big biopsy', thereby allowing the pathologists to confirm or refute the presence of any cancerous cells.

Following a period of 4 weeks of maximal medical treatment you re-endoscope the patient with high resolution endoscopy and find generalised improvement in the appearance of the Barrett's segment. The nodule at 28cm persists and you perform an EMR. The EMR result confirms the presence of HGD but no cancerous cells. How will you treat her?

The treatment options to some extent are dictated by local expertise. Some centres would continue with high dose PPI and re-endoscope the patient at frequent intervals. Radiofrequency ablation (RFA) is an increasingly popular and efficacious treatment modality in these patients. In the context of HGD there is good evidence from RCTs that RFA can significantly reduce progression of HGD to cancer with minimal procedure-related morbidity.

Once visible lesions have been removed by EMR and confirmation obtained that disease is limited to the mucosa, then the treatment of choice is endoscopic ablation. As per BSG guidelines the presence of HGD without visible lesions should be managed with an endoscopic ablative technique. Of all the ablative procedures available RFA has a better safety profile and high efficacy. Other ablative techniques include photodynamic therapy (PDT) and Argon Plasma Coagulation (APC).

Are you aware of the evidence base for using RFA for HGD?

A number of studies revealed that RFA has been shown to reduce the risk of progression to cancer in patients with HGD (Shaheen 2009; Pouw RE 2010). Follow up studies displayed a durable response to treatment. Molecular studies show the newly formed squamous epithelium (neosquamous epithelium) appears to be biologically stable.

What are the complications of RFA?

RFA is not free of morbidity. There is an approximately 10% incidence of oesophageal stricture formation (mainly with circumferential RFA), bleeding and rarely perforation. Recurrence and treatment failure are also recognised complications. Stricture formation is generally easily treated with serial endoscopic dilatation.

To what extent should endoscopic ablation be performed?

Ablation should not be limited to just the site of HGD. More than 20% of patients treated with EMR of visible lesions will develop metachronous lesions within 2 years. Therefore eradication of residual BE reduces the risk of metachronous neoplastic lesions developing.

What do you understand by the term 'buried glands'?

With ablative techniques concern has been raised about the development of metaplasia within glands 'buried' beneath the neosquamous epithelium. Current data suggest that the incidence of buried gland cancer following RFA is low at approximately 0.9%. The incidence is much higher with PDT (14.2%). Until the long term outcome of RFA is fully established, the follow up of patients is vital to detect recurrence.

For patients treated with HGD endoscopic follow up is recommended 3 monthly for 1 year and yearly thereafter. As per NICE guidelines in the UK patients who undergo RFA for Barrett's oesophagus should enter all details onto the UK National HALO Patient Registry, and review outcomes locally.

Are you aware of any national audits on the management of Barrett's HGD?

From 1st April 2012 the National Oesophagogastric cancer audit has included patients with oesophageal HGD in Barrett's oesophagus. The main audit questions for these patients are:

1) Have two expert pathologists confirmed the diagnosis of HGD?

2) Characteristics of HGD at diagnosis e.g. endoscopic appearance

3) Has the patient with HGD been discussed in an oesophagogastric MDM?

4) Outcomes of treatment

What are the Prague Criteria? Can you draw a diagram to explain how you would measure BE?

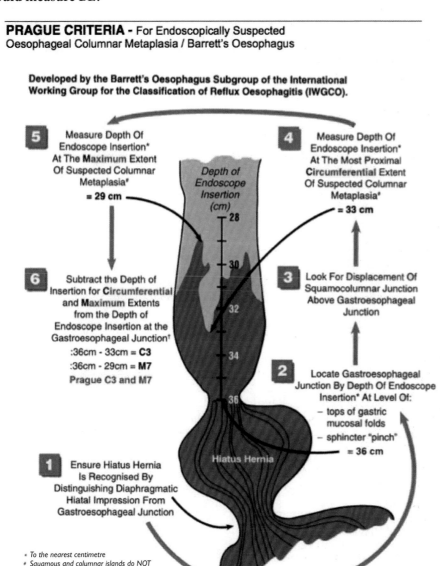

PRAGUE CRITERIA - For Endoscopically Suspected Oesophageal Columnar Metaplasia / Barrett's Oesophagus

Developed by the Barrett's Oesophagus Subgroup of the International Working Group for the Classification of Reflux Oesophagitis (IWGCO).

5 Measure Depth Of Endoscope Insertion* At The **Maximum** Extent Of Suspected Columnar Metaplasia* = 29 cm

4 Measure Depth Of Endoscope Insertion* At The Most Proximal **Circumferential** Extent Of Suspected Columnar Metaplasia* = 33 cm

Depth of Endoscope Insertion (cm)

6 Subtract the Depth of Insertion for **Circumferential** and **Maximum** Extents from the Depth of Endoscope Insertion at the Gastroesophageal Junction†
:36cm - 33cm = **C3**
:36cm - 29cm = **M7**
Prague C3 and M7

3 Look For Displacement Of Squamocolumnar Junction Above Gastroesophageal Junction

2 Locate Gastroesophageal Junction By Depth Of Endoscope Insertion* At Level Of:
– tops of gastric mucosal folds
– sphincter "pinch"
= 36 cm

1 Ensure Hiatus Hernia Is Recognised By Distinguishing Diaphragmatic Hiatal Impression From Gastroesophageal Junction

Hiatus Hernia

* To the nearest centimetre
* Squamous and columnar islands do NOT contribute to measures of extent
† To the nearest centimetre, except when areas of columnar metaphasis are estimated to be less than 1cm: report this as <1cm

Supported by an educational grant from AstraZeneca

Prague criteria are used to standardize a method for measuring BE. It is obtained by measuring the most proximal circumferential extent (C) and the maximal extent (M) of the visible columnar epithelium in relation to the gastro-oesophageal junction (GOJ). The GOJ is taken as the proximal extent of the gastric folds. For a GOJ at 38cm with a maximum circumferential distance to 34 cm and a tongue of Barrett's extending to 31cm, it is given as C4M7.

What is the natural history of low grade dysplasia (LGD)?

In Barrett's LGD the glandular architecture is relatively preserved but cytological atypia may be seen in the deeper glands. It can be a difficult diagnosis to make and is subject to much inter-observer variation between pathologists. It is now accepted that a diagnosis of LGD is associated with an increased risk of progression to cancer.

Is there any evidence for the role of ablative therapy in the management of LGD?

There are RCTs and NICE guidelines that support the use of RFA for the treatment of LGD in expert hands. The recently reported SURF (Surveillance vs Radiofrequency Ablation) trial was a multi-centre RCT of 136 patients comparing RFA (n=68) with endoscopic surveillance (n=68) in patients with Barrett's LGD. The progression rate to adenocarcinoma was significantly less in the RFA group (2% vs 27% p<0.0001) at 3 year follow up.

How would you take biopsies from a patient with Barrett's as part of surveillance endoscopy?

Biopsies should be taken from all four quadrants at 2cm intervals as per the Seattle protocol along the length of the segment. In addition biopsies of any mucosal lesions should be taken particularly from suspected nodular areas or abnormal surface architecture.

References

Fitzgerald RC1, di Pietro M, Ragunath K et al. British Society of Gastroenterology Guidelines on the diagnosis and management of Barrett's oesophagus. Gut. 2014 Jan;63(1):7-42.

Shaheen NJ1, Sharma P, Overholt BF,N Engl J Med. 2009 May 28;360(22):2277-88. doi: 10.1056/NEJMoa0808145. Radiofrequency ablation in Barrett's oesophagus with dysplasia.

Bennett C1, Vakil N, Bergman J et al. Gastroenterology. 2012 Aug;143(2):336-46. doi: 10.1053/j.gastro.2012.04.032. Epub 2012 Apr 24. Consensus statements for management of Barrett's dysplasia and early-stage oesophageal adenocarcinoma, based on a Delphi process.

Phoa KN1, van Vilsteren FG1, Weusten BL et al JAMA. 2014 Mar 26;311(12):1209-17. doi: 10.1001/jama.2014.2511. Radiofrequency ablation vs endoscopic surveillance for patients with Barrett's oesophagus and low-grade dysplasia: a randomized clinical trial.

Shaheen NJ, Bergein F et al. Durability of Radiofrequency Ablation in Barrett's Oesophagus_ with Dysplasia. Gastroenterology; 141(2): 460–468.

Early Oesophageal Cancer

A normally fit and well 50 year old gentleman with known Barrett's oesophagus is found to have a nodular lesion at 37cm on surveillance endoscopy (figure 1). The lesion is less than 2cm in size on a 5cm segment of Barrett's. Biopsies of this lesion came back suspicious of at least intramucosal adenocarcinoma.

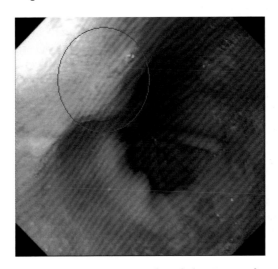

Figure 1: Endoscopic appearance of nodular Barrett's oesophagus

How would you proceed?

Firstly the patient needs to be informed that the endoscopic findings are suggestive of a cancer. His case needs to be discussed at the next upper GI MDT, and in the meantime I would obtain a staging CT scan of his chest/abdomen/pelvis as well as an EUS if locally available. The CT would help rule out distant metastatic disease and an EUS may help provide staging information on the depth of tumour invasion.

A CT scan shows no evidence of metastatic disease and no evidence of lymphadenopathy. CT staging is TxN0M0 as the primary lesion could not be seen. EUS is performed and is reported as a probable T1b lesion. What are the limitations of EUS in this setting?

EUS is not considered to be a good staging modality for early stage oesophageal cancer. EUS has a poor sensitivity differentiating a T1a from T1b tumour and is only 20% accurate in doing so. EUS can however reliably identify T3 disease. Therefore the finding of T1b in this setting may not be accurate and the lesion could still be T1a or vice versa.

How would you proceed from here?

Endoscopic resection of the lesion followed by microscopic pathological assessment would provide the most accurate staging. Given the uncertainty of whether this is a T1a or T1b lesion it would be reasonable to offer this man an endoscopic submucosal resection (EMR) of the lesion. This would provide a 'big biopsy' and may be curative if the lesion is a pure intramucosal adenocarcinoma (T1a).

What type of lesions are amenable to EMR?

EMR should only be performed if the lesion can be safely 'lifted' off the muscularis propria. Lesions which are less than 2cm in size, non ulcerated and moderate/well differentiated are potentially suitable for EMR. Any ulcerated lesion or poorly differentiated lesion would not be suitable. Furthermore if at EMR the lesion does not lift then it should not be attempted.

Describe how EMR is performed.

EMR is usually a day case procedure performed under sedation with opiate analgesia. First the lesion to be removed is marked in the periphery with APC, following which it is injected with a mixture of adrenaline/gelofusine. If the nodule 'lifts' up easily it is amenable to EMR. This is then performed using a multi-band mucosectomy device whereby a rubber band is fired around the lesion creating a pseudopolyp. This is then snared and removed using diathermy. The specimen is retrieved and placed on a corkboard in the correct orientation. A careful inspection must be made to exclude perforation or bleeding. Circumferential biopsies from the resected area may then be taken as evidence of complete or incomplete resection margins.

What are the complications of EMR?

EMR is associated with an immediate risk of perforation as well as bleeding. Late complications include stricture formation, particularly with extensive circumferential EMR. Perforation and bleeding should be carefully looked for at the end of the procedure and may require further endoscopic or surgical intervention.

What are the other disadvantages of EMR?

EMR may not be locally available and needs expertise in performing it to a high standard. Local resection margins (particularly the deep margin) may be involved, in which case further EMR may be required. Although one should always strive for intact specimen retrieval this may at times be piecemeal. This is against surgical oncological principles and negates meaningful pathological assessment. Endoscopic interventions do not allow lymphadenectomy to be performed.

What is the significance of a T1b tumour?

A T1b tumour implies invasion of the submucosal layer which is rich in lymphatic channels. This represents an approximately 20% chance of lymph node i.e. systemic involvement.

The risk of lymph node metastasis increases with the depth of cancer invasion.

Are you aware of any other endoscopic techniques for resecting tumours?

Endoscopic submucosal dissection (ESD) can be performed but has limited availability in the west. In contrast to EMR, procedural times may be significantly longer as well as higher incidence of complications such as perforation. It is a technique commonly performed in the Far East where a higher proportion of patients present with earlier stage lesions.

Reference

Griffin SM, Burt AD, Jennings NA. Lymph node metastasis in early oesophageal adenocarcinoma. Ann Surg. 2011 Nov;254(5):731-6;

Gastric Cancer

Scenario 1

A 70 year old man is referred to you with epigastric pain. A transnasal endoscopy was performed in a private treatment centre and this showed a suspicious ulcer on the lesser curve. Only small biopsies were taken and these have come back to be 'suspicious of malignancy'. He is reasonably fit with a history of mild COPD only.

How would you manage this patient?

In the first instance I need to repeat the endoscopy and obtain further biopsies to prove whether this is a carcinoma or not. Biopsies from a gastric ulcer should be taken from the ulcer edge in a 'drill' manner by which deeper biopsies are taken through the same spot.

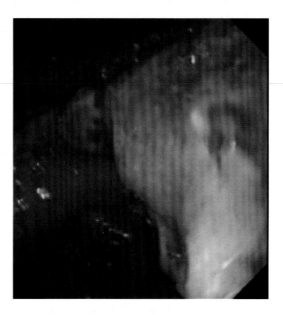

The endoscopy shown above confirms a suspicious ulcer at the incisura angularis extending towards the greater curve. There is no proximal involvement. Biopsies have come back showing a poorly differentiated adenocarcinoma.

What would you do next for the patient?

I would arrange to speak to the patient and his family ideally with a nurse specialist being present to explain the diagnosis and the importance of correctly staging him. I would obtain an urgent CT scan of his chest/abdomen and pelvis in the first instance and book him for the oesophagogastric MDT.

The CT scan did not show any significant lymphadenopathy or metastases. What are the treatment options?

The evidence so far would suggest that this is an early stage gastric cancer. Given its poor differentiation and ulcerative morphology it would not be suitable for a local endoscopic resection such as EMR. Therefore it is best dealt with surgically and the operation of choice would be a subtotal gastrectomy, as a proximal resection margin of 5cm can be easily achieved between the tumour and the OGJ. Established criteria for EMR are mucosal cancers <2 cm size and which are histologically differentiated and not ulcerated.

An early gastric cancer is defined as one which is confined to either the mucosa or submucosa irrespective of lymph node status. These carcinomas have a much better 5 year survival compared with advanced gastric cancer.

Are there any further tests that need to be performed before embarking on a curative treatment?

All gastric cancers should undergo a staging laparoscopy mainly to exclude peritoneal disease. With an early gastric cancer such as this it is unlikely that there will be peritoneal involvement, but it is not impossible. This should ideally be performed prior to surgical resection and the findings discussed in conjunction with the remaining staging tests before committing to radical surgery. Some surgeons would routinely perform peritoneal cytology during laparoscopy, which if positive constitutes metastatic (M1) disease.

What is the role of PET scanning for gastric cancer?

PET scanning has a limited role as most gastric cancers are not PET avid, particularly the diffuse and mucinous varieties. Therefore PET is not routinely used to stage gastric cancer.

How do you perform a subtotal gastrectomy?

I would do a midline laparotomy and confirm the resectability of the primary lesion. Once a decision is made to proceed the operation then begins with an omental bursectomy separating the transverse mesocolon from the greater omentum. This will bring the dissection onto the level of the right gastroepiploic vessels which can then be ligated and divided. The gastrohepatic ligament is then dissected and the right gastric vessels ligated and divided. A plane is developed below the first part of the duodenum staying clear of the pancreas, and is then divided with a linear stapler and oversewn. Posterior gastric adhesions are divided and the left gastric vessels ligated and divided. The dissection is taken up the lesser curve and the right paracardial tissue taken down. A level of division on the greater curve is chosen usually just below the first short gastric vessels. The stomach is then divided with a linear stapler. A roux loop of jejunum is fashioned and delivered in a retrocolic manner and a 2 layer hand sewn gastrojejunostomy constructed. At 50cm downstream the biliopancreatic limb is anastomosed to the efferent roux limb as a jejunojejunostomy. Finally I would leave a single drain to cover the duodenal stump and anastomosis before closing. Lymphadenectomy should be carried out, but a pragmatic approach should be taken.

The patient makes an uneventful recovery from surgery. His post operative histology confirms a grade 3 gastric adenocarcinoma invading into the submucosa but not through the muscularis propria with lymphovascular invasion, R0 and 4/15 nodes involved with tumour (pT1bN2). What further treatment would you consider for him?

Although he has undergone radical surgery with a node positive gastric cancer there is a significant risk that the cancer will recur due to the presence of micrometastases. As we know that in node positive gastric cancer chemotherapy will improve the cure rate, it is logical to assume that adjuvant chemotherapy with ECX would provide a similar benefit in this situation, though there is less evidence to back it up.

The current TNM recommends that for reliable staging a minimum of 15 nodes should be resected.

What is the evidence for the use of chemotherapy in the curative setting for gastric cancer?

The MAGIC/UK Medical Research Council (MRC) trial set the standard of care for the UK and most parts of Europe for the treatment of resectable gastric (and junctional adenocarcinoma), demonstrating that perioperative chemotherapy with epirubicin, cisplatin and 5-fluorouracil (ECF) confers a 5 year survival benefit over surgery alone (23% with surgery alone versus 36% with surgery and chemotherapy).

Capecitabine (X) is the oral pro-drug of 5-fluorouracil (5-FU) and has been demonstrated to be as efficacious and obviates the need for a central venous access device. Therefore many centres use ECX in the perioperative setting.

What is the subdivision of the mucosa and submucosa for staging purposes?

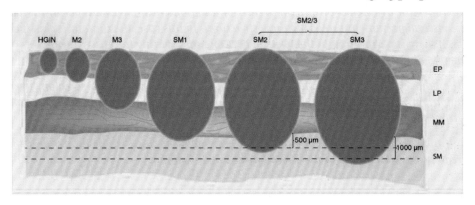

For staging purposes the mucosa and submucosa are divided into thirds:

Level	Incidence of positive nodes
M1 – epithelium	3%
M2 – lamina propria	3%
M3 – muscularis mucosae	3%
SM1	10%
SM2	19%
SM3	33%

Primary Tumour (T)

TX   Primary tumour cannot be assessed.

T0   No evidence of primary tumour.

Tis   Carcinoma *in situ*: intraepithelial tumour without invasion of the lamina propria.

T1   Tumour invades lamina propria, muscularis mucosae, or submucosa.

T1a   Tumour invades lamina propria or muscularis mucosae.

T1b   Tumour invades submucosa.

T2   Tumour invades muscularis propria.[a]

T3   Tumour penetrates subserosal connective tissue without invasion of visceral peritoneum or adjacent structures.[b,c]

T4   Tumour invades serosa (visceral peritoneum) or adjacent structures.[b]

T4a   Tumour invades serosa (visceral peritoneum).

T4b   Tumour invades adjacent structures.

[a] A tumour may penetrate the muscularis propria with extension into the gastrocolic or gastrohepatic ligaments, or into the greater or lesser omentum, without perforation of the visceral peritoneum covering these structures. In this case, the tumour is classified T3. If there is perforation of the visceral peritoneum covering the gastric ligaments or the omentum, the tumour should be classified T4.

[b] The adjacent structures of the stomach include the spleen, transverse colon, liver, diaphragm, pancreas, abdominal wall, adrenal gland, kidney, small intestine, and retroperitoneum.

[c] Intramural extension to the duodenum or oesophagus is classified by the depth of the greatest invasion in any of these sites, including the stomach.

Regional Lymph Nodes (N)

NX   Regional lymph node(s) cannot be assessed.
N0   No regional lymph node metastasis.[a]
N1   Metastases in 1–2 regional lymph nodes.
N2   Metastases in 3–6 regional lymph nodes.
N3   Metastases in ≥7 regional lymph nodes.
N3a   Metastases in 7–15 regional lymph nodes.
N3b   Metastases in ≥16 regional lymph nodes.

[a] A designation of pN0 should be used if all examined lymph nodes are negative, regardless of the total number removed and examined.

Distant Metastasis

M0   No distant metastasis.
M1   Distant metastasis.

References

Cunningham et al. Perioperative chemotherapy versus surgery alone for resectable gastric cancer. NEJM 2006. 355:11-20.

Edge SB, Byrd DR, Compton CC, et al., eds.: AJCC Cancer Staging Manual. 7th ed. New York, NY: Springer, 2010, pp 117-26.

Gastric Lymphoma

An 80 year old lady is referred to your outpatient clinic with a history of vague abdominal pain and melaena. Gastroscopy showed a gastric ulcer and biopsies taken confirm dense lymphoid infiltration consistent with low-grade gastric MALT lymphoma.

What is a MALT lymphoma?

These are low grade lymphomas that arise from the gastric mucosa-associated lymphoid tissue (MALT). They are a form of B cell non-Hodgkin's lymphoma as per the WHO classification. Occasionally T cell lymphomas and Hodgkin's disease are also seen.

How commonly do gastric lymphomas occur?

Primary gastric lymphomas are rare but are one of the commonest sites for 'extranodal' lymphoma. The stomach is also the commonest site for gastrointestinal lymphomas.

MALT lymphomas often present with the same vague non–specific symptoms of dyspepsia, vague epigastric discomfort and may be associated with weight loss. Patients may present acutely with peritonitis from perforation or bleeding.

How is gastric lymphoma staged?

Staging CT of chest, abdomen and pelvis should be performed to assess the extent of disease. EUS to assess depth of invasion and regional lymph node involvement may also be of value.

What is the treatment of MALT lymphoma?

As they are generally low grade lymphomas they behave in an indolent manner. They are usually associated with *H.pylori* infection and often regress with eradication therapy (antibiotics and PPI). In *H. pylori*-negative cases or patients who fail antibiotic therapy, irradiation and systemic therapies should be considered depending on the stage of the disease.

What is the treatment of more advanced MALT lymphoma?

More advanced tumours may not respond to *H.pylori* eradication and may require either chlorambucil and rituximab or CHOP chemotherapy (Cyclophosphamide, doxorubicin, vincristine and prednisolone) and rituximab. Surgery has not been shown to have favourable outcomes when compared with irradiation or systemic chemotherapy in more advanced cases.

Gastro Intestinal Stromal Tumour (GIST)

A 45 year old fit and well lady has been referred with a history of melaena and anaemia. At gastroscopy the following is seen within the proximal stomach.

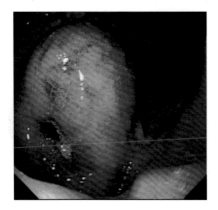 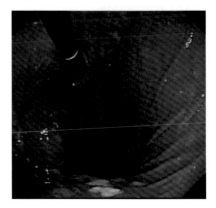

What is your diagnosis?

This image shows a pedunculated, smooth, spherical, likely submucosal lesion with a prominent ulcerated region which would account for the history of GI bleeding. These appearances are consistent with a gastric GIST. The lesion appears to be in the gastric fundus and well away from the OG junction.

Would you biopsy this?

If the appearance is convincing of a gastric GIST as in the picture, then a biopsy is not recommended by current guidelines. The majority of these lesions (60%) are submucosal so biopsy will often reveal normal mucosa. If there is diagnostic uncertainty then an EUS with core biopsy may be considered (see GIST guidelines in the references section). Furthermore percutaneous or laparoscopic biopsies should not be performed for resectable disease due to the risk of tumour rupture or seeding.

How and where do these tumours typically present?

The commonest anatomical site is the stomach (50%) followed by small bowel (25%) and colorectum (10%). Oesophageal, mesenteric, and omental GISTs are rare. Presentation can be symptomatic or asymptomatic. Symptomatic presentation is most commonly with bleeding, abdominal pain, and weight loss. Asymptomatic incidental presentation may be from radiological scans for other conditions (CT, MRI) or found incidentally during OGD or intra-operatively (e.g. laparoscopy).

How would you further investigate this?

Formal staging investigations are essential to exclude distant disease and determine loco-regional disease. A CT scan of the chest / abdomen / pelvis should be ordered to exclude distant disease such as liver metastases. In selected cases EUS may be used to confirm the submucosal origin if the diagnosis is uncertain (in this scenario, it can also be used with FNA to obtain biopsies). EUS is also able to accurately characterise the diameter of the GIST (an important prognostic indicator) and may also examine regional lymph nodes (although GISTs tend not to metastasise to lymph nodes).

Her CT scan confirms the presence of a lesion within the proximal stomach. There is no evidence of lymphadenopathy or distant metastases. How would you proceed?

As the lesion is localised and she is symptomatic she should be offered surgical resection. The majority of these are resectable laparoscopically. As the lesion is endoscopically clear of the OGJ it should be suitable for a wedge resection rather than an anatomical resection such as a total gastrectomy. I would laparoscope the patient and, given its position in the fundus, would expect to secure the short gastric vessels followed by stapling the lesion ensuring that we stay well clear of the OG junction.

What are the principles for treating these tumours?

Asymptomatic small (2cm or less) GISTs can be managed by surveillance through annual endoscopy +/- EUS. Symptomatic or growing GISTs may require surgical excision after staging. Surgery is considered as the primary treatment modality in those fit for resection. The principal goal of surgery is to achieve a R0 resection as this is known to be associated with the most favourable outcomes.

Surgical options include either a local excision or anatomical resection. In the majority of cases a local "wedge excision" can be performed allowing adequate resection margins. For tumours close to or invading proximally to the OGJ or involving pylorus an anatomical resection such as total gastrectomy or distal gastrectomy may be required.

The postoperative histology confirms a GIST 5.8cm in maximum dimension with 9 mitoses per 50 high power fields. How would you proceed from here?

This places her in a high risk of recurrence category. There is good evidence that adjuvant treatment with imatinib increases disease-free survival for high risk GISTs. Once she has made a full recovery from surgery this can be considered, and in the meantime the specimen should be sent for immunotyping, which is done in specific centres only. This would confirm whether the lesion is sensitive to a tyrosine kinase inhibitor or not.

All high risk and intermediate risk GISTs and small bowel GISTs should have mutational analysis performed.

The mutational analysis reveals an exon 11 mutation that is sensitive to imatinib. What is the histopathology of these tumours and how does this influence treatment?

GISTs arise from the interstitial cells of Cajal (ICC) which are the pacemaker cells in the gastrointestinal tract (GIT) located in the myenteric plexus. They have a characteristic immunostaining pattern which is important in confirming the histological diagnosis. Expression of the KIT proto-oncogene is essential in the development of ICC cells. The product of the KIT proto-oncogene, KIT, is a member of the tyrosine kinase receptor family and a transmembrane receptor for growth factors. This is also closely related to the platelet derived growth factor receptor (PDGFR). The growth of many GISTs is dependent on KIT expression and activation. Such activation involves a mutation in the c-KIT gene, the commonest of which is in exon 11.

The majority (95%) of GISTs will stain positive for *c-kit* (CD117) as well as the recently discovered DOG1 (Discovered On GIST1 and encodes for a chloride channel). This staining pattern has implications for treatment as TKI may be used in C-kit positive GISTs. The remaining 5% of GISTs that are c-kit negative should undergo mutational analysis as some may still be TKI sensitive.

What is the mechanism of action of imatinib?

Imatinib is a tyrosine kinase inhibitor and it represents a major breakthrough in the treatment of GISTs as these lesions are resistant to conventional chemotherapy. There is good evidence for the use of adjuvant imatinib (400mg/day) for high risk GISTs following surgical resection. A Scandinavian study randomised patients to adjuvant imatinib for either 1 or 3 years after surgery for high risk GIST. They found overall survival and disease-free survival was higher in the 3 year treatment group (92.0% vs 81.7% for overall survival – Joensuu et al). Data is still awaited from the largest study, conducted by the European Organisation for Research and Treatment of Cancer (EORTC), in which 908 patients were randomly assigned to receive either 2 years of adjuvant imatinib or no imatinib. Based on the current evidence, 3 years of imatinib at a daily dose of 400 mg should be considered in patients with a 50% or higher risk of relapse within 5 years after surgery. In patients where surgical resection is deemed high risk, primary treatment with imatinib should be considered. If there is progression on imatinib then consideration to switching to second line treatment (sunitibib 50mg/day) should be made.

How are surgically excised GISTs classified on histopathology?

Surgically resected tumours are assigned into one of a number of risk groups depending on size and mitotic index and site of tumour (see table below). This is based on data derived from a large dataset on GIST patients know as the Miettenen and Lasota dataset. This replaces the previous National Institute of Health (NIH) classification which underestimates the risk of small bowel GISTs and overestimates for gastric GISTs.

Tumour parameters		Risk of progressive disease (metastasis or tumour-related death)			
Mitotic index	Size	Gastric	Duodenum	Jejunum/ileum	Rectum
$\leq$5 (in 5mm^2)*	$\leq$2 cm	None (0%)	None (0%)	None (0%)	None (0%)
	>2–$\leq$5 cm	Very low (1.9%)	Low (8.3%)	Low (4.3%)	Low (8.5%)
	>5–$\leq$10 cm	Low (3.6%)	(Insufficient data)	Moderate (24%)	(Insufficient data)
	>10 cm	Moderate (10%)	High (34%)	High (52%)	High (57%)
>5 (in 5mm^2)*	$\leq$2 cm	(Insufficient data)	(Insufficient data)	High (limited data)	High (54%)
	>2–$\leq$5 cm	Moderate (16%)	High (50%)	High (73%)	High (52%)
	>5–$\leq$10 cm	High (55%)	(Insufficient data)	High (85%)	(Insufficient data)
	>10cm	High (86%)	High (86%)	High (90%)	High (71%)

How would you follow this patient up?

All patients following resection should be discussed in a MDM. As she has a high risk of recurrence she should have a CT at 3 months and then 3 monthly for 2 years –see below.

Following baseline clinic review post op, the follow up depends on histology:

- *Very low risk tumours – no imaging required*

- *Low risk tumours – CT at 3 months following surgery then clinical follow up*

- *Intermediate risk tumours – CT at 3 months post surgery then 6 monthly for 2 years then annually for 5 years*

- *High risk tumours – CT at 3 months post surgery then 3 monthly for 2 years then 6 monthly for 2 years then annually*

Are they associated with any syndromes?

The majority of GISTs are not associated with any syndromes but rare associations do exist:

These include - a familial association – with multiple small bowel GISTs

Carney's syndrome/triad (GIST, pulmonary chondroma and extra adrenal paraganglioma)

Von Recklinghausen's disease (Neurofibromatosis Type 1)

In those deemed to have non-resectable metastatic disease is there a role for surgery?

There is no role for debulking surgery in these patients. However surgery may be required to alleviate symptoms in those having problems with bleeding or obstruction.

In those commenced with imatinib surgery may be considered if there is sufficient improvement to consider the tumour operable. There is increasing recognition of so-called "induction chemotherapy". This is the use of neoadjuvant imatinib to "down-size" the disease, which may render an initially unresectable tumour resectable.

References

Casali PG, Blay J-Y. Gastrointestinal stromal tumours: ESMO Clinical Practice Guidelines for diagnosis, treatment and follow-up. *Ann Oncol (2010) 21 (suppl 5): v98-v102*

Guidelines for the management of gastrointestinal stromal tumours (GIST). http://www.britishsarcomagroup.org.uk/guidelines/4556224410

Joensuu H, Eriksson M, Sundby Hall K et al One vs three years of adjuvant imatinib for operable gastrointestinal stromal tumour: a randomized trial. JAMA. 2012 Mar 28;307(12):1265-72.

Gastro-oesophageal Reflux Disease

The gastroenterologists refer to you a 35 year old man with severe heartburn, to consider anti-reflux surgery. He has been taking regular pantoprazole 40mg twice a day with limited success and is unhappy about taking tablets. How would you proceed?

The history, examination and investigations that have already been carried out should be revisited. The presence of typical symptoms of reflux alone such as heartburn, regurgitation and dysphagia are not enough to make a firm diagnosis of GORD. The patient may have atypical symptoms such as cough, hoarseness and chest pain. Response to PPIs and their effect on symptom relief are important to ascertain.

Lifestyle factors should also be considered: smoking and alcohol intake can contribute towards symptoms, and these should also be addressed. Also if the patient is overweight this will contribute towards the problem.

The endoscopic diagnosis should be confirmed and whether or not there was any evidence of oesophagitis. The results of any oesophageal physiology studies and radiological investigations such as barium swallow should be reviewed.

Proper evaluation of patients with suspected GORD is essential for a correct diagnosis and treatment plan. Response of symptoms to proton pump inhibitors (PPIs), together with typical symptoms, and abnormal pH monitoring are important predictors of successful anti-reflux surgery. Confirmation of the objective presence of reflux by demonstrating abnormal distal oesophageal acid exposure and correlation of reflux events on pH monitoring with the symptoms experienced by the patient are essential.

An upper GI endoscopy on this patient was last performed a few years ago. Therefore you decide to repeat it. What are the aims of upper GI endoscopy in this patient?

The aims of the upper GI endoscopy in the evaluation of suspected GORD are:

1) Detect complications of reflux such as Barrett's oesophagus, high grade erosive oesophagitis (LA classification grades C/D) and stricture.

2) Exclude other diseases (e.g., gastritis, peptic ulcer disease) which may mimic the symptoms of GORD.

What proportion of patients with GORD symptoms have evidence of reflux at endoscopy?

Less than two-thirds of patients with reflux symptoms have endoscopic evidence of oesophagitis i.e. a normal endoscopy does NOT exclude a diagnosis of GORD. Endoscopy can diagnose complications of GORD e.g. the development of oesophageal ulceration, stricture, Barrett's epithelium and most importantly it can exclude neoplasia.

What further investigations would you request?

I would request a 24 hour ambulatory pH monitoring as this is the gold standard in diagnosing GORD. This may provide objective evidence of abnormal reflux. The test has a high specificity and sensitivity. Anti-secretory medications such as PPI should be withheld for 7 days prior to testing. Results may help correlate with typical and atypical symptoms of reflux. This is particularly important for atypical symptoms such as cough, hoarseness and chest pain.

A barium swallow is useful to look at anatomical abnormalities and will also give an idea about oesophageal motility.

An upper GI endoscopy is performed and this shows a small hiatus hernia (<5cm) along with grade A oesophagitis. How would you classify oesophagitis?

This is done using the Los Angeles classification:

Grade A	One (or more) mucosal break no longer than 5 mm that does not extend between the tops of two mucosal folds
Grade B	One (or more) mucosal break more than 5 mm long that does not extend between the tops of two mucosal folds
Grade C	One (or more) mucosal break that is continuous between the tops of two or more mucosal folds but which involve less than 75% of the circumference
Grade D	One (or more) mucosal break which involves at least 75% of the circumference

What is the purpose of performing manometry?

Manometry is very important to help exclude motility disorders such as achalasia. Performing a fundoplication on a patient with poor peristalsis can be disastrous. Other conditions such as scleroderma may also cause poor peristalsis. Manometry also confirms the level of the lower oesophageal sphincter thereby allowing accurate positioning of the pH catheter.

What is the purpose of 24 hour pH monitoring?

Ambulatory pH monitoring provides objective evidence of abnormal reflux. It has a high specificity and good sensitivity. It serves as an important outcome predictor of surgery and is able to correlate both typical and atypical symptoms with episodes of reflux. Anti-secretory medications are withheld for at least 7 days before the test.

Manometry shows 90% oesophageal peristalsis with a distal oesophageal amplitude of 70mmHg. A 24 hour pH monitoring test off PPIs showed a pathologic amount of reflux (DeMeester score of 78). What is the Demeester score?

This is a score calculated using six parameters to give a surrogate measure of GORD severity.

A score >14.72 indicates significant reflux. The parameters are:

- Supine reflux

- Upright reflux

- Total reflux

- Number of episodes

- Number of episodes longer than 5 minutes

- Longest episode

How is oesophageal manometry performed? Can you draw the typical tracings obtained from manometry in a normal patient?

Generally this is a test which involves placement of a manometry catheter transnasally using a water-perfused catheter. These catheters typically have eight pressure sensing side holes at 3cm intervals and are perfused with bubble free water by a pump. Pressure changes are recorded as the flow of water through the side hole of a tube is impeded by circumferential contraction of the wall of the oesophagus.

Initially a 'station pull through' manoeuvre is used to locate a high pressure zone created by the lower oesophageal sphincter and diaphragmatic contractions. The catheter is pulled back in 1cm increments from the low pressure gastric lumen until the high pressure zone is reached (Figure 1).

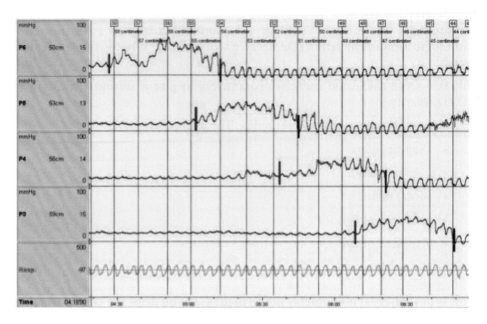

Figure 1: Example of station pull through technique to locate position of the LOS. Taken from *GI Motility online* (2006) doi:10.1038/gimo90

Five wet swallows involving delivery of 5mls of water through a syringe are used to assess swallow-induced LOS relaxation. Normally the pressure at the LOS will fall to approximate with intra-gastric pressure. The function of the oesophageal body is assessed with 10 wet swallows. These swallows should normally produce a peristaltic wave along the length of the oesophagus with an amplitude of at least 20mmHg. The amplitude and duration of the waves are assessed as well as the percentage of wet swallows that produced a normal peristaltic response (Figure 2).

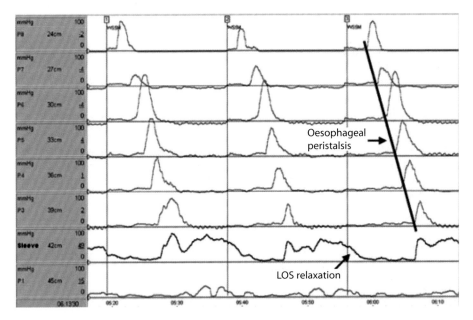

Figure 2: Examples of oesophageal peristalsis and LOS relaxation during three swallows each of 5 mL of water. Taken from *GI Motility online* (2006) doi:10.1038/gimo90

What is impedance monitoring?

Impedance monitoring is an increasingly used method of detecting intraluminal bolus movement. It is often performed in combination with pH testing and allows for the identification of both acid and non-acid reflux. In brief it relies upon measurement of changes in resistance to an electric current when a bolus passes between two sensors. Liquid containing boluses have an increased number of ions therefore have a higher conductivity and when entering the impedance measuring segment will lower the impedance. Gas passing will produce a rapid rise in the impedance since it has poor electrical conductance.

What are the indications for anti-reflux surgery?

1) Patients who have failed to respond to medical therapy. PPIs are most effective at controlling heartburn rather than volume regurgitation. Failed medical therapy is most often seen in patients with the latter symptoms.

2) Patients whose symptoms are fully controlled by medications such as PPIs but wish to discontinue these medications.

What are the pros and cons of a partial versus total fundoplication?

The long term outcome of a partial anterior 180° versus Nissen fundoplication has been reported recently by two studies. The first study was a prospective RCT that looked at symptomatic and pH outcomes 14 years after treatment. The results of this study showed that after an anterior fundoplication rates of recurrent reflux were higher but dysphagia scores were lower. The second study was from the same group in Adelaide and evaluated 2,261 patients with a mean follow-up of 7.6 years and found that after an anterior fundoplication, heartburn was slightly worse (while reoperation was more common) and dysphagia was lower (while reoperation was less common). The conclusion from these studies was that both operations provide good long-term results with similar rates of control of reflux and dysphagia rates at ten years.

References

Jobe BA, Richter JE, Hoppo T, et al. Preoperative diagnostic work-up before antireflux surgery: an evidence and experience-based consensus of the Esophageal Diagnostic Advisory Panel. J Am Coll Surg. 2013;217(4):586–97

Broeders JA, Broeders EA, Watson DI, Devitt PG, Holloway RH, Jamieson GG. Objective outcomes 14 years after laparoscopic anterior 180-degree partial versus Nissen fundoplication: results from a randomized trial. Ann Surg. 2013 Aug;258(2):233–9

Engström C, Cai W, Irvine T, Devitt PG, Thompson SK, Game PA, Bessell JR, Jamieson GG, Watson DI. Twenty years of experience with laparoscopic antireflux surgery. Br J Surg. 2012 Oct;99(10): 1415–21.

Iatrogenic Oesophageal Perforation

You are called by the gastroenterology team to the endoscopy suite where an 86 year old lady has just sustained a perforation of the oesophagus during intubation for an ERCP. She has severe pain in her neck and mild surgical emphysema. She is apyrexial but tachcycardic at 110 bpm. She has no significant past medical history.

How do perforations of the cervical oesophagus present?

Cervical perforations commonly present with neck pain and hoarseness. Dysphagia and odynophagia are also common. Systemic features are not always apparent as mediastinitis is uncommon.

How would you manage this lady?

The immediate priority is to ensure that the patient is fully resuscitated with IV fluids, analgesia and broad spectrum intravenous antibiotics. As the perforation has only just occurred it will be fresh and amenable to surgical repair. I would proceed to get the patient seen urgently by the anaesthetic team with a view to urgent surgery.

The patient has consented for surgical intervention. What operation would you do?

Firstly I would endoscope the patient myself under GA to ascertain the size and site of the perforation. At the same time this would allow passage of a nasogastric tube as well as a nasojejunal feeding tube under direct vision.

You endoscope the patient and find a significant full thickness defect just below the cricopharyngeus leading into a false passage all the way down towards the oesophageal hiatus.

Prompt surgical drainage is the best option and reduces morbidity, mortality and hospital stay. Generally the left side of the neck is approached via an incision along the lower third anterior to sternocleidomastoid (SCM). The SCM muscle is dissected posteriorly off the underlying sternohyoid muscle until the lateral surface of the internal jugular vein is well seen. The anterior belly of the omohyoid muscle is identified and may be divided. The deep cervical fascia is incised along the anterior border of the internal jugular vein after taking the middle thyroid vein between ligatures and then more deeply and slightly anteriorly along the common carotid artery. The carotid sheath can then be retracted laterally. The inferior thyroid artery is ligated where it courses medially from behind the carotid artery. Blunt dissection is used to access the retrovisceral space posterior to the oesophagus. Dissection may be facilitated by feeling the nasogastric tube within the oesophagus. If the perforation is visualised an attempt can be made to close it with absorbable sutures but this is not absolutely necessary as adequate drainage usually leads to healing. Blunt finger dissection along the retrovisceral plane allows entry into the posterior superior mediastinum for irrigation and insertion of a drain.

What are the essential steps of managing this patient post-operatively?

- Strictly Nil by Mouth

- Intravenous fluids

- Nasogastric decompression at endoscopy or via radiology

- Enteral nutrition via endoscopically placed nasojejunal tube

- Intravenous PPI as antisecretory agent

- Broad spectrum antimicrobials

- Frequent clinical reassessment

- Follow up CT scans to assess collections / contamination

- Targeted radiological drains as appropriate

- Multidisciplinary approach involving intensivists, radiologists, dietician, physiotherapists and nursing staff

- Contrast study at weekly intervals to assess for ongoing leak and communication into a cavity

Why might the outcome from iatrogenic oesophageal perforation be better than following other causes?

The injury may be recognized at the time of the procedure, therefore treatment delay tends to be minimised and the degree of contamination less as the stomach was prepared prior to the procedure. As a principle management decisions should be guided primarily by the degree of contamination rather than the aetiology of the perforation.

Reference

Nirula R. Esophageal perforation. Surg Clin North Am. 2014 Feb;94(1):35-41.

Ivor Lewis Complications

Your registrar calls you to the ward due to high output from the chest drains 24 hours after a two-phase oesophagectomy. What is the most likely diagnosis?

There are a number of causes - I would want to establish that the patient was stable and there was not an active bleed, however change of position can lead to drainage of fluid from the chest. If it has been ongoing and is not blood then my concern would be a chyle leak. It may appear serosanguinous but can turn milky in colour if enteral feeding has commenced.

What is the aetiology of chylothorax following oesophagectomy?

The thoracic duct may be damaged during mobilization of the oesophagus. The incidence of chylothorax is about 2%-3%.

Chylothorax usually presents in the first 7 days when the patient has commenced enteral intake, especially of fat-containing nutrients. A massive increase in chest drainage may be seen that can lead to significant malnutrition and immune suppression from loss of CD4+ white cells.

What are the treatment steps for a chylothorax?

- If the volume is 800mls> on 3-4 consecutive days (not everyone agrees on this) then operative intervention may be considered. For major leaks immediate re-exploration is best as the damaged thoracic duct is easily identified at re-exploration

- Enteral feed by medium chain triglycerides thereby absorbed directly into portal circulation bypassing lymphatics

- Cotrimoxazole to prevent pneumocystitis infection

- Monitor CD4 white cell count for lymphopenia

- Pleuroperitoneal shunt may be considered for refractory cases in which abnormal lymphatic anatomy may account for the persistence of leakage despite operative and conservative intervention

If you were re-operating what steps would you follow?

- If there has been a large output (usually >800mls on 3-4 consecutive days), then reoperation should be considered, or if greater than 1-2l on the first morning after surgery

- Position and reopening of chest as per initial surgery

- Introduction of cream via the feeding jejunostomy at the introduction of anaesthesia. If this is done too early it may hinder identification of the leak.

- Close below and above the leak: clips may be used or pledgeted sutures.

What evidence is there to show a difference in leak rates between hand sewn and stapled anastomoses?

No significant difference has been shown between hand sewn and stapled anastomoses. This was demonstrated in a small study by Law et al, but a higher rate of anastomotic stricture was seen with the stapled anastomosis.

What is the evidence for routine use of contrast radiology following oesophagectomy or total gastrectomy?

There is no evidence to show that there is improved survival or outcome following routine contrast radiology. Practices vary with some surgeons electing to perform contrast radiology routinely whereas others do so selectively.

Why is it essential to ensure that the gastric conduit is fully within the chest?

It is vital to ensure that the gastric conduit sits well within the mediastinum without excessive tortuosity. This is particularly important for those patients with a good long term outlook. Otherwise these patients can have significant trouble with reflux, regurgitation and gastric emptying. Occasionally this requires conduit revisional surgery which is a complex undertaking.

What is dumping syndrome?

Patients may complain of postprandial nausea, vomiting, bloating, cramping, diarrhoea and dizziness. This is due to rapid post surgery movement of food into the small intestine. The hyperosmolar nature of this leads to a fluid shift which causes the above symptoms.

Many of the symptoms may be alleviated by addressing eating habits e.g smaller more frequent meals rather than three large ones, or avoiding foods that have been noticed to precipitate symptoms (usually carbohydrates). Symptoms usually resolve 12 months after surgery.

This patient sees you in outpatients and is complaining of dysphagia and vomiting 12 weeks after surgery. What is your plan?

This patient needs a repeat endoscopy, although a barium swallow may be of some diagnostic use. They are likely to have an anastomotic stricture, although patients who have not had a pyloroplasty may also complain of similar problems and require pyloric dilatation.

What is the best treatment for benign anastomotic strictures following oesophagectomy?

These strictures are not uncommon but usually respond to a single dilatation performed by endoscopy and image intensifier. Practices vary but dilation can be performed with balloon dilators or Savary-Gilliard® dilators.

What is the adequate size of staple gun for a CEEA stapled oesophagogastric anastomosis?

There is evidence that a staple gun head diameter of <25mm may lead to increased incidence of benign anastomotic stricture.

Reference

S Law, M Fok, K M Chu, and J Wong Comparison of hand-sewn and stapled oesophagogastric anastomosis after esophageal resection for cancer: a prospective randomized controlled trial Ann Surg. 1997 August; 226(2): 169^173

Obesity Surgery

Scenario 1

A 45 year old woman is referred to your outpatients clinic by her GP. She is overweight and has tried a variety of diets with varying success but now wishes to be considered for weight-loss surgery. What are the qualification criteria for bariatric surgery in the UK?

There are a number of criteria that are set out by the recent (November 2014) NICE guidelines – Obesity: identification, assessment and management of overweight and obesity in children, young people and adults [CG189]. These include:-

- Morbid obesity i.e. BMI > 40

- BMI 35-40 with obesity related co-morbidity e.g. diabetes, hypertension etc.

- All appropriate non-surgical measures have been tried but the person has not achieved or maintained adequate, clinically beneficial weight loss.

- The person has been receiving or will receive intensive management in a tier 3 service.

- Committed to treatment and follow up.

- Expedited assessment BMI>35 or over with recent-onset type 2 diabetes.

- Consider an assessment for people with a BMI of 30–34.9 who have recent-onset type 2 diabetes.

- Consider an assessment for bariatric surgery for people of Asian family origin who have recent-onset type 2 diabetes at a lower BMI.

However, some Clinical Commissioning Groups will set up their own qualifying criteria which often include a higher BMI.

How do you define Body Mass Index and what are the advantages and disadvantages of using BMI?

BMI is a convenient and reproducible method of defining whether an individual is overweight. It is essentially a ratio of weight to height and is defined as (weight (kg)/ height^2 (m)).

However, it does not accurately allow for the calculation of percentage of body fat, possibly a more useful tool. In adults who are extremely active, and carrying a high muscle mass, the BMI may label them as overweight when in fact they have a low level of body fat.

BMI is a poor predictor of cardiovascular risk and mortality. Other scores assessing metabolic risk or comorbidity (such as the Edmonton obesity staging system, which takes into account the severity of comorbidities and functional status) predict obesity related risk more accurately. Although BMI is widely used as a method for identifying patients who may benefit from weight loss surgery, focusing on obesity-associated morbidity, particularly in a multidisciplinary team environment, may be a more effective way to stratify individual patient risk and use healthcare resources.

How do you define obesity?

Currently almost **2.5%** of the adult population in the UK are morbidly obese with a BMI > 40

BMI (Kg/m2)	Category
20 or less	Underweight
20-25	Ideal
25-30	Overweight
>30	Obese
>40	Morbid (clinically severe) obesity
>50	Super obesity

A further "super" is added for each additional 10 in BMI after 50 (eg >60 is super super obese, >70 is super super super obese)

What co-morbidities are associated with morbid obesity?

- Diabetes mellitus
- Arterial hypertension
- IHD/ stroke
- Obstructive sleep apnoea
- Gallstones
- Non-Alcoholic Fatty Liver Disease/Non-Alcoholic Steatohepatosis (NAFLD/NASH)
- Polycystic ovarian syndrome and subfertility
- GORD/Cancer
- Arthritis
- Psychological disorders

Which operation is your preferred bariatric procedure?

In my practice, patient choice determines the type of procedure performed. Most patients are very well informed and have already formed an opinion regarding the operation they prefer. If not, I encourage them to attend a patient support group where they can meet patients who have already undergone different procedures.

The most common weight loss procedure performed in the UK according to the National Bariatric Surgery Registry is the laparoscopic roux en y gastric bypass. Weight loss outcomes are excellent and the effect on diabetes often leading to improvement in glycaemic control and remission is impressive. Sleeve gastrectomy is gaining popularity with similar results, however the long-term data are still being collected. The laparoscopic Adjustable Gastric Band is associated with the lowest mortality, but the reoperation rate in the long term can be 10%-20%. In addition regular band consultations are required, ideally at a frequency of 8 per year, which is not achievable in today's NHS.

What is the impact of surgery on diabetes mellitus?

The impact of surgery on DM is dramatic and seen most profoundly following biliary pancreatic diversion and duodenal switch (BPD and DS) and bypass which results in remission of DM in 97% and 85% respectively. The effect of gastric banding on diabetes is greatest in lighter patients (BMI 30-40). According to the National Bariatric Surgery Register (NBSR) 2014 report, at two years 65.1% of patients with type 2 diabetes returned to a state of no indication of diabetes, meaning, in practice, that they were able to stop their diabetic medications.

What are the theories behind how diabetes is improved?

The mechanism of the improvement in diabetes after weight loss surgery has not been fully elucidated and is most likely multifactorial. In addition to the reduced food intake and the weight loss, both of which have a positive effect on glucose metabolism, it has been demonstrated that some improvements in diabetes occur in the very early postoperative period, prior to any meaningful weight loss. The change in the route of nutrients with the associated hormonal changes mainly in GLP-1 may explain in part some of this improvement.

What are the quoted figures for weight loss following bariatric surgery?

A meta-analysis of 22,000 patients from 136 studies showed a mean percentage excess weight loss for BPD/DS 70.1%, gastric bypass 61.6% and gastric banding 47.5%. According to the 2014 NBSR report, at 12 months postoperatively patients lost 58.4% of their excess weight (36.6% for gastric banding, 68.7% for gastric bypass and 58.9% for sleeve gastrectomy).

What are the quoted mortality rates for bariatric surgery?

The same meta-analysis has quoted a mortality rate of 0.1% for banding, 0.5% gastric bypass and 1.1% for BPD/DS.

In the second report of the UK National Bariatric Surgery Registry (2011-2013), the in-hospital mortality rate after primary weight loss surgery was 0.07% overall (and 0.07% for gastric bypass).

There is a substantial reduction in mortality from other co-morbidities including diabetes and hypertension, as shown by a number of studies including the Swedish Obese Subjects study.

Interestingly in the gastric bypass group the greatest reduction in mortality is from reduction in cancer related death (60% reduction at 7 years).

References

Padwal RS1, Pajewski NM, Allison DB, Sharma AM. Using the Edmonton obesity staging system to predict mortality in a population-representative cohort of people with overweight and obesity. CMAJ. 2011 Oct 4;183(14):E1059-66. doi: 10.1503/cmaj.110387. Epub 2011 Aug 15

The UK National Bariatric Surgery Registry Second Registry Report 2014

Suter MI, Calmes JM, Paroz A, Giusti V. A 10-year experience with laparoscopic gastric banding for morbid obesity: high long-term complication and failure rates. Obes Surg. 2006 Jul;16(7):829-35.

Buchwald H,Avidor Y, Braunwald E, Jensen MD, Pories W, Fahrbach K, Schoelles K Bariatric surgery: a systematic review and meta-analysis. JAMA. 2004 Oct 13;292(14):1724-37.

Sjöström L, Narbro K, Sjöström CD, Karason K, Larsson B, Wedel H, Lystig T, Sullivan M, Bouchard C, Carlsson B, Bengtsson C, Dahlgren S, Gummesson A, Jacobson P, Karlsson J, Lindroos AK, Lönroth H, Näslund I, Olbers T, Stenlöf K, Torgerson J, Agren G, Carlsson LM; Swedish Obese Subjects Study. Effects of bariatric surgery on mortality in Swedish obese subjects. N Engl J Med. 2007 Aug 23;357(8):741-52.

Obesity Surgery

Scenario 2

You are seeing a super morbidly obese patient in clinic who has been discussed at the bariatric MDM. The feeling was that a sleeve gastrectomy may be most appropriate for this patient, given her lifestyle and multiple comorbidities. Counsel the patient as to the options and the nature of a sleeve gastrectomy.

A sleeve gastrectomy is an irreversible procedure and works by creating a long, narrow gastric tube through laparoscopic stapling and by removing the gastric fundus. It has the advantage of being often a safer and quicker procedure than a gastric bypass, and may be used as an intermediate step before progressing on to a gastric bypass in some cases. In this patient the extreme obesity and comorbidities mean that a sleeve gastrectomy would be a safer route, and the possibility of converting the operation to a gastric bypass exists if this should required in future.

The complications of a sleeve gastrectomy include:

Immediate

- Staple line leakage
- Venous thromboembolism

Long-term

- Stenosis of the gastric tube
- GORD: reflux symptoms tend to predominate in the first year but reduce thereafter
- Weight regain

What is ghrelin?

Ghrelin is an orexigenic hormone produced by the gastric fundus. Ghrelin is therefore reduced in a sleeve resection which is associated with reduced hunger. Initially it was thought that the effect of roux-en-y gastric bypass on appetite was mediated via ghrelin. However subsequent studies did not show a consistent change on ghrelin. Furthermore it has been demonstrated that an increase in the postprandial response of the satiety gut hormones PYY and GLP-1 contribute to appetite control.

What are the steps of a roux-en-y gastric bypass?

The RYGB is the commonest operation worldwide for morbid obesity.

- Creation of a gastric pouch based on high lesser curve of <30ml

- Gastrojejunostomy. In my practice I prefer the use of a (state your preference) circular stapler/linear stapler with suturing of the defect/completely hand-sewn) in retrocolic/antecolic, antegastric fashion.

- Jejunojejunostomy. My preferred choice is (state your preference) linear stapler with suturing of the defect/fully stapled technique/completely hand-sewn.

- I close the mesocolic, Petersen's and JJ mesenteric defects.

How does weight loss occur following roux-en-y gastric bypass?

- Profound impact on gut hormone profiles with elevated satiety hormones such as peptide YY and GLP-1.

- Some new data suggest changes in food preference and taste as well as a paradoxical increase in energy expenditure.

What is the rationale for performing a concurrent cholecystectomy?

1) Development of gallstones seems to be accelerated following rapid weight loss. Gallstones may develop in 30% of such cases.

2) Adhesions may make subsequent cholecystectomy difficult to perform.

3) Endoscopic access to the biliary tree is challenging due to the anatomical changes.

In the open era, it was common to perform a cholecystectomy during the gastric bypass procedure. However with laparoscopic bypass, a cholecystectomy is not routinely performed currently as the risk of the cholecystectomy is not justified. A complication from the cholecystectomy during the catabolic period after gastric bypass may lead to mortality risk, which is not justified.

Oesophageal Cancer

Scenario 1

A 71 year old man presents with a history of progressive dysphagia and weight loss. He undergoes an endoscopy which reveals a circumferential obstructing oesophageal stricture from 34cm which is non-traversable. Biopsies confirm this to be a poorly differentiated adenocarcinoma. He is generally fit and active cycling up to 8 miles on some days and gardening 3 times per week.

How would you proceed from this stage?

Once the patient has been informed of the diagnosis I would complete his staging investigations by obtaining a CT scan of his chest/abdomen/pelvis to exclude any metastatic disease. Provided the CT scan shows no evidence of metastatic disease then I would next request a positron emission tomography (PET) scan. An endoscopic ultrasound (EUS) will have a limited role in a non-traversable stricture but may provide limited information. Given that the patient sounds fit for a surgical resection then all these tests are justifiable. The case will also need to be discussed in the oesophagogastric MDM.

On CT scan this lesion extends beyond the OG junction for about 3cm. On CT scan and PET scan there is no metastatic disease. The EUS confirms a T3N1 lesion.

What is a T3N1 lesion?

T3 tumours invade into but not beyond the muscularis propria layer. N1 implies that 1-2 nodes are involved. The stage is given according to the American Joint Cancer Committee (AJCC)/Union for International Cancer Control (UICC) TNM system (7th edition).

How would you proceed?

Given that the tumour extends into the stomach I would complete staging investigations by doing a staging laparoscopy. This is because laparoscopy can be used to exclude peritoneal metastases, which can be missed on CT scan when there is a gastric component to the tumour. In addition the staging laparoscopy may give a 'feel' of how stable the patient is under GA and highlight any potential anaesthetic issues prior to a major resection.

Staging laparoscopy does not show any evidence of metastatic disease. What would you do next?

This patient's treatment should continue on a curative intent pathway and he needs to be seen by an oncologist and assessed for suitability for neoadjuvant chemotherapy prior to surgical resection.

What is the evidence for a benefit from neoadjuvant chemotherapy for operable oesophageal cancer?

The MRC OEO2 trial is the largest and most significant trial to demonstrate the benefits of neoadjuvant chemotherapy for locally advanced cancer of the oesophagus. For locally advanced oesophageal cancer (T2-4 N0-3 M0) surgery alone may be associated with unacceptably high R1 resection rates and compromised long term survival. OE02 was a RCT of 802 patients in 42 European centres – randomised to either chemotherapy (Cisplatin and 5-FU) for 2 cycles then surgery (CS) or immediate surgery (S) (n=402). Survival benefit was demonstrated in the CS group over the surgery alone group (median survival 16.8 months vs 13.3 months p=0.04). Disease free survival was also prolonged in the CS group. Surgical resection was more complete and tumours were smaller with less extension into surrounding tissue and less nodal involvement in the CS over S group (p<0.0001). Patients with all histological types of oesophageal and cardia cancer were included in this group (squamous/adeno/undifferentiated).

The oncology team commence chemotherapy for this patient. After one cycle he presents with pain and swelling in his left arm. A Doppler scan reveals a DVT of the axillary vein. How would you manage him?

There is an appreciable incidence of thromboembolic events (venous and arterial) in patients receiving cisplatin-based chemotherapy. In the event of a proven DVT the patient will need treatment dose LMWH.

The superiority of LMWH over vitamin K antagonists such as warfarin for reduction in the risk of recurrent cancer-associated VTE was established in the randomized CLOT trial. Dalteparin significantly reduced the risk of recurrent VTE with no significant differences in bleeding or 6-month overall mortality. In some units newer oral anticoagulants such as rivaroxaban are used in the prophylaxis of VTE during chemotherapy. The ease of administration, lack of required monitoring or dose-adjustments make agents such as rivaroxaban particularly attractive to use.

Five weeks following completion of chemotherapy a re-staging CT was performed which showed a partial response. Five weeks after chemotherapy you perform an Ivor Lewis oesophagectomy.

At 8 week follow up in clinic he is complaining of dysphagia and vomiting. How would you proceed?

This patient needs a repeat endoscopy as he is likely to have an anastomotic stricture. Hold up at the level of the pylorus should be suspected if a pyloroplasty was not performed during oesophagectomy although these patients tend not to have dysphagia. Both can be treated with endoscopic balloon dilatation. If in doubt a contrast swallow may help to demonstrate the level of hold up prior to any intervention.

You endoscope the patient and find a significant non-traversable stricture at 24cm corresponding to an anastomotic stricture. How would you treat this?

The patient would benefit from an endoscopic dilatation. This may be easily performed with a through the scope (TTS) balloon dilator in a step by step manner, ensuring that over zealous dilatation is not performed.

Take me through the basic steps of how to perform an endoscopic balloon dilatation.

The patient should ideally be given intravenous opiate based analgesia as well as sedation (e.g. 50mg pethidine, 3mg midazolam) depending on their age and renal function. Generally a size 12mm balloon is a reasonable starting size and should be inserted through the scope into position. The ideal position would be one that allows half of the balloon above and below the stricture. The minimal inflation pressure should be initially applied and maintained for one minute. Following dilatation a check endoscopy should be performed to check the result as well as exclude perforation and bleeding. The procedure may need to be repeated after a few weeks, depending on the patient progress and severity of stricture. The patient may need to be kept nil orally for two hours and monitored in recovery prior to discharge.

Do you know of any other alternative methods of performing oesophageal stricture dilatation?

An alternative method incorporates image intensifier screening and bougienage dilatation e.g. Savary-Gilliard® dilators. Generally bougienage dilatation is more forceful as it exerts a radial as well as a shearing force, unlike a balloon dilator which exerts a radial force only.

Oesophageal Cancer

Scenario 2

You are referred a 59 year old patient who presents with dysphagia to solids. At endoscopy a circumferential obstructing lesion was found at 25cm to 34cm – 2cm above the OG junction. The lesion could only be traversed with a paediatric scope. Histology from this lesion confirms a poorly differentiated squamous cell carcinoma. The patient has been informed of the diagnosis.

What staging investigations would you organise at this stage?

My immediate priority would be to obtain a staging CT scan of the chest, abdomen and pelvis. The purpose of obtaining the CT would be to help exclude distant metastatic disease as well as provide some information on the local extent of disease.

What are the limitations of CT staging of oesophagogastric cancers?

CT provides limited information of the presence of peritoneal and pleural disease. However, the presence of ascites, pleural effusion or nodules in the omentum or pleura may suggest involvement of mesothelial surfaces.

One of the other main limitations of CT is correctly identifying malignant lymph nodes. Size criteria are used to help differentiate benign nodes from malignant nodes. The short axis of lymph nodes can be easily measured. Enlarged lymph nodes in the intrathoracic and abdominal regions are defined as greater than 1 cm. However not all enlarged lymph nodes are malignant. Inflammatory nodes are the most common cause of a false-positive examination.

On CT there is a suspicious looking left supraclavicular lymph node measuring 16mm. There is also destruction of the lateral aspect of the left 6th rib with an associated 46mm x 18 mm soft tissue mass demonstrating extra-pleural extension. Your MDM decides to obtain a PET scan.

How would a PET help confirm metastases?

PET images would be acquired from the orbits to the upper thighs and co-registered with low dose CT for anatomical localisation. This would demonstrate increased fludeoxyglucose (FDG) uptake in keeping with the known oesophageal malignancy and FDG avid left supraclavicular lymph nodes. There would also be a focal increase of FDG uptake associated with the lateral aspects of the left 6th rib where there is a metastasis. Although the CT findings are convincing, a CT-PET scan may also confirm the presence of metastases in the neck and rib cage. Alternatively ultrasound guided FNAC of the left supraclavicular nodes may confirm metastatic disease. If ultrasound FNAC was to be done then it should be deferred until after CT-PET scan as an FNAC may lead to a false positive result on a subsequent PET scan.

How good is CT at detecting liver metastases?

Hepatic metastases appear as ill-defined, low-density lesions of variable size. Conventional CT imaging with intravenous contrast is excellent in the detection of hepatic metastases greater than 2cm. However CT frequently does not recognize sub-centimetre metastases - the main cause of false-negative examinations. Therefore CT has limitations, and for these reasons further staging tests (e.g. MRI liver) are necessary if CT shows potentially curable disease.

Having confirmed metastatic disease the oncologists offer him palliative chemoradiotherapy. He remains severely dysphagic though he is managing some soft diet only. The dieticians are concerned about ongoing weight loss as well as feeding access. What are the best options for feeding access in his case?

As this patient has incurable disease he will proceed down a palliative route of care. He is going to have progressive dysphagia to the point of obstruction in the very near future, at which point he is best served with a palliative stent or brachytherapy. However he may have a reasonable response to palliative chemoradiotherapy, in which case a stent can be deferred until he obstructs. Feeding options include endoscopically placed nasoenteric feeding tube, surgical or radiological gastrostomy or a feeding jejunostomy.

A nasoenteric tube (NG or NJ) is feasible but unpleasant for the patient, particularly given his poor prognosis. A gastrostomy tube allows feed to be delivered at a reasonable rate but may be associated with severe reflux and nausea / vomiting. Gastrostomy may be placed radiologically (Radiologically Inserted Gastrostomy - RIG tube) but in a patient with previous abdominal surgery may require open surgical insertion. A feeding jejunostomy is placed surgically but feed can only be given at slower rates compared to a gastrostomy. In this case I would simply place an NG or NJ feeding tube to optimise his nutrition and start his chemoradiotherapy.

Further reading

Li Z, Rice TW. Diagnosis and staging of cancer of the oesophagus and oesophagogastric junction. Surg Clin North Am. 2012 Oct;92(5):1105-26.

Kelsen DP, Ginsberg R, Pajak TF et al. Chemotherapy followed by surgery compared with surgery alone for localized oesophageal cancer. N Eng J Med 1998; 339;1979-84.

Surgical resection with or without preoperative chemotherapy in oesophageal cancer: a randomised controlled trial. Medical Research Council Oesophageal Cancer Working Group. Lancet. 2002 May 18;359(9319):1727-33.

Para-oesophageal Hiatus Hernia

A 66 year old lady presents with upper abdominal pain and retching and is suspected of having gallstones. The junior spots a retro-cardiac air fluid level on a CXR from a large hiatus hernia and passes down an NG tube, which drains over one litre of dark gastric content. This gives her immediate symptom relief. She is not known to have had any previous upper GI investigations. Blood tests show a CRP of 350 and WCC $21 \times 10^9/l$. She has no metabolic acidosis on a blood gas.

What other investigations would you order for her?

Given that the nasogastric tube has provided immediate symptom relief it is highly likely that the hiatus hernia was obstructed. I would obtain an urgent CT scan of her chest and abdomen with iv contrast to define the hernia in more detail e.g. any volvulus, and to exclude other differential diagnoses. Oral contrast is best not given due to the risk of aspiration which is common with these herniae. The CT may also give information on evidence of complications such as perforation or strangulation.

Obtaining a contrast swallow would also be a risky investigation due to the risk of aspiration should there be underlying obstruction.

What is the role of upper GI endoscopy for this patient?

If the patient is comfortable and not septic then an upper GI endoscopy needs to be performed within 24 hours of admission. In this patient although she looks well she has significantly raised inflammatory markers and my concern would be whether she has any gastric wall ischaemia. An endoscopy would be the best way to exclude this and would also provide an assessment of the degree of volvulus and gastric outlet obstruction. It would also allow passage of a nasojejunal feeding tube and correctly positioned nasogastric tube. In addition there may be Cameron's ulcers or stasis ulcers evident. Evidence of gastric mucosa swelling and congestion would be of concern and may indicate some degree of ischaemia.

You decide to perform an OGD on her. What do the images show?

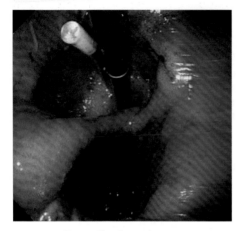 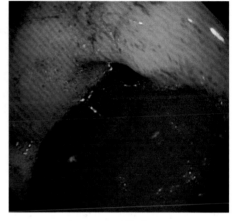

Retroflexion view   **Antrum / Pylorus**

On retroflexion there is evidence of a twist in the lining of the stomach as well as visualisation of the antrum/pylorus next to the fundus. There is also a nasogastric tube just beyond the OG junction. In the antrum/pyloric forward view there is a large fluid level just proximal to the pylorus with stagnant looking fluid in keeping with gastric outlet obstruction. All of these endoscopic features are in keeping with an obstructed gastric volvulus.

What is the incidence of strangulation in these herniae?

Acute complications such as gastric volvulus with incarceration or strangulation are rare (approximately 1%). However, gastric ischaemia leading to perforation is the main cause of mortality.

Endoscopically the hernia is obstructed but you are able to pass an NJ feeding tube. There is no evidence of ischaemia and the patient remains stable. However the bloods indicate an ongoing high CRP and WCC. How would you proceed?

If the gastric mucosa appears healthy on OGD an alternative septic source needs to be considered. Often these patients aspirate from the obstructed stomach leading to an aspiration pneumonia. This may be evident on the lung windows of the CT. Intravenous antibiotics and chest physiotherapy must be commenced without delay as an undertreated pneumonia may complicate surgical intervention. The patient should also be nursed at 45 degrees and a PPI commenced.

How would you classify hiatus herniae?

These are usually classified from I-IV:

Type I is a sliding hiatus hernia representing the majority (90%) of hiatus herniae.

II-IV are variations of paraoesophageal herniae:-

Type II is regarded as a true paraoesophageal hiatus hernia (3%). In this hernia part of the fundus herniates through the hiatus but the OGJ remains in its normal place.

Type III involves a combination of I and II with a sliding OGJ and herniated fundus.

Type IV represents a large defect in the hiatus with accompanying other viscera (usually transverse colon).

What are Cameron's ulcers?

Repeated movement and abrasion of the gastric mucosa across the hiatus leads to gastric erosions with a subsequent iron deficiency anaemia from chronic blood loss.

What are the surgical principles of operating on these herniae?

Laparoscopic repair is the technique of choice for repair of large hiatal herniae whether elective or emergency. I would place the patient in a supine position, reverse Trendelenburg, with the operator standing between the patient's legs. A five-port technique with liver retractor placed just to the left of falciform ligament is used. Dissection begins at the anterior crura, dividing the phreno-oesophageal ligament, everting the hernia sac and dissecting the sac off surrounding mediastinal structures. Complete reduction of the sac is essential for the long-term success of surgery. Care is taken during this dissection to maintain the integrity of the crural lining and to avoid damage to the crural muscle. Ensure an adequate length of oesophagus is mobilised – it may be possible to see the longitudinal fibres of the oesophagus merge with cardia of the stomach thereby returning the OG junction to an intra-abdominal position. Generally most surgeons would perform an anti-reflux procedure as well.

What is the role of using mesh in repairing these herniae?

Paraoesophageal hernia repair has a high radiologic recurrence rate although symptomatic recurrence is much lower. Although many have used biologic mesh as a prosthetic buttress to reinforce the primary crural repair, concerns exist about mesh infection and oesophageal erosion by mesh. Although there are several encouraging reports from case series there are very few RCTs to prove its efficacy and safety.

Reference

Koetje JH, Irvine T, Thompson SK, Devitt PG, Woods SD, Aly A, Jamieson GG, Watson DI Quality of Life Following Repair of Large Hiatal Hernia is Improved but not Influenced by Use of Mesh: Results From a Randomized Controlled Trial. World J Surg. 2015

Peptic Ulcer Disease

A 51 year old man has been referred to you for a second opinion by his GP. He presents with nine months of post prandial abdominal pain and intermittent vomiting. He has a history of long term diclofenac use for a spinal cord injury. Endoscopically an ulcer was seen in the pre-pyloric area which looks like a malignancy, but repeated biopsies have been benign. A CT scan of his abdomen shows pre-pyloric thickening and some lymphadenopathy around the left gastric territory but no ascites. Treatment to date has been omeprazole 40mg od.

How would you proceed in managing this patient?

My main immediate concern is whether he has a neoplastic gastric ulcer. Although repeated biopsies have been benign they may have been too superficial. I would repeat his endoscopy and aim to take deeper 'drill biopsies' whereby the ulcer edge is biopsied deeper and deeper so as to obtain a truly representative sample. I would also get an assessment of the degree, if any, of gastric outlet obstruction.

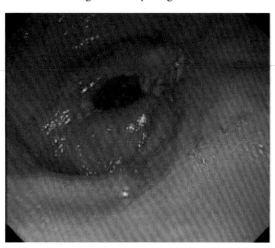

You endoscope the patient yourself (see above image). There is no significant gastric outlet obstruction as there is no food residue and there is bile reflux. You visualise a pre-pyloric ulcer but this is traversable into the duodenum. How would you manage this patient from now on?

I would request the biopsies to be processed urgently due to the concern of neoplasia. In the meantime I would commence maximal anti-secretory treatment with an aim to healing the ulcer rather than rush into operative intervention unless histology is neoplastic. I would commence the patient on omeprazole 80mg bd and empirically treat him with *H.pylori* eradication treatment (a regime such as PPI / clarithromycin / metronidazole). As there is no significant gastric outlet compromise I would not insert a feeding tube. The patient should cease diclofenac and cease any smoking or alcohol intake. I would repeat his endoscopy in 6 weeks time.

The patient is compliant to all medication and measures. Biopsies have come back reassuringly benign and *H.pylori* negative. He re-attends for an endoscopy in 6 weeks time. He is still symptomatic. On repeat endoscopy there is now a progressively worsening ulceration at the same position which you are unable to traverse. How would you proceed?

He has a non-healing gastric ulcer despite maximal medical treatment and conservative measures. I am concerned about the nature of the ulcer despite benign biopsies. I would discuss surgical options with the patient and in the meantime consider measuring his serum fasting gastrin levels as well as serum chromogranin A levels. Intractable peptic ulcers, failure to comply with or tolerate medical therapy, and rare cases of gastrinoma or Zollinger-Ellison Syndrome (ZES), are indications for elective surgery for peptic ulcer disease.

Why would you measure serum fasting gastrin and chromogranin A?

In a patient with refractory peptic ulcer disease one has to consider the possibility of ZES as being a potential cause. Other causes include idiopathic gastric acid hypersecretion or persistent *H.pylori* infection.

As the use of PPI (and H.pylori) can elevate gastrin levels to obtain a more accurate fasting gastrin, a plan to discontinue PPI therapy and convert to high-dose histamine receptor antagonist (ranitidine, 450 mg every 6 hr) for 10 days may be considered. If the serum gastrin was elevated in the face of an acidic pH in the gastric lumen, then this would be more suggestive of a gastrinoma.

What is Zollinger-Ellison syndrome?

ZES is characterized by severe peptic ulcer disease due to gastric acid hypersecretion that results from gastrin secreting tumours (gastrinomas) of the GI tract. Gastrin stimulates the parietal cells to secrete acid directly and indirectly by releasing histamine from enterochromaffin-like cells. It should be suspected in patients with severe ulcerative oesophagitis, multiple peptic ulcers, peptic ulcers in unusual locations, refractory peptic ulcers, peptic ulcers associated with diarrhoea, and a family history of multiple endocrine neoplasia type 1 (MEN-1). Patients with ZES have two problems that require treatment—the hypersecretion of gastric acid and the gastrinoma itself which may be malignant.

The patient's serum fasting gastrin is within normal limits. What are the operative options you would consider?

The most effective operation would be a distal gastrectomy / antrectomy with Roux en Y reconstruction. An alternative would be to bring up a Roux loop of jejunum to the stomach thereby bypassing the ulcerated area, which should lead to healing. However this would not provide any histology and risks leaving behind a potential neoplastic ulcer.

Post Oesophagectomy Anastomotic Leak

A 55 year old man is day 6 following a radical subtotal oesophagectomy. He develops fast AF but is haemodynamically stable. He is short of breath and has a temperature of 39°C. A single apical chest drain is draining a moderate amount of bile. What do you suspect and how do you proceed?

My immediate concern at this stage following surgery is the possibility of an anastomotic leak. The priority is to resuscitate the patient fully and stabilise the atrial fibrillation. I would discuss his case with the critical care team who may recommend insertion of a central line and administering amiodarone or intravenous beta blocker. The aim would be to cardiovert the patient back to sinus rhythm. He would be best managed on a monitored bed as he is at risk of becoming unstable.

With regards to the possibility of a leak a full septic screen including blood cultures should be taken. It is still possible that he may be having a severe chest infection rather than a leak. All possible sources of sepsis should be examined including urine. I would discuss his case with the on call radiologist and obtain an urgent CT scan of his chest and abdomen with some oral contrast.

A chest x-ray is performed during the resuscitation phase prior to endoscopy. What does this show and what action should be taken?

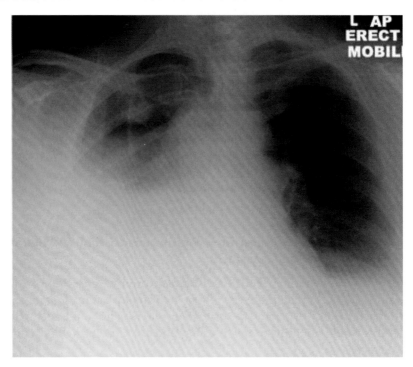

The CXR shows a large right sided hydropneumothorax which may indicate an anastomotic leak. I would insert a size 28F intercostal chest drain prior to performing endoscopy, otherwise there is a risk of tension pneumothorax from air insufflation during endoscopy.

The CT scan shows evidence of flecks of air around the anastomosis and a moderate sized right pleural effusion. The radiologist reports this to be consistent with an anastomotic leak. How would you proceed?

I would immediately treat the patient with broad spectrum intravenous antibiotics (e.g. meropenem and metronidazole) and antifungals (e.g. fluconazole) because mediastinitis can be rapidly progressive. In the meantime once the AF is stabilized an upper GI endoscopy should be performed to visualise the integrity of OG anastomosis, gastric staple line and conduit vascularity. This can be done with sedation and can provide valuable information in experienced hands.

What is the role of an upper GI endoscopy for anastomotic leak?

Upper GI endoscopy in the hands of an experienced oesophagogastric surgeon is a highly valuable means of assessing the oesophagogastric anastomosis, vascularity of the gastric conduit and integrity of the gastric resection staple line. When correctly performed the risk of causing anastomotic disruption is minimal. It also provides the option of ensuring adjuncts are placed for feeding such as nasojejunal or NG tube. A contrast swallow may demonstrate a leak but will not provide any useful information on the gastric conduit.

At endoscopy you find evidence of a small defect in the gastric resection staple line. How would you proceed?

Provided the gastric conduit does not show any evidence of frank ischaemia this can usually be managed conservatively, provided the defect is not major. This would involve antibiotics, as well as targeted radiological drains to any pleural/mediastinal collection. In this case there is a well placed apical drain that is serving its purpose. If a nasogastric tube is not already present then at the time of endoscopy one should be inserted under direct vision.

How would you feed this patient?

The provision of adequate enteral nutrition is of major importance in this patient. Practice varies but this can be achieved either with an endoscopically placed nasojejunal tube or a feeding jejunostomy which may require operative intervention. However many units routinely place a feeding jejunostomy for oesophagectomies.

The patient continues to be septic in the coming days and a repeat CT shows significant worsening, with marked stranding around the gastric conduit, with ongoing gas and fluid collections in the mediastinum. A further upper GI endoscopy is performed which confirms significant gastric necrosis.

How would you proceed?

In this situation the patient will need emergency surgery for formation of a cervical oesophagostomy and to close the viable component of the gastric remnant. A thorough mediastinal and pleural debridement should be performed and large drains left in situ.

Principles of Oesophagectomy

What are the surgical approaches for an oesophagectomy?

Surgical approaches for an oesophagectomy can be either open or minimally invasive.

Open approaches for an oesophagectomy include:-

Transthoracic Ivor Lewis – this is a two stage operation with an abdominal and a chest component (via right thoracotomy)

Transhiatal – completely avoids a thoracotomy but anastomosis in the neck

Left thoraco-abdominal

'Three phase' McKeown oesophagectomy – this has an abdominal, thoracotomy and neck phase

Minimally invasive approaches include:-

Laparoscopic transhiatal

Hybrid: Laparoscopic abdomen and open right thoracotomy

Minimally Invasive Oesophagectomy (MIO) – Ivor Lewis: Laparoscopic abdomen and thoracoscopic chest phase with intra-thoracic anastomosis

Minimally Invasive Oesophagectomy (MIO) – McKeown: Laparoscopic abdomen and thoracoscopic chest with open left neck for anastomosis

Robotic oesophagectomy

According to the most recent NOGCA audit report the most commonly performed minimally invasive method in the UK is the hybrid operation. However, the open abdomen and open chest approach remains the most popular. The Ivor Lewis MIO involves an intra-thoracic anastomosis which is technically challenging and has been associated with significant complications in some centres.

Is there any evidence for superiority of minimally invasive approaches over open?

There is a limited amount of good quality data on this contentious issue. There is some evidence to show MIO is associated with reduced blood loss, reduced post-operative pain, decreased time in the intensive care unit, and shortened length of hospital stay. Some high volume centres report excellent outcomes in expert hands. However sceptics argue that radicality of resection is compromised with minimally invasive approaches, thus oncological outcome may be compromised. However the results of RCTs and long term data are awaited on this topic. Randomized trials comparing MIO versus open resection in oesophageal cancer are in progress with two phase III trials recruiting, the TIME and the MIRO trials.

What is the role of enhanced recovery (ERAS) after oesophageal surgery?

The evidence base for ERAS following oesophagectomy is limited. However, these have demonstrated favorable morbidity, mortality, and length of stay. With the increasing popularity of minimally invasive oesophagectomy the evidence for ERAS should improve.

How does the trans-hiatal (TH) approach compare with transthoracic approach (TT)?

RCTs have compared the trans-hiatal with trans-thoracic approach for oesophagectomy. Although the transhiatal approach obviates the need for a thoracotomy, no significant differences have been demonstrated between the two. The evidence suggests a better lymph node yield with the TT approach albeit more pulmonary complications. However there was a trend to better long term survival with the TT group, particularly in lymph node positive patients.

What do you know of the National Oesophago-gastric cancer audit?

The National Oesophago-gastric cancer audit (NOGCA) was started in 2006 and is an audit based on prospectively collected data to measure the quality of care received by patients with OG cancer and high grade dysplasia in England and Wales. The most recent audit was based on a two year data collection period up to March 2013. Amongst many other findings the audit showed an increase in the percentage of patients with OG cancer that were managed with curative intent (37%). It demonstrated steady improvement in mortality rates. Mortality rates are now lower than those reported when the audit started (2008-2010), with a decrease in 30 day mortality from 4.1% to 2.3% and a decrease in 90 day mortality from 6.5% to 4.5%.

NOGCA also details the number of operations individual surgeons have performed on patients diagnosed with OG cancer and also publishes adjusted 30 and 90-day postoperative mortality rates, as well as median length of stay, for individual surgeons and hospital trusts. The results showed that the 30 and 90-day postoperative mortality for all NHS trusts and surgeons were within the range expected, taking into account the variation in patients treated.

References

Luketich JD1, Pennathur A, Awais O et al Outcomes after minimally invasive esophagectomy: review of over 1,000 patients. Ann Surg. 2012 Jul;256(1):95-103

Findlay JM1, Gillies RS, Millo J, Sgromo B, Marshall RE, Maynard ND. Enhanced recovery for esophagectomy: a systematic review and evidence-based guidelines. Ann Surg. 2014 Mar;259(3):413-31.

Briez N, Piessen G, Bonnetain F et al, Open versus laparoscopically-assisted esophagectomy for cancer: a multicentre randomised controlled phase III trial - the MIRO trial. BMC Cancer. 2011 Jul 23;11:310

van der Sluis PC, Ruurda JP, van der Horst S, Verhage RJ, Robot-assisted minimally invasive thoraco-laparoscopic esophagectomy versus open transthoracic esophagectomy for resectable esophageal cancer, a randomized controlled trial (ROBOT trial). Trials. 2012 Nov 30;13:230

Swallowed Foreign Body / Corrosive Ingestion

Scenario 1

You are asked to see a 15 year old child with learning difficulties who has ingested a disk battery. A plain x-ray shows evidence that the battery seems to be lodged in the oesophagus. The child is asymptomatic. How would you proceed?

Ingestion of disk batteries represents a special case. There is a real danger of liquefaction necrosis and perforation if left alone untreated. An urgent endoscopy needs to be performed. A stone retrieval basket is most often successful. The endoscopy is best performed under a general anaesthetic given the child's predisposition and would also allow airway protection when the battery is being withdrawn.

The oesophageal mucosa of the oesophagus does not tolerate retained foreign bodies well. Complications are higher with impaction for >24 hours and with sharp objects. Oedema, necrosis and perforation may ensue over time. Other complications include airway compression, retropharyngeal abscess as well as vascular complications such as aorto-oesophageal fistula. Inability to swallow saliva and drooling are suggestive of complete oesophageal obstruction. Airway complications are commoner in children as their airways are softer and more compressible.

Where are foreign bodies likely to lodge in the oesophagus?

There are three anatomic areas of narrowing where foreign bodies are most likely to impact in the oesophagus. These are at the cricopharyngeus muscle, the aortic arch and the lower oesophageal sphincter. Foreign bodies preferentially become lodged at the cricopharyngeus in children and at the LOS in adults.

At endoscopy there is no evidence of perforation or damage. The button battery could not be retrieved from the oesophagus but is pushed into the stomach. What would you do?

Although once in the stomach most disk batteries will pass without consequence it would be ideal to try once with the stone retrieval basket.

Button batteries contain an alkaline solution that can rapidly cause liquefaction necrosis of the oesophageal mucosa within 4 hours. They can be catastrophic. They are not easy to remove endoscopically due to their smooth edge – endoscopic removal may fail in a significant proportion. Should endoscopic removal fail the battery can be pushed distally to the stomach where it will likely pass through the gastrointestinal tract without difficulty. Once past the duodenum 85% are passed within 72 hours. An x-ray to follow progress every 3 days is sufficient.

What pharmacological therapies do you know of in the management of retained foreign bodies?

Glucagon is often considered as a first line agent. Intravenous glucagon has been used and acts through relaxation of the smooth muscle found in the distal oesophagus and a decrease in the lower oesophageal resting pressure. Glucagon has no effect on the striated muscle of the proximal oesophagus, where children often have impacted foreign bodies. As vomiting is a potential side effect of rapid administration it should be given slowly to minimise the risk of oesophageal perforation from an obstructed oesophagus. The patient should be nursed upright and given water to sip one minute after injection in order to stimulate peristalsis.

Carbonated beverages may act through producing carbon dioxide which distends the oesophagus and so relaxes the LOS which may push the object into the stomach.

Scenario 2

A 35 year old lady has ingested oven cleaner as part of an act of deliberate self harm. She has no obvious signs of oesophageal perforation but has significant swelling of the oropharynx. Her observations are stable. How will you proceed?

The priority in this patient is to ensure she has a patent airway. I would ask the anaesthetist to come and see her urgently as she is at risk of developing acute airway obstruction over time. If intubation is not possible by conventional means then a surgical airway may be required.

With regard to the oesophagus I would organise an urgent upper GI endoscopy which will provide an assessment of the extent of oesophaegeal involvement as well as exclude any underlying perforation. In the meantime she should have a CXR looking for any pneumoperitoneum which would suggest a gastric perforation, but it would also serve as a baseline in the event she develops aspiration pneumonia. The poisons centre should also be contacted for more information on the agent ingested.

Caustic injury has a bimodal peak of occurrence. The first peak is in children and most commonly due to accidental ingestion. The second peak is in adults due to suicide attempts. Short term complications are perforation and death. Long term complications include stricture and lifetime risk of oesophageal carcinoma. Oesophageal injury in adults attempting deliberate self harm tends to be significant as they deliberately consume large amounts.

At endoscopy you find extensive circumferential ulceration from 30cm to 34cm but no evidence of necrosis or perforation. The stomach and duodenum appear to be normal. What else would you do at this point?

I would insert a nasojejunal feeding tube as the patient needs to be kept on minimal oral intake for the next week or so and this would provide enteral feeding access. The patient needs to be kept on a high dose PPI and monitored for any evidence of oesophageal perforation which can occur up to one week following the incident.

Alkaline substances can be lethal. They are able to cause full thickness injury and liquefactive necrosis within seconds. Lye is the general term for alkali found in cleaning products. Acidic substances have a poor taste and are irritating. They lead to coagulative necrosis and an eschar which limits penetration into the oesophagus.

What are the indications for surgical intervention in these patients?

Perforation of the oesophagus may present with sepsis and mediastinitis requiring emergency oesophagectomy with cervical oesophagostomy and gastrostomy. Gastric or duodenal perforation may require laparotomy. Airway complications may require a surgical tracheostomy.

What are the longer term complications that occur following corrosive injury to the oesophagus?

Recalcitrant oesophageal strictures can be a major problem requiring lifelong dilatation. These can also lead to nutritional problems. There is a long term risk of oesophageal carcinoma with an estimated increase by a factor of 1,000.

Reference

Lupa M, Magne J, Guarisco JL, Amedee R. Update on the diagnosis and treatment of caustic ingestion. Ochsner J. 2009;9(2):54-9.

VASCULAR SURGERY

Michael Delbridge Peng Wong

Contents

Abdominal Aortic Aneurysm

A 64 year old gentleman has been referred to you with an incidental finding of a 5.5cm infra-renal abdominal aortic aneurysm on USS. He would like to know more about aneurysms and his treatment options. As he drives a bus, he would like to know if he could continue working.

What is an aneurysm?

An aneurysm is defined as an abnormal dilatation of a vessel that is more than 50% of its adjacent diameter. The normal diameter of an abdominal aorta is about 2cm and therefore 3cm is used as the normal cut off point for defining an abdominal aortic aneurysm (AAA). 90% of AAA are infra-renal and the remaining 10% are juxta-renal [<1cm below the renal artery(s)] and para-renal [involving the renal artery(s)].

What causes an aneurysm?

The majority of AAAs are due to degeneration of the wall of the aorta resulting in loss of its wall integrity. A combination of other factors such as genetic predisposition, ageing and damage to the aorta from risk factors such as hypertension and smoking further perpetuate the injury. AAA can also be caused by infection (termed mycotic aneurysms), trauma, arteritis and connective tissue disorders (such as Ehlers-Danlos, Marfan's and Loeys-Dietz syndrome). The most important implicating factor in AAA formation is smoking, with an eightfold increase in risk.

AAA is four times more common in men than women and the prevalence increases with age. Around 4% of men aged between 65 and 74 in England have an AAA (approximately 80,000 men). It is uncommon in people under the age of 60. The exact genetic predisposition has not been defined but it is strongest in men, with male siblings having a 20-30% absolute risk. Caucasian men are more likely to be affected, and AAA is rare in Asian and African populations. An AAA screening programme is now running in the UK. All men at the age of 65 are invited for an USS. Men over the age of 65 can request an USS.

What are the annual risks of AAA rupture?

Risk of AAA rupture increases with size as follows (Brewster 2003):

Size of AAA, cm	Annual rupture rate, %
< 4.0	<0.5
4.1 – 4.9	0.5 – 5
5.0 – 5.9	3 – 15
6.0 – 6.9	10 – 20
7.0 – 7.9	20 – 40
> 8.0	30 – 50

The rate of AAA expansion increases with size, and on average the rate of growth is about 0.3 to 0.4 cm per year. Aneurysms that expand rapidly (> 0.5 cm over 6 months, or > 1cm per year) are at high risk of rupture.

Apart from rupture, what are the other complications of AAA?

Complications of AAA can be divided into - within the lumen, within the wall and outside the wall. Within the lumen, the aneurysm can embolise distally or thrombose. Within the wall, the AAA can rupture, become inflamed (with raised ESR and symptoms of abdominal or back pain, and weight loss) or rarely dissect. Outside the wall, AAA can cause extrinsic compression of the duodenum resulting in gastric outlet obstruction; rarely it may fistulate into the inferior vena cava (aorto-caval fistula) or duodenum (aorto-enteric fistula).

What treatment options are available for him?

The main aim of treatment is to prevent death from rupture. As his AAA has reached the threshold of treatment (5.5 cm), I would offer him surgical treatment. This is based on results from the UK Small Aneurysm Trials and the Aneurysm Detection and Mortality (ADAM) trial (patients with AAA between 4.0 – 5.5 cm were randomised to either USS surveillance or surgery) whereby patients with small (< 5.5 cm) AAA who received early surgery did not show demonstrable significant survival benefit compared to patients who had USS surveillance.

Open surgery with replacement of the AAA with prosthetic graft has the benefit of long term durability with low secondary re-intervention rate. However, it has a slightly higher peri-operative mortality rate.

Endovascular abdominal aortic aneurysm repair (EVAR) can be done under local or regional anaesthesia with lower mortality risk and shorter critical care unit and in-patient stay. The biggest limiting factor for EVAR is the morphology of the AAA. There are various aortic stent grafts currently available. Generally, the infra-renal aortic neck length must be at least 10-15 mm; with a diameter of less than 30 mm; with minimal thrombus or atheroma; and parallel wall (instead of conical or barrel shaped) to allow for proximal sealing of the stent graft. The neck also needs to be minimally angulated (<60°) in relation to the aneurysm. In order to facilitate access to the aneurysm for the sheath of the stent graft, the iliac arteries need to be at least 7-8 mm in size with minimal tortuosity.

The long term results of the EVAR I trial (comparing open repair with EVAR) showed that the 30 day mortality for EVAR was less than half that of open repair (1.8% compared to 4.3% respectively). There was also a shorter in-patient stay with quicker recovery. The long term results, however were less favourable for EVAR. The early benefit of EVAR in terms of reduced mortality rate is lost with all cause mortality and aneurysm related mortality converging at two years and six years respectively. This is due to late rupture in the EVAR group. In addition, up to 10% of patients who had EVAR will require re-intervention on an annual basis.

What are the specific complications related to EVAR?

The stent graft may migrate, fracture or leak (endoleak). Endoleak is seen when there is persistent blood flow to the aneurysm sac instead of staying within the stent. There are five types of endoleak:

I: leak at either proximal (Ia) or distal (Ib) endograft attachment site

II: retrograde flow into the aneurysm sac, usually from either the lumbar artery or the inferior mesenteric artery

III: leak at either the junctions of the graft components or a defect within the graft fabric itself

IV: due to porosity of the fabric of the stent graft

V: endotension, no visible leak seen but the aneurysm sac continues to expand

For this reason, EVAR patients will need long term follow up. The follow up modality will depend on the preferences of each individual unit. This can be in the form of annual CT angiogram; or abdominal X-ray and USS.

What treatment would you offer this patient?

The type of treatment offered to him will need to take into consideration the patient's overall fitness and health, anatomical suitability and the patient's choice. I will send him for a CT angiogram to delineate the anatomy of the AAA, and pre-assessment to ascertain his general fitness of health. As he is relatively young and if he is fit, I would offer him open surgery due to the long term benefits of open surgery compared to EVAR. I will explain the slightly higher risk of sexual dysfunction in open surgery to him.

What are the DVLA's (Driver and Vehicle Licensing Agency) recommendations in patients with AAA?

DVLA policy states that:

For motor car drivers: DVLA should be notified once an AAA reaches 6cm. Patients should be suspended from driving once the AAA reaches 6.5 cm.

Drivers of lorries and buses should be suspended from driving once an AAA reaches 5.5 cm. Therefore our patient is automatically disqualified from driving.

Further reading

Brewster DC, Cronenwett JL, Hallett JW Jr, et al. Guidelines for the treatment of abdominal aortic aneurysms. Report of a subcommittee of the Joint Council of the American Association for Vascular Surgery and Society for Vascular Surgery. J Vasc Surg 2003; 37(5): 1106-1117.

Greenhalgh RM, Brown LC, Powell JT, et al. United Kingdom EVAR Trial Investigators. Endovascular versus open repair of abdominal aortic aneurysm. N Engl J Med. 2010; 362: 1863-1871.

Lederle FA, Wilson SE, Johnson GR et al; Aneurysm Detection and Management Veterans Affairs Cooperative Study Group. Immediate repair compared with surveillance of small abdominal aortic aneurysms. N Engl J Med. 2002; 346(19): 1437-44.

United Kingdom Small Aneurysm Trial Participants. Long-term outcomes of immediate repair compared with surveillance of small abdominal aortic aneurysms. N Engl J Med 2002; 346: 1437-44.

Carotid Disease

A 76 year old, right-handed gentleman has been referred by the stroke physician from a peripheral hospital with symptoms of expressive dysphasia a week ago which resolved within 24 hours. CT head has not shown any acute infarction. Carotid duplex has shown bilateral internal carotid artery 70-89% stenosis.

He has enquired about the bilateral carotid stenosis and their relation to his symptoms. What are you going to explain to him?

This gentleman by definition had an episode of carotid territory (altered motor or sensory signs, visuo-spatial neglect, dysphasia or amaurosis fugax) TIA (an acute loss of focal cerebral function with symptoms lasting less than 24 hours, with no other apparent cause other than of a vascular origin). In more than 95% of right-handed men and 90% of right-handed women, the left hemisphere is dominant. In left-handed people, the incidence of left hemispheric dominance is reported as 73% and 61% respectively for men and women respectively. The left carotid is therefore considered symptomatic and the contralateral right carotid asymptomatic.

What are his further risks from cerebral events?

ABCD^2 score is a good risk predictor of stroke following the initial cerebral event and can be calculated as below for TIA patients:

Age	≥ 60	1 point
Blood pressure	>140/90 (either systolic or diastolic)	1 point
Clinical features	Speech disturbance only	1 point
Unilateral weakness	2 points	
Duration of symptoms	10-59 min	1 point
≥60 min	2 points	
Diabetes	Diagnosed	1 point

ABCD^2 score can range between 0-7 and is stratified into low (score 0-3), moderate (4-5) and high (6-7). The 2-day (7-day) stroke risk for the category of patients with low, moderate and high risks are 1.0% (1.2%), 4.1% (5.9%) and 8.1% (11.7%) respectively. Therefore, patients with an ABCD^2 score of >4 should be assessed and investigated within 24 hours of index symptoms (NICE 2008 CG 68).

How would you investigate him?

I would organise a confirmatory duplex scan at my hospital to confirm the degree of carotid stenosis. Both the North American Symptomatic Carotid Endarterectomy Trial (NASCET) and European Carotid Surgery Trials (ECST) measurement methods are currently being used to diagnose the severity of carotid disease. The ECST method generates a higher grade of stenosis compared to the NASCET measurements. Duplex ultrasound however, may be confounded by heavily calcified plaque and high bifurcation. Depending on the internal validation of the centres, it is acceptable for surgery to be performed on the basis of ultrasound provided the first scan has been concurred by a different vascular technologist. CTA or MRA have been commonly used as confirmatory imaging depending on their availability in each centres. CTA and MRA have the advantages of assessing the arch aorta for suitability of carotid stenting (CAS), inflow, distal disease, and the intracranial circulation for tandem lesions. Catheter directed angiography (previously the gold standard) is now not routinely performed due to the stroke related risk associated with it (1-2%) which would have accounted for >50% of the overall stroke risk associated with carotid endarterectomy (CEA).

What treatment will he require and when?

The initial treatment will entail best medical therapy (optimal blood pressure control, antiplatelet agents – clopidogrel now replacing aspirin and dipyridamole, cholesterol lowering through diet and drugs, and lifestyle advice). As he has significant stenosis (50-99% according to NASCET and 70-99% according to ECST criteria), he should be considered for carotid intervention (CEA or CAS). The timing of intervention is crucial. The NICE guideline recommends that all patients with TIA should be referred within 1 week of onset of symptoms and, if appropriate, they should have CEA within 2 weeks of onset and up to 3 months of symptoms.

What is the evidence behind it?

The 5 year combined data of NASCET, ECST and Veteran's Affairs (VA) trials as reported by the Carotid Endarterectomy Trialists Collaboration (CETC) has shown that CEA confers modest but significant benefits in patients with NASCET stenosis of between 50-69% (corresponding to ECST 70-85% stenosis). The absolute risk reduction (ARR) at 5 years is 7.8% and number-needed-to-treat (NNT) to prevent 1 stroke at 5 years is 13. This benefit is more pronounced in patients with NASCET stenosis between 70-99% (corresponding to ECST 86-99% stenosis) where the ARR increases to 15.6% at 5 years and NNT to prevent 1 stroke at 5 years is only 6. There is no long term benefit in performing CEA in patients with near occlusion (string-sign) or occlusion. The maximum benefit in terms of late stroke prevention is seen when surgery was performed within 2 weeks of initial symptoms as the stroke risk is at its highest between 7-14 days of the initial symptom. At < 2 weeks from index symptoms, CEA confers an ARR at 5 years of 18.5% with NNT of 5. If surgery was delayed beyond 12 weeks, only 8 ipsilateral strokes were prevented at 5 years by performing 1000 CEAs (as opposed to 185 if patients were treated with < 2 weeks), and the NNT to prevent 1 stroke at 5 years is equivalent to 125 with an ARR at 5 years of only 0.8%. Most surgeons will therefore consider patients who are more than 3 months from the index symptom as being asymptomatic.

What about carotid stenting (CAS)?

Careful patient selection is required in patients undergoing CAS. They will need imaging of the arch aorta and views of the intracranial arteries. An occluded ICA or presence of thrombus are absolute contraindications to CAS. Tortuosity of the common and internal carotid arteries are relative contraindications. CAS can be performed under local anaesthesia and has extra advantage in patients with significant co-morbidities. Distal ICA filter, flow reversal devices and common carotid artery cutdown as access for CAS (avoid plaque embolisation from aortic arch) are methods available to prevent distal embolisation during CAS. CAS is however associated with a slightly higher risk of stroke (odds ratio, OR 1.72, P = 0.0003) compared to CEA based on a recent Cochrane review (2012) of 16 trials. CAS has a slightly lower risk of cranial nerve injury (OR 0.08; P < 0.00001), MI (OR 0.44, P = 0.02) and access site haematoma (OR 0.37, P = 0.008) compared to CEA. Patients who are fit should therefore be offered CEA. CAS can be reserved for patients who had previous neck radiotherapy, neck surgery, short neck or high bifurcation which will make CEA difficult.

He would like to know his risks from the procedure, and what peri-operative measures are available to reduce them?

The risk of death and stroke following CEA is between 2-3% and overall cranial nerve injury (mandibular branch of VII, X and XII nerve) can be as high as 8%. The risk of stroke or death within 30 days following CEA in a recent Cochrane review (2013) comparing local versus general anaesthesia (incorporating results from the GALA trial - General Anaesthetic versus Local Anaesthetic for carotid surgery) did not show any significant differences. There is limited data to either support or refute the use of routine or selective shunting in CEA to prevent stroke. Performing CEA under loco-regional anaesthesia can obviate the need for shunting but surgeons must still be prepared to use a shunt if the patient shows any signs of cerebral deterioration during the procedure. A carotid patch appears to confer advantage in reducing risk of peri-operative stroke compared to primary closure (OR 0.31, P = 0.001) based on a meta-analysis. Eversion endarterectomy does not appear to provide any additional benefit over standard endarterectomy as long as the arteriotomy is patched.

What would you do with the contralateral carotid stenosis?

The surgical treatment of asymptomatic carotid stenosis remains controversial. The Asymptomatic Carotid Artery Stenosis (ACAS) and Asymptomatic Carotid Surgery Trial (ACST) (5 year risk of any stroke and any perioperative stroke/ death reduced from 11.8% with best medical therapy compared to 6.4% with CEA, p < 0.0001) showed that CEA conferred a small but significant benefit in asymptomatic patients who are <75 years old. Asymptomatic female patients gain less benefit from CEA than men. The key factor remains in indentifying the sub-group of asymptomatic patients with significant stenosis who will benefit most from CEA. There is no role for CAS in treatment of asymptomatic patients. Due to this patient's age, I would recommend best medical therapy for his contralateral carotid stenosis.

An asymptomatic patient was found to have bilateral carotid stenosis whilst being preassessed for coronary artery bypass graft (CABG) for severe angina. What would you recommend to the cardiothoracic team?

Whilst carotid artery disease is an important risk factor for post-CABG stroke, the most important cause in this group of patients is due to embolism from an atherosclerotic arch. CEA followed by staged CABG carries highest risk of MI (6.5%), but lowest risk of stroke (2.7) with mortality of 3.9%. Conversely CABG followed by CEA carries the lowest risk of risk of MI (0.9%) but highest risk of stroke (6.3%) with mortality of 2.0%. Synchronous CEA and CABG carry the highest risk of mortality (4.6%) with an MI rate of 3.6% and stroke risk of 4.6%. I would recommend that the cardiothoracic team proceed to CABG as planned.

Further reading

Bonati LH, Lyrer P, Ederle J, Featherstone R, Brown MM. Percutaneous transluminal balloon angioplasty and stenting for carotid artery stenosis. Cochrane Database Syst Rev. 2012; 9: CD000515.

GALA Trial Collaborative Group, Lewis SC, Warlow CP, Bodenham AR, Colam B, Rothwell PM, Torgerson D, Dellagrammaticas D, Horrocks M, Liapis C, Banning AP, Gough M, Gough MJ. General anaesthesia versus local anaesthesia for carotid surgery (GALA): a multicentre, randomised controlled trial. Lancet. 2008; 372(9656): 2132-2142.

National Institute for Health and Care Excellence (2008). Stroke: Diagnosis and initial management of acute stroke and transient ischaemic attack (TIA) (CG68). London: National Institute for Health and Care Excellence.

Rothwell PM, Eliasziw M, Gutnikov SA, Fox AJ, Taylor DW, Mayberg MR, Warlow CP, Barnett HJ; Carotid Endarterectomy Trialists' Collaboration. Analysis of pooled data from the randomised controlled trials of endarterectomy for symptomatic carotid stenosis. Lancet. 2003; 361(9352): 107-116.

Rothwell PM, Eliasziw M, Gutnikov SA, Warlow CP, Barnett HJ; Carotid Endarterectomy Trialists Collaboration. Endarterectomy for symptomatic carotid stenosis in relation to clinical subgroups and timing of surgery. Lancet. 2004; 363(9413): 915-924.

Vaniyapong T, Chongruksut W, Rerkasem K. Local versus general anaesthesia for carotid endarterectomy. Cochrane Database Syst Rev. 2013; 12:CD000126/

Claudication (Suprainguinal Disease)

A 55 year old gentleman has complained of intermittent claudication in his bilateral buttocks, thighs and calves after about 200 yards of walking. He is unable to work as a rubbish collector or walk his dog. He is asking for your advice.

What are your thoughts?

Due to the distribution of his symptoms, he is most likely to have aorto-iliac artery disease. I would expect to find completely absent lower limb pulses bilaterally. Occasionally, patients with inflow disease may still have palpable lower limb pulses and almost normal ABPI. In these patients, there will be a significant drop in ABPI after exercise.

On clinical examination, you noticed that his pulse was regular with no expansile pulsatile mass in his abdomen. Indeed he has completely absent lower limb pulses. What investigations would you consider?

As his symptoms are affecting his lifestyle and livelihood, I would organise a CT angiogram (CTA) or MR angiogram (MRA) peripherals depending on local availability. CTA has the advantage of visualising the degree of thrombus within the aorta and calcifications to plan aorto-iliac intervention. Dual energy CTA has an extra advantage of removing calcified plaque from the images, reducing the radiation dose and improving diagnostic accuracy. MRA has the benefit of avoiding radiation and iodinated contrast (with risk of contrast nephropathy) but carries the risk of gadolinium related nephrogenic systemic fibrosis apart from its other specific MRI related contraindications. An arterial duplex will be difficult due to the overlying bowel gas and calcification to visualise the iliac arteries sufficiently.

CTA has shown right common iliac artery stenosis and left iliac artery occlusion. What are your initial treatment options?

The initial treatment will entail best medical therapy (antiplatelet agent with clopidogrel replacing aspirin based on NICE guideline (TA 210) and recent Cochrane review (2012), statin and optimisation of risk factors) with alterations in lifestyle (stop smoking and exercise). Supervised exercise programme with three sessions of 30 minutes each per week for at least six months has been shown in a meta-analysis of 21 studies to improve walking distance by 122%. Naftidrofuryl is the only vasodilator by NICE guideline (TA 223) and has been shown to be cost-effective in improving walking distance.

He returned 3 months later and did not find any difference with his symptoms. What would you offer him and why?

I will at this stage counsel him regarding the risk and benefits of surgery. The TASC (Trans-Atlantic Inter-Society Consensus) II classified lesions in the aorto-iliac and femoro-popliteal segments and reviewed the evidence for the treatment options. Surgically, the options are 1) right iliac angioplasty and right to left femoro-femoral crossover, 2) aorto-bifemoral bypass or 3) axillo-bifemoral bypass. If the patient is fit and as he is relatively young, I would consider offering him an aorto-bifemoral bypass. This has the best primary patency rate of 85% at 5 years with an operative mortality of 5%. The risk of graft infection and pseudoaneurysm is 1% at 10 years. A femoro-femoral crossover would not be ideal as it will rely on the durability of the iliac angioplasty/stent to ensure its patency. An axillo-bifemoral graft should be reserved for the unfit patients or hostile abdomen due to its variable long term patency (40-80% at 5 years).

After the discussion, he was deemed fit for an aorto-bifemoral bypass. What are your surgical options?

There is no evidence to favour either a transverse or vertical incision, or transperitoneal or retroperitoneal approach. A transverse approach has the benefit of fewer respiratory complications due to avoidance of an incision over the epigastrium which may sometimes 'escape' an epidural. End-to-end anastomosis is used if there is flush occlusion below the renal arteries, but in this patient's case I will consider an end-to-side anastomosis preserving blood flow to the inferior mesenteric artery and/or internal iliac artery, therefore reducing the risk of pelvic ischaemia. The types of graft used will depend on the preference of the surgeon. I will consider using a Dacron graft over PTFE, due to its better handling and suturing characteristics with lower risk of suture hole bleeding. PTFE however does carry a lower risk of infection but this has been overcome with use of rifampicin soaked or silver impregnated Dacron on in vitro studies. The superficial femoral vein as graft does carry significant morbidity and adds extra time to the procedure and is therefore not widely used.

Further reading

Gardner AW, Poehlman ET. Exercise rehabilitation programs for the treatment of claudication pain. A meta-analysis. JAMA. 1995; 274(12): 975-980.

Norgren L, Hiatt WR, Dormandy JA, Nehler MR, Harris KA, Fowkes FG; TASC II Working Group. Inter-Society Consensus for the Management of Peripheral Arterial Disease (TASC II). J Vasc Surg. 2007; 45 Suppl S: S5-67.

West CA Jr, Johnson LW, Doucet L, et al. A contemporary experience of open aortic reconstruction in patients with chronic atherosclerotic occlusion of the abdominal aorta. J Vasc Surg. Nov 2010; 52(5): 1164-1172

Wong PF, Chong LY, Mikhailidis DP, Robless P, Stansby G. Antiplatelet agents for intermittent claudication. Cochrane Database Syst Rev. 2011; (11): CD001272.

Critical Limb Ischaemia

A 76 year old gentleman presented with a 2 week history of constant pain in his right foot and necrosis overlying his 5th toe. He is a smoker with past medical history of ischaemic heart disease and non-insulin dependent diabetes. He has palpable femoral pulses bilaterally with absent bilateral popliteal and pedal pulses.

Are you aware of any classifications for severity of peripheral arterial disease?

There are the Fontaine and Rutherford's classifications. The former is simpler and more widely used in clinical practice.

Fontaine:

I: Asymptomatic

II: Intermittent claudication

III: Rest pain

IV: Tissue loss

Rutherford:

Grade:	Category:	
0	0	Asymptomatic
I	1	Mild claudication
I	2	Moderate claudication
I	3	Severe claudication
II	4	Ischaemic rest pain
II	5	Minor tissue loss
III	6	Major tissue loss

What is critical limb ischaemia (CLI)?

It is defined as symptoms of rest pain > 2 weeks unremitting to analgesia, or tissue loss (ulcer or gangrene), or ankle pressure < 50mmHg, or toe pressure < 30 mmHg. It implies a chronic aetiology. Majority of patients with CLI have significant cardiovascular risk and the outcome is often poor. At 1 year following presentation, 25% of patients have resolved CLI, 20% with ongoing CLI, 30% are alive amputees and 20% are dead.

How would you investigate him further?

Patients with CLI often have multilevel disease and investigation will depend on the patient's overall health and fitness and salvageability of the lower limb. The types of radiological investigations also depend on ease of access to either duplex, CTA or MRA. In this patient, I will organise an arterial duplex as it does not involve radiation or contrast, and is easily accessible. Duplex has a sensitivity of 84-87% and specificity of 92-98%. In addition, as this patient has an absent popliteal pulse, the most likely level of proximal disease is the superficial femoral artery (SFA) or popliteal artery. If the ultrasound scan showed a short SFA occlusion, this can be treated with an angioplasty and at the same time treatment of any crural disease could be performed. If there is a long SFA or popliteal occlusion, this patient will require a lower limb bypass and will then require either CTA/MRA or catheter angiography to visualise the run-off vessels. In the author's unit, the next modality will be the latter, to allow better visualisation of the crural arteries to plan the bypass. If a bypass is contemplated, apart from the usual blood tests, I will also organise ECG, echocardiogram, respiratory function test, and venous duplex to assess suitability of underlying greater saphenous vein (GSV) as bypass conduit (will require minimum diameter of 3mm).

This patient has a long length SFA occlusion (10cm) with 2 vessel posterior tibial and peroneal run off. What treatment would you recommend?

The TASC (Trans-Atlantic Inter-Society Consensus) II classified lesions in the aorto-iliac and femoro-popliteal segments and reviewed the evidence for the treatment options. The BASIL trial (Bypass versus Angioplasty in Severe Ischaemia of the Leg) compared angioplasty against infrainguinal bypass. Overall 30 day mortality was low with 5% in surgery and 3% in angioplasty. Surgery was associated with a higher morbidity (57% with surgery compared to 41% with angioplasty), mainly due to MI and wound infection. At 1 year, surgery is more expensive due to longer in-patient stay. However, at 3 year follow up, there was no significant difference in costs between the 2 modalities as patients who initially had angioplasty needed reintervention (28% for angioplasty group versus 17% for surgery group) due to the higher failure rate (20% for the angioplasty group versus 3% for surgery at 12 months). There were no differences in quality of life, amputation free survival and all cause mortality at 2 years. In patients who are fit and with suitable veins, sub-group analysis suggests that surgery will be the best option. If the echocardiogram and respiratory function test in this patient shows that he is fit, I will consider offering him a femoro-above knee popliteal bypass.

What graft would you consider and why?

The GSV (> 3mm) would be the best conduit if there is adequate length. Using a prosthetic graft in this patient's case will be high risk (of infection) due to the toe gangrene, and less durable. Results from a meta-analysis showed primary patency of 66% for vein (any level) compared to 47% for above knee PTFE and 33% for below knee PTFE at 5 years. The 5 year pooled weighted data for primary patency of femoro-distal bypass with vein are 80% and 70% at 3 and 5 years, and 35% and 25% for the same time-frame with prosthetic graft. In the absence of GSV, the short saphenous vein or cephalic vein could be harvested. If a prosthetic graft is used especially in a below knee bypass, a vein cuff (examples are Miller cuff,

Taylor's patch, St Mary's boot) is used at the distal anastomosis to improve graft patency.

Are you aware of any non-interventional treatment which may help to improve his symptoms?

Lumbar sympathectomy (limited use in patients with both tissue loss and rest pain), spinal cord stimulator (no evidence that it improves the ulcer healing rate, limb salvage or mortality), iloprost infusion (an intravenous vasodilator, expensive and long term results remain unclear) and gene therapy (to improve angiogenesis, still at an experimental stage) are options in patients with non-reconstructable disease.

Further reading

Adam DJ, Beard JD, Cleveland T, Bell J, Bradbury AW, Forbes JF, Fowkes FG, Gillepsie I, Ruckley CV, Raab G, Storkey H; BASIL trial participants. Bypass versus angioplasty in severe ischaemia of the leg (BASIL): multicentre, randomised controlled trial. Lancet. 2005; 366 (9501): 1925-34.

Bradbury AW, Adam DJ, Bell J, Forbes JF, Fowkes FG, Gillespie I, Raab G, Ruckley CV.

Multicentre randomised controlled trial of the clinical and cost-effectiveness of a bypass-surgery-first versus a balloon-angioplasty-first revascularisation strategy for severe limb ischaemia due to infrainguinal disease. The Bypass versus Angioplasty in Severe Ischaemia of the Leg (BASIL) trial. Health Technol Assess. 2010; 14(14): 1-210, iii-iv.

Hunink MG, Wong JB, Donaldson MC, Meyerovitz MF, Harrington DP. Patency results of percutaneous and surgical revascularization for femoropopliteal arterial disease. Med Decis Making. 1994; 14(1): 71-81.

Norgren L, Hiatt WR, Dormandy JA, Nehler MR, Harris KA, Fowkes FG; TASC II Working Group. Inter-Society Consensus for the Management of Peripheral Arterial Disease (TASC II). J Vasc Surg. 2007; 45 Suppl S: S5-67.

Hyperhidrosis

A 21 year old student nurse has complained of excessive bilateral axillary sweating which she finds debilitating and embarrassing. She is having to change her clothes 4 times a day during the summer time as a result and has asked you for your opinion on her treatment options.

What are the causes of hyperhidrosis?

Hyperhidrosis is defined as excessive sweating beyond that required for thermoregulation. Primary hyperhidrosis (PH) (idiopathic or essential) is often localised to either the palms, axillae, feet or face. PH tends to occur symmetrically, often starts during adolescence or even in childhood, and can be made worse by anxiety. Typically it is absent during sleep and can be hereditary (autosomal dominant). It is attributable to a disorder of the eccrine sweat glands, and is associated with excessive sympathetic activity. PH affects up to half a million people in the UK.

Secondary hyperhidrosis can be generalised to the whole body or localised to specific areas of the body. It often occurs during sleep and can be asymmetrical. Secondary hyperhidrosis can be due to infection, obesity, endocrine disorders (hyperthyroidism, hyperpituitarism, menopause, diabetes, neurological disorders and phaeochromocytoma), and drug induced (SSRI antidepressants).

What treatment options are available?

The simple treatment options start with antiperspirants containing aluminium chloride. Failing that, anticholinergic agents such as oxybutynin and menthatheline bromide, and alpha-adrenergic agonist (for example clonidine) have been shown to be effective. These oral agents have side-effects of dry mouth, blurred vision, tiredness and dizziness. Other options include either inotophoresis (used more for palmar and plantar hyperhidrosis), botulinum toxin injection, thoracoscopic sympathectomy and axillary sweat gland excision.

Tell us more about botox injections.

Botulinum A is a natural protein derived from *Clostridium botulinum* toxin, which has been purified and refined. Its anticholinergic effect at the neuromuscular junction and in the postganglionic sympathetic cholinergic nerves in the sweat glands helps alleviate PH. It is often given intradermally in the axilla to relieve localised axillary hyperhidrosis. Its use in palmar and plantar hyperhidrosis is limited. Its effects are only localised to the area injected and are often medium lasting (up to 4-7 months), and currently it is not readily available on the NHS. A maximum dose of 50 units are injected into each axilla in 0.1 to 0.2 ml aliquots, evenly distributed 1 cm apart. The commonest side effects of axillary botox injections include pain, haemorrhage, compensatory hyperhidrosis, pharyngitis and flu-like symptoms. Distant spread of toxin effect can result in dyspnoea, muscle weakness, or dysphagia. Botox injections are not recommended for pregnant women or mothers who are breastfeeding, nor patients with neuromuscular disorders. Studies in pregnant animals are limited and suggest that botox does not cross the placenta, however there have been no studies on pregnant women. Similarly, there have been no studies on breastfeeding women. The safety of botox in patients under 18 years old is also not established. Residual botox should be disposed of by mixing with hypochlorite solution (0.5%).

What surgical treatment options are available?

Surgical approaches include the excision of sweat glands or subcutaneous curettage for axillary hyperhidrosis, and should be reserved for patients who have failed conservative and medical treatment. The more established approach, especially for palmar hyperhidrosis, is endoscopic thoracic sympathectomy (ETS).

Please tell us more about endoscopic thoracic sympathectomy.

The patient is positioned supine in a semi-seated position. Following induction of general anaesthesia, two incisions are made (anterior axillary line at level of 4th or 5th intercostal space, and mid-axillary line in 2nd or 3rd intercostal space) to facilitate 5 mm port insertions after partial deflation of the lung. The 2nd rib is identified. The sympathetic chain is identified as a whitish, longitudinal cord that forms a slight prominence in the latero-posterior region of the thoracic vertebra. The T2 ganglion is located between the 2nd and 3rd ribs, and T3 ganglion is located between 3rd and 4th ribs. The ganglion is denervated with diathermy, avoiding damage to the periosteum of the rib, which may produce severe chest pain. The procedure is then repeated on the contralateral side. For palmar hyperhidrosis, T2 and T3 ganglia were commonly denervated, but this led to increased risk of Horner's syndrome and compensatory hyperhidrosis. Some experts would currently advocate T3 denervation alone for palmar hyperhidrosis. For axillary hyperhidrosis, denervation of T2, T3 and T4 ganglia are recommended but T4 denervation alone does appear to confer a high level of satisfaction, with less severe compensatory hyperhidrosis. Success rates vary and can range between 96% -100% for palmar hyperhidrosis, and 63%-100% for axillary hyperhidrosis. Symptom recurrence has also been reported in 1%-13% of patients.

What are the complications of thoracoscopic sympathectomy?

Compensatory hyperhidrosis is the commonest side-effect and has been reported to be as high as 92%. It commonly affects the back, abdomen and thigh, and can be more debilitating than the original palmar or axillary hyperhidrosis. Compensatory hyperhidrosis has a high correlation with the level and extent of denervation. The higher the level of denervation, the more severe the compensatory hyperhidrosis due to more afferent fibres being affected. Horner's syndrome (0.5%), gustatory hyperhidrosis, neuralgia and pneumothorax are the other more serious adverse events encountered. Patients should therefore be forewarned of the risk of irreversible compensatory hyperhidrosis prior to embarking on the procedure.

References

Benson RA, Palin R, Holt PJ, Loftus IM. Diagnosis and management of hyperhidrosis. BMJ. 2013;347:f6800

Li X, Tu YR, Lin M, Lai FC, Chen JF, Dai ZJ. Endoscopic thoracic sympathectomy for palmar hyperhidrosis: a randomized control trial comparing T3 and T2-4 ablation. Ann Thorac Surg. 2008; 85(5): 1747-1751.

National Institute for Health and Care Excellence (2014). Endoscopic thoracic sympathectomy for primary hyperhidrosis of the upper limb. IPG487. London: National Institute for Health and Care Excellence.

Lower Limb Ulcer

A 65 year old lady presented with a recurrent ulcer above the right medial malleolus. This is on a background of longstanding varicose veins. She has also acknowledged to having trouble walking with cramps in her right calf.

What is the likely aetiology of her lower limb ulcer?

She most likely has mixed arterial venous ulcer especially with her history of claudication. Venous ulcers tend to occur around the gaiter area. Arterial ulcers are commonly distributed peripherally in the digits, heels and bony prominences of the foot.

How would you clinically assess the lower limbs?

I would ascertain the nature of her calf claudication to rule out spinal (pain with prolonged standing or lying flat, relieved only by sitting down or leaning forward; claudication worse on going downhill; associated symptoms of paraesthesia or numbness) or venous (pain relieved by foot elevation, nocturnal rest pain alleviated by walking) claudication. I would elicit for history of previous deep venous thrombosis suggestive of underlying deep venous incompetence or even venous outflow obstruction. On clinical examination, I would assess the lower limb pulses with measurement of ABPI. ABPI < 0.9 would highly suggest underlying peripheral arterial disease as a co-contributor to her ulcer. I would examine for presence of varicose veins (and its distribution) and changes of chronic venous insufficiency (pigmentation around gaiter area, oedema, lipodermatosclerosis, varicose eczema and ulceration). Using the handheld doppler, I would test for reflux in the sapheno-femoral and sapheno-popliteal junctions.

How would you investigate this further?

I would organise an arterial and venous duplex of the lower limb. Due to the changes of chronic venous insufficiency, it is important to ensure that the deep veins are patent and competent without any venous outflow obstruction (stenosis or occlusion). It is also important to ascertain the site of superficial venous reflux to plan treatment. Arterial duplex will help determine site and severity of arterial disease and suitability for endovascular treatment.

The arterial duplex has shown a full length superficial femoral artery (SFA) occlusion which reconstitutes at the level of the adductor hiatus with two vessels: anterior tibial and peroneal run off. Venous duplex showed patent and competent deep veins with reflux in the saphenofemoral junction and long saphenous vein. Her ABPI was 0.6. How would you manage this patient?

Endovascular treatment for the long SFA occlusion is not a feasible option, and the only solution will be a femoro-above knee popliteal bypass. Treatment for her venous component at present will entail reduced compression bandaging. The exact level of arterial insufficiency that warrants modified compression is debatable but most people would recommend reduced compression to reduce risk of compression related complications including pain and necrosis. The important consideration is balancing the perfusion of the capillaries against the external compression exerted by the bandaging. High strength compression bandaging has a graduated pressure of 40 mmHg at the ankle and 30 mm around the calf and should be avoided in patients with ankle pressure of less than 80 mmHg or ABPI below 0.7. Modified compression bandaging (20 – 26 mmHg) in patients with ankle pressure of more than 60 mmHg or ABPI between 0.5 – 0.8 has been shown to be acceptable. In a study by Mosti *et al* (2012) using inelastic compression bandaging has been shown to improve laser Doppler flowmetry at the ulcer level. The compression bandaging needs to be supervised closely and to be discontinued if the patient reports increased discomfort or worsening ulceration.

Is there any evidence in treating the superficial venous reflux at this stage?

The ESCHAR trial showed that surgery to abolish superficial venous reflux in addition to compression bandaging does not improve ulcer healing but reduces the recurrence of ulcer at four years and gives a greater proportion of ulcer free time. In addition, superficial venous surgery also helps to abolish segmental deep venous reflux. Therefore, I will consider treating the ulcer at present with compression bandaging and once the ulcer has healed, consider venous surgery to obliterate superficial venous reflux to prevent ulcer recurrence.

The patient returned 3 months later and the ulcer appears to have deteriorated. What is your treatment option?

If the ulcer does not heal or the patient's ABPI is < 0.5 or ankle pressure is less than 60 mmHg, I may need to assess the patient's general fitness for suitability of femoro-above knee popliteal bypass with a venous conduit to allow for ulcer healing. This may however increase the risk of post-operative oedema following revascularistion and runs the risk of wound infection. Keeping the foot elevated post-operatively may be impractical and intermittent pneumatic compression applied to the foot and calf may be used in these patients with deeply tunnelled graft to reduce the risk of post-operative oedema.

Further reading

Gohel MS, Barwell JR, Earnshaw JJ, Heather BP, Mitchell DC, Whyman MR, Poskitt KR. Randomized clinical trial of compression plus surgery versus compression alone in chronic venous ulceration (ESCHAR study)--haemodynamic and anatomical changes. Br J Surg. 2005; 92(3): 291-297.

Gohel MS, Barwell JR, Taylor M, Chant T, Foy C, Earnshaw JJ, Heather BP, Mitchell DC, Whyman MR, Poskitt KR. Long term results of compression therapy alone versus compression plus surgery in chronic venous ulceration (ESCHAR): randomised controlled trial. BMJ. 2007; 335(7610): 83.

Mosti G, Iabichella ML, Partsch H. Compression therapy in mixed ulcers increases venous output and arterial perfusion. J Vasc Surg. 2012; 55(1): 122-128.

O'Meara S, Cullum N, Nelson EA, Dumville JC. Compression for venous leg ulcers. Cochrane Database Syst Rev. 2012; 11: CD000265.

Symptomatic Varicose Veins

A 48 year old woman presented to your outpatient clinic with a painful and itchy right lower limb associated with prominent varicose veins. She claimed that her varicose veins had been present since her first pregnancy and became worse after her ankle fracture 5 years ago.

What important part of her history will you elicit?

In treating superficial venous reflux, it is important to enquire for history suggestive of previous venous surgery and underlying deep venous disease, especially a history of deep vein thrombosis (DVT), pelvic tumour and congenital malformations. I would be slightly concerned that her varicose veins had deteriorated following her presumed period of immobilisation after her ankle fracture, and would enquire if she had symptoms of DVT around that time.

What classification system is commonly used for varicose veins?

The CEAP (Clinical, Etiological, Anatomical and Pathological) classification is currently being widely used. The clinical (C) component of the classification is defined as follows:

C0: no visible or palpable signs of venous disease

C1: telangiectasia or reticular veins

C2: varicose veins

C3: oedema

C4a: pigmentation or eczema

C4b: lipodermatosclerosis or atrophie blanche

C5: healed venous ulcer

C6: active venous ulcer

How will you assess and investigate her underlying venous disease?

It is important to note the distribution of the varicose veins i.e long or short saphenous vein, and presence of features of chronic venous insufficiency (CVI) (eczema, pigmentation, lipodermatosclerosis and ulceration). Hand held Doppler during clinic consultation can help ascertain for saphenofemoral or saphenopopliteal junctions (SPJ) reflux. False positives are commonly seen at SPJ and therefore reflux here should be further investigated with venous duplex. Venous duplex will assess truncal reflux, incompetent perforators, deep venous patency and competency. Duplex will also assess suitability of the truncal veins for endovenous surgery (relatively straight vein, adequate diameter > 0.5 cm, > 1 cm deep to avoid skin burn).

What treatment options are available?

Conventional surgery – high tie, stripping of long saphenous vein and multiple stab avulsions, can be offered to patients with long saphenous vein territory varicosities. Saphenopopliteal junction ligation and multiple stab avulsions are performed in patients with short saphenous vein distribution varicosities. The short saphenous vein is rarely stripped to avoid damaging the sural nerve.

Endovenous thermal ablation [radiofrequency ablation (RFA) or laser] – mainly treats the truncal reflux and will require multiple stab avulsions to treat the residual varicosities. This will involve tumescence anaesthesia to allow the truncal vein to collapse during the procedure. The success rate has been quoted as high as 93% at 3 years for RFA.

Ultrasound guided foam sclerotherapy (UGFS) – sodium tetradecyl sulphate solution is agitated with air using the Tessari method (ratio of 1 part of solution to 3 part of air to create the foam, using a three way tap and two 2ml syringes).

What are the advantages and disadvantages of each modality?

Conventional surgery:

Advantages - reduced recurrence rate

Disadvantages - groin wound infection, prolonged recovery time, increased risk of haematoma from stripping, saphenous nerve injury during stripping of long saphenous vein, sural nerve or peroneal nerve injury with saphenopopliteal junction ligation

Endovenous thermal ablation:

Advantages - can be done under local anaesthesia, avoidance of groin wound and its potential complications, quicker recovery time and return to normal activities

Disadvantages – risk of saphenous and sural nerve injury with LSV and SSV treatment respectively resulting in chronic pain

UGFS:

Advantages – done under local anaesthetic avoiding groin incision, stripping or use of thermal energy

Disadvantages – most patients will need to return for multiple sessions to completely occlude the varicosities due to the limit on the amount of foam that can be injected each time, risk of haemosiderin pigmentation and ulceration in event of extravasation (thereby making it less ideal in young women with fair complexion), risk of transient blurring of vision. There have been reported cases of stroke.

What are the current recommendations for managing symptomatic varicose veins?

The current NICE guideline (CG168) recommended the following for patients with varicose veins and truncal reflux:

Endovenous thermal ablation (either RFA or laser) is suitable.

If endovenous thermal ablation is unsuitable, offer UGFS.

If UGFS is unsuitable, offer conventional surgery.

Compression hosiery is only used if interventional treatment is unsuitable.

What grades of compression stockings are available?

There are 4 classes of compression stockings

Class	Pressure at ankle (mmHg)	Indications
I	<25	Mild varicosities, DVT prophylaxis
II	25-35	Marked varicose vein, oedema, CVI
III	35-45	CVI, lymphoedema, following venous ulceration to prevent recurrence
IV	45-60	Severe lymphoedema and CVI

What would you recommend to this patient?

If her veins are not too tortuous and of suitable calibre and depth, I would recommend endovenous thermal ablation of her truncal vein with multiple stab avulsions.

Further reading

National Institute for Health and Care Excellence (2013) Varicose veins in the legs: The diagnosis and management of varicose veins (CG168). London: National Institute for Health and Care Excellence.

Rasmussen LH, Lawaetz M, Bjoern L, Vennits B, Blemings A, Eklof B. Randomized clinical trial comparing endovenous laser ablation, radiofrequency ablation, foam sclerotherapy and surgical stripping for great saphenous varicose veins. Br J Surg. 2011; 98(8):1079-87.

Synchronous AAA and Tumour

A 70 year old gentleman was recently diagnosed with a sigmoid colon tumour (T2N1M0). As part of his staging investigations, a CT scan has shown a 6.0 cm AAA.

What are the important considerations?

Incidence of AAA and concomitant malignancy is difficult to ascertain but is reported to range between 0.5% and 2.1%. There is no consensus with regards to the optimal management of these patients. When surgery is contemplated, it is important to decide on whether a combined or staged procedure is the appropriate approach. If a staged procedure is being planned, the order of treatment should be considered with regards to their advantages and disadvantages. It is important to understand the stage of the cancer, the proposed cancer treatment, the life expectancy of the patient and the risk/benefit of AAA repair. It is also vital to be aware of the risk of AAA rupture at this stage and the option of open versus EVAR. The main aim is to treat the most life-threatening and symptomatic lesion first. It is also important to bear in mind the National Cancer Strategy timeframe.

What are the advantages and disadvantages of treating the colonic tumour first in a two stage procedure?

The proteolytic enzymes released during the colonic resection, postoperative nutritional depletion and inflammatory response to surgery could lead to potential risk in increased AAA growth and rupture. Chemoradiotherapy with corticosteroids may also contribute to AAA enlargement, possibly due to inhibition of smooth muscle proliferation, and collagen and elastin synthesis. Of the 80 reported cases of staged repair where colonic resection was performed first, there were nine (11%) interval AAA ruptures. The median size of these aneurysms was > 6.0 cm. There were no cases of interval ruptures in AAA < 5.0 cm. There was no reported incidence of sigmoid colon ischaemia in patients undergoing right sided colonic resection followed by AAA repair. The risk of anastomotic complications appeared to be lower in patients undergoing colonic resection first followed by AAA repair (1%), and higher in patients undergoing combined repair (4%) and staged AAA followed by colonic resection (4%).

What are the advantages and disadvantages of treating the AAA first?

AAA treatment could either be open or EVAR. Open surgery will be a bigger physiological insult with a higher mortality rate (5-7% with open compared to 2% with EVAR) and length of recovery. Due to the increased risk of cardiovascular events in this age group of patients, if the patient had an MI following the initial procedure, the second stage procedure may have to be postponed for at least 3 months. This will not only delay curative cancer surgery but also adjuvant therapy, thereby increasing risk of cancer progression.

EVAR has the advantage of shorter in-patient stay, faster recovery, and reduced morbidity and mortality. EVAR can also be performed percutaneously or under loco-regional anaesthesia. Colonic resection following EVAR has been reported as soon as 2 weeks post EVAR. The initial benefit of EVAR however is not sustained in the long run due to risk of late rupture from endoleak or stent failure (migration or fracture).

In a review of 269 cases, mortality appeared to be highest in patients treated with AAA first (25%), followed by colonic resection (23%) and combined repair (7%).

There were no reported instances of colorectal cancer progressing to an unresectable stage after delay in cancer surgery following AAA repair.

What about the one stage procedure?

Performing both procedures simultaneously has the advantage of only going into the abdomen once and avoiding dense adhesions. The risk of cancer progression and AAA rupture are also kept to a minimum.

The main risks of combined procedure are AAA graft infection, duration of procedures and risk of decreased bowel perfusion. The reported rate of graft infection in the literature, however, was low.

What would you do for this patient?

If this patient's aneurysm is anatomically suitable, and the colonic tumour is not urgently symptomatic, I will consider offering this patient an EVAR under loco-regional anaesthesia and plan the colonic resection 2 weeks later provided he has not developed any major complications. This will reduce his mortality risk compared to an open AAA repair either performed concurrently or staged, and will facilitate early colonic resection and adjuvant treatment.

Further reading

Lin PH, Barshes NR, Albo D, Kougias P, Berger DH, Huynh TT, LeMaire SA, Dardik A, Lee WA, & Coselli JS. Concomitant colorectal cancer and abdominal aortic aneurysm: evolution of treatment paradigm in the endovascular era. J Am Coll Surg 2008; 206: 1065-1073.

Shalhoub J, Naughton P, Lau N, Tsang JS, Kelly CJ, Leahy AL, Cheshire NJ, Darzi AW, Ziprin P. Concurrent colorectal malignancy and abdominal aortic aneurysm: a multicentre experience and review of the literature. Eur J Vasc Endovasc Surg. 2009 May;37(5):544-56. doi: 10.1016/j.ejvs.2009.01.004. Epub 2009 Feb 23.

Thoracic Outlet Syndrome

A 35 year old mechanic has presented with paraesthesia and pain in his right ring and little fingers and ulnar aspect of the right forearm. This has affected his work and he is finding it difficult when needing to work with his arms above his head.

What is the most likely diagnosis?

This mechanic has evidence of neurogenic thoracic outlet syndrome (TOS). This is the commonest manifestation of TOS (up to 90%) which is a compilation of upper limb symptoms and signs attributed to compression of the neurovascular bundle in the thoracic outlet region (bordered by scalene muscles, clavicle and first rib). Apart from neurogenic TOS, the other causes of TOS can be arterial (involving subclavian artery) or venous (subclavian vein) in aetiology, all with their distinct symptoms and signs. Patients with neurogenic TOS have symptoms attributable to compression of the lower trunk of the brachial plexus (C8, T1). They may develop wasting of the intrinsic muscles of the hand. Arterial TOS may present with a discoloured hand or symptoms of claudication with the upper limb elevated above the head. Occasionally, they may present with an acutely ischaemic upper limb. Venous TOS, on the other hand, can present with upper limb swelling, venous distension, upper limb DVT (Paget-Schroetter syndrome) or pain.

What are the causes of TOS?

TOS could be due to cervical ribs, hypoplastic first rib, fibrous bands, and hypertrophied scalene muscles. Repetitive stress injuries or trauma can lead to the formation of scarring in the scalene muscles. In fact, repetitive stress and trauma (resulting in haematoma, myositis ossificans, callus formation or malunion of fractured clavicle) are the commonest causes of TOS. Cervical ribs are seen in up to 0.1% of adults and only 5%-10% of them become symptomatic.

What signs would you elicit?

Adson's test - where the radial pulse is abolished in the upper limb (held in slight abduction and extension) when the patient takes a deep breath, extends and turns his head towards the ipsilateral arm. The test is 79% sensitive and 76% specific.

Wright's test – progressive hyperabduction and external rotation of the shoulder joint resulting in absent ipsilateral radial pulse or development of paraesthesia.

Roos test – the patient's upper limbs are held in an abducted and external rotated (90°) and elbow flexed (90°) ("surrender") position. The patient then opens and closes his hands for several minutes. A positive result occurs if the manoeuvre reproduces the upper limb symptoms, sensation of fatigue or heaviness. The test is 84% sensitive and 30% specific.

How would you investigate his symptoms further?

An X-ray of thoracic inlet and chest X-ray will rule out underlying cervical rib, lung lesion or clavicular abnormality. Dynamic arterial and venous duplex with the upper limbs in abducted and externally rotated positions will help to rule out arterial or venous TOS. It is also important to rule out aneurysmal change of the subclavian artery due to external compression. CT scan and MRI may help to assess underlying soft tissue abnormality (fibrous bands and abnormal muscle). MRA with the upper limbs in an abducted and externally rotated position may help with the diagnosis of arterial TOS. Nerve conduction studies can be helpful in neurogenic TOS when it is positive. Neurogenic TOS may be intermittent and therefore a negative test does not rule that out.

This patient's X-ray showed evidence of bilateral cervical ribs and his arterial and venous duplex were both normal. What are his treatment options?

Conservative management – correcting postural abnormalities and avoiding overhead arm position while sleeping. Physiotherapy with emphasis on improving range of movement, pain control, stretching exercises and shoulder muscle strengthening have also been shown to help.

Surgical treatment in the presence of cervical ribs will entail their excision together with anterior scalenectomy and removal of any fibrous bands. This can be done preferably via the supraclavicular approach (alternative route will be infraclavicular). Complications of this approach include injury to the brachial plexus, phrenic nerve and lymphatic leakage. In the absence of cervical rib, it will be prudent to consider 1st rib excision (via the transaxillary route). The transaxillary route allows for good exposure of the anterior end of the first rib and prevents damage to the collaterals. It has the disadvantage of poor views and hence difficulty with managing intra-operative haemorrhage. The success rates vary and have been reported as high as 75%.

What would you do if he had concomitant venous or arterial TOS?

Venous TOS often presents with upper limb DVT. The treatment option these days will include upper limb catheter directed venous thrombolysis (+/- venous stenting) and 1st rib or cervical rib excision to decompress the thoracic outlet and prevent re-thrombosis. The timing of thoracic outlet decompression remains controversial. Early decompression (<1 week) prevents re-obstruction of vein and earlier resumption of activities. Late decompression (between 6 weeks and 6 months), has the advantage of allowing for selective decompression and reducing unnecessary procedures and their peri-operative complications.

Arterial TOS often will have changes of post-stenotic dilatation and will need repair of the aneurysmal subclavian artery. Treatment has to cover three elements: thoracic outlet decompression (as described above), removing the source of embolus (in most cases, this will be thrombus within the aneurysmal segment) and restoring the distal circulation. Planning for arterial TOS will be dictated by the status of distal circulation. A supraclavicular approach is required to control the subclavian artery and an infraclavicular incision may be required to access the axillary artery to perform the bypass. A reinforced Dacron is commonly used as conduit.

References

Degeorges R, Reynaud C, Becquemin JP. Thoracic outlet syndrome surgery: long-term functional results. Ann Vasc Surg. 2004; 18(5): 558-565.

Huang JH, Zager EL. Thoracic outlet syndrome. Neurosurgery. 2004; 55(4): 897-902.

Illig KA, Doyle AJ. A comprehensive review of Paget-Schroetter syndrome. J Vasc Surg. 2010 Jun; 51(6): 1538-1547.

SUGGESTED PAPERS BY SUBJECT

While there are countless papers that could be referenced for each area within each sub-specialty, we have tried to list a few that might be worth knowing, with a short précis of what the paper is about to help act as an aide memoire.

Critical Care:

Rivers E, Nguyen B, Havstad S, et al. Early goal-directed therapy in the treatment of severe sepsis and septic shock. N Engl J Med. 2001;345:1368-1377.

Comparison of early goal directed therapy for severe sepsis and septic shock patients. 263 enrolled patients split between groups. In hospital mortality 30.5% in goal-directed therapy versus 46.5% in standard therapy. Also lower APACHE II scores at each post admission time interval.

Hébert PC, Wells G, Blajchman MA, Marshall J, Martin C, Pagliarello G, Tweeddale M, Schweitzer I, Yetisir E. A multicenter, randomized, controlled clinical trial of transfusion requirements in critical care. Transfusion Requirements in Critical Care Investigators, Canadian Critical Care Trials Group. N Engl J Med. 1999 Feb 11;340(6):409-17.

TRICC trial looking at transfusion requirements. 838 critically ill patients with Hb <9 within 72 hours of admission to ICU randomised to a restrictive strategy of transfusion if Hb<7g/dl and maintained at 7-9 g/dl and a liberal strategy of transfusions when Hb <10g/dl and maintained at 10-12g/dl.. 30 day mortality was 18.7% (restrictive) versus 23.3% (liberal) P=0.11. However in those with APACHE II of ≤ 20 this was 8.7% and 16.1% (p=0.03), and among those less than 55 years (5.7% versus 13% p=0.02). Overall mortality rate was 22.3% versus 28.1% (p=0.05). No difference in those with a cardiac history. They concluded that restrictive strategy was superior to liberal transfusion in critically ill patients except for those with acute MIR or unstable angina.

Snowden CP, Prentis JM, Anderson HL, Roberts DR, Randles D, Renton M, Manas DM. Submaximal cardiopulmonary exercise testing predicts complications and hospital length of stay in patients undergoing major elective surgery. Ann Surg. 2010 Mar;251(3):535-41.

This study investigated CPET in comparison with a questionnaire for assessing functional capacity. CPET and an algorithm-based activity assessment were used in 171 consecutive patients. Lower anaerobic threshold (AT) was associated with increased complications and preoperative AT improved outcome prediction when compared with questionnaire based assessment.

Heyland DK, Novak F, Drover JW, Jain M, Su X, Suchner U. Should immunonutrition become routine in critically ill patients? A systematic review of the evidence. JAMA. 2001;286(8):944-53.

A systematic review looking at the impact of immunonutrition on infectious complications and mortality within critically ill patients. This study suggested that immunonutrition had no impact on mortality rates but was associated with fewer infectious complications. In particular high arginine content was associated with fewer complications and a trend towards lower mortality.

Emergency Surgery:

Myers E, Hurley M, O'Sullivan GC, Kavanagh D, Wilson I, Winter DC. Laparoscopic peritoneal lavage for generalized peritonitis due to perforated diverticulitis. Br J Surg. 2008; 95:97-101

A prospective study evaluating laparoscopic peritoneal lavage for 100 consecutive cases of perforated diverticulitis. Hartmann's procedure was required for those with Hinchey 4 diverticulitis (8), however remaining patients were managed with laparoscopic lavage with a morbidity rate of 4% and mortality of 3%.

Hansson J, Körner U, Khorram-Manesh A, Solberg A, Lundholm K. Randomized clinical trial of antibiotic therapy versus appendicectomy as primary treatment of acute appendicitis in unselected patients. Br J Surg. 2009 May;96(5):473-81.

Randomised trial evaluating antibiotics to surgery in patients with acute appendicitis. Recurrent appendicitis occurred in 15 patients (13.9%), after 1 year. Further, 96 of the 202 patients randomised to antibiotics had surgery either through patient preference or clinical requirement. Major complications were higher within the surgical cohort (p=0.05).

Antibiotic Therapy

Salminen P, Paajanen H, Rautio T et al. Antibiotic Therapy vs Appendectomy for Treatment of Uncomplicated Acute Appendicitis. The APPAC Randomized Clinical Trial. JAMA 2015;313(23):2340-2348.

Antibiotic treatment versus surgery for CT diagnosed uncomplicated appendicitis in adults 18-60 years. Patients were randomised to surgery (95% open 5% laparoscopic) or iv antibiotics for 3 days followed by 7 days of oral antibiotics. 273 patients in surgery group 257 antibiotics group. In antibiotic group 70 patients (27.3%) needed surgery within a year. Concluded that most patients with uncomplicated appendicitis who received antibiotics did not require surgery, however antibiotic treatment did not meet their pre-specified non-inferiority margin of 24%. (NB 849 of 1379 patients excluded. Interestingly the complication rate for the "failed" antibiotic group who went on to have surgery was 7% versus 20.5% in the group that were randomised to surgery).

General Surgery:

The MRC Laparoscopic Groin Hernia Trial Group. Laparoscopic versus open repair of groin hernia: a randomised comparison. Lancet. 1999 Jul 17;354(9174):185-90.

928 patients were randomised to laparoscopic or open repair. There were more complications in the open group at one week (43.5% versus 29.9%), however all three serious complications were in the laparoscopic group. Return to activities was swifter in the laparoscopic group, 10 versus 14 days. Persistent groin pain at 1 year was lower in the laparoscopic group, 28.7% versus 36.7%. However, all seven recurrences at one year were in the laparoscopic group.

O'Dwyer PJ, Serpell MG, Millar K, Paterson C, Young D, Hair A, Courtney CA, Horgan P, Kumar S, Walker A, Ford I. Local or general anaesthesia for open hernia repair: a randomized trial. Ann Surg. 2003 Apr;237(4):574-9.

Randomised control trial comparing LA and GA for primary repair of groin herniae. 279 patients were randomised. There was no difference in vigilance, memory, and cognitive function post operatively between groups. Return to social activity was similar in both groups. Those in the LA group had less pain on moving at 6 hours but were less likely to recommend surgery.

Livhits M, Ko CY, Leonardi MJ, Zingmond DS, Gibbons MM, de Virgilio C. Risk of surgery following recent myocardial infarction. Ann Surg. 2011 May;253(5):857-64.

Retrospective population analysis of the impact of recent MI on outcomes after subsequent surgery (including hip surgery, cholecystectomy, colectomy, AAA repair, and amputation). Risk of postoperative further MI decreased as length of time from MI to surgery was increased. Risk under 30 days was 32.8%, 31-60 days was 18.7%, 61-90 days was 8.4% and 91-180 days was 5.9%. MI within 30 days of an operation also increased the 30 day mortality and 1 year mortality.

Darouiche RO, Wall MJ Jr, Itani KM, Otterson MF, Webb AL, Carrick MM, Miller HJ, Awad SS, Crosby CT, Mosier MC, Alsharif A, Berger DH. Chlorhexidine-Alcohol versus Povidone-Iodine for Surgical-Site Antisepsis. N Engl J Med. 2010 Jan 7;362(1):18-26.

This is a randomised control trial comparing chlorhexidine-alcohol with povidone-iodine as a skin preparation for clean-contaminated surgery. 849 patients were randomised between groups which demonstrated significantly fewer wound infections in the chlorhexidine-alcohol group (9.5% versus 16.1%; relative risk 0.59l 95% confidence interval 0.41 to 0.85). This included both superficial (4.2% versus 8.6% p=0.008) and deep (1% versus 3% p=0.05) infections within incisions. There was no difference in organ space infections.

Breast Surgery:

Davies C et al Long-term effects of continuing adjuvant tamoxifen to 10 years versus stopping at 5 years after diagnosis of oestrogen receptor-positive breast cancer: ATLAS, a randomised trial Lancet. 2013 Mar 9;381(9869):805-16.

Adjuvant Tamoxifen: Longer against Shorter (ATLAS) trial- comparison of 10 years versus 5 years treatment with tamoxifen in ER positive early breast cancer. 12,894 women were randomised between groups. Continuing tamoxifen to 10 years rather than stopping at 5 produces a further reduction in recurrence and mortality, particularly after year 10. These results, taken together with results from previous trials of 5 years of tamoxifen treatment versus none, suggest that 10 years of tamoxifen treatment can approximately halve breast cancer mortality during the second decade after diagnosis.

Giuliano AE, Hunt KK, Ballman KV, Beitsch PD, Whitworth PW, Blumencranz PW, Leitch AM, Saha S, McCall LM, Morrow M. Axillary dissection versus no axillary dissection in women with invasive breast cancer and sentinel node metastasis: a randomized clinical trial. JAMA. 2011 Feb 9;305(6):569-75.

Randomised trial to determine if complete axillary lymph node dissection (ALND) effects survival in patients with sentinel lymph node metastasis. 991 patients receiving lumpectomy and whole breast radiation were randomised between groups at median follow up of 6.3 years. 5 year survival was 91.8% with ALND and 89.1% with just sentinel lymph node dissection. Five year disease free survival was 82.2% (ALND) and 83.9% (SLND). Use of SLND alone in patients with SLN metastatic breast cancer did not result in inferior survival.

de Boer M, van Deurzen CH, van Dijck JA, Borm GF, van Diest PJ, Adang EM, Nortier JW, Rutgers EJ, Seynaeve C, Menke-Pluymers MB, Bult P, Tjan-Heijnen VC. Micrometastases or isolated tumour cells and the outcome of breast cancer. N Engl J Med. 13;361(7):653-63

A study determining the outcome of micrometastases in regional lymph nodes on clinical outcome in breast cancer. Patients with favourable primary tumour characteristics and isolated tumour cells or micrometastases who did not receive systemic adjuvant therapy were compared with those found to be node negative, and a third cohort with isolated tumour cells or micrometastases who did receive systemic adjuvant therapy. They found that those who had received adjuvant therapy had improved survival over those who did not, and that the finding of isolated tumour cells or micrometastases was associated with reduced 5-year disease free survival.

Colorectal Surgery:

Sebag-Montefiore D, Stephens RJ, Steele R, Monson J, Grieve R, Khanna S, Quirke P, Couture J, de Metz C, Myint AS, Bessell E, Griffiths G, Thompson LC, Parmar M. Preoperative radiotherapy versus selective postoperative chemoradiotherapy in patients with rectal cancer (MRC CR07 and NCIC-CTG C016): a multicentre, randomised trial. Lancet. 2009 Mar 7;373(9666):811-20.

Short Course Preoperative RT versus surgery with selective chemoradiotherapy in operable rectal adenocarinoma. 1,350 patients randomised between the two. A 61% reduction in RR of local recurrence in those receiving SCRT and absolute difference of 6.2% at 3 years. However, overall survival did not differ between groups.

Jayne DG, Guillou PJ, Thorpe H, et al: Randomized trial of laparoscopic-assisted resection of colorectal carcinoma: 3-year results of the UK MRC CLASICC trial Group. 2007. *J Clin Oncol 25:3061-3068, 2007*

Conventional versus laparoscopic assisted colorectal surgery for cancer. 794 patients randomised 2:1 in favour of laparoscopic arm. There were no differences in long term outcomes. Higher positive CRM positivity in the laparoscopic arm for anterior resections, but this did not translate to increased local recurrence.

Green BL, Marshall HC, Collinson F, Quirke P, Guillou P, Jayne DG, Brown JM. Long-term follow-up of the Medical Research Council CLASICC trial of conventional versus laparoscopically assisted resection in colorectal cancer. Br J Surg. 2013 Jan;100(1):75-82. doi: 10.1002/bjs.8945.

Long-term outcome from CLASICC trial. No significant difference in overall survival or disease free survival at median 62 months follow up. However, in colonic cancer intraoperative conversions to open surgery were associated with worse overall survival and disease free survival. At 10 years there was increased propensity for local recurrence in right sided colonic cancers versus left colonic cancers, irrespective of resection method.

Quasar Collaborative Group, Gray R, Barnwell J, McConkey C, Hills RK, Williams NS, Kerr DJ. Adjuvant chemotherapy versus observation in patients with colorectal cancer: a randomised study. Lancet. 2007 Dec 15;370(9604):2020-9.

Quasar study to determine size and duration of adjuvant chemotherapy in colorectal patients at low risk for recurrence. 3,239 patients (91% stage II node negative) 71% colonic cancer. Adjuvant chemotherapy was 5-FU and folinic acid or observation. 293 recurrences in the chemotherapy group versus 359 in the observation group. Five-year survival may be improved in stage II colorectal cancer with adjuvant chemotherapy and an absolute improvement survival of 3.6%.

Hepatobiliary Surgery:

Neoptolemos JP, Dunn JA, Stocken DD, Almond J, Link K, Beger H, Bassi C, Falconi M, Pederzoli P, Dervenis C, Fernandez-Cruz L, Lacaine F, Pap A, Spooner D, Kerr DJ, Friess H, Büchler MW; European Study Group for Pancreatic Cancer. Adjuvant chemoradiotherapy and chemotherapy in resectable pancreatic cancer: a randomised controlled trial Lancet. 2001 Nov 10;358(9293):1576-85

ESPAC1 evaluates the roles of chemoradiotherapy and chemotherapy. Clinicians could randomise patients into a two-by-two factorial design (observation, chemoradiotherapy alone, chemotherapy alone, or both) or into one of the main treatment comparisons (chemoradiotherapy versus no chemoradiotherapy or chemotherapy versus no chemotherapy). The primary endpoint was death, and all analyses were by intention to treat. Findings: 541 eligible patients with pancreatic ductal adenocarcinoma were randomised: 285 in the two-by-two factorial design (70 chemoradiotherapy, 74 chemotherapy, 72 both, 69 observation); a further 68 patients were randomly assigned chemoradiotherapy or no chemoradiotherapy and 188 chemotherapy or no chemotherapy. 541 patients were randomised looking at chemoradiotherapy (20 Gy in ten daily fractions over 2 weeks with 500 mg/m(2) fluorouracil intravenously on days 1-3, repeated after 2 weeks) or chemotherapy (intravenous fluorouracil 425 mg/m(2) and folinic acid 20 mg/m(2) daily for 5 days, monthly for 6 months). Overall results showed no benefit for chemoradiotherapy (median survival 15.5 months versus 16.1 months without). There was evidence of survival benefit for adjuvant chemotherapy 19.7 months versus 14 months without.

Neoptolemos JP, Moore MJ, Cox TF, Valle JW, Palmer DH, McDonald AC, Carter R, Tebbutt NC, Dervenis C, Smith D, Glimelius B, Charnley RM, Lacaine F, Scarfe AG, Middleton MR, Anthoney A, Ghaneh P, Halloran CM, Lerch MM, Oláh A, Rawcliffe CL, Verbeke CS, Campbell F, Büchler MW; European Study Group for Pancreatic Cancer. Effect of adjuvant chemotherapy with fluorouracil plus folinic acid or gemcitabine vs observation on survival in patients with resected periampullary adenocarcinoma: the ESPAC-3 periampullary cancer randomized trial. JAMA. 2012 Jul 11;308(2):147-56

ESPAC 3- randomised trial evaluating adjuvant chemotherapy (fluorouracil or gemcitabine) in periampullary adenocarcinomas. 428 patients recruited (297 ampullary, 96 bile duct and 35 other cancers). Patients split between observation, folinic acid and fluorouracil or gemcitabine. Median survival was 35.2 months in the observation group versus 43.1 months in the two chemotherapy groups. Eighty-eight patients (61%) in the observation group, 83 (58%) in the fluorouracil plus folinic acid group, and 73 (52%) in the gemcitabine group died. After adjusting for prognostic variables a statistically significant survival benefit was conferred with adjuvant chemotherapy.

Oettle H, Neuhaus P, Hochhaus A, Hartmann JT, Gellert K, Ridwelski K, Niedergethmann M, Zülke C, Fahlke J, Arning MB, Sinn M, Hinke A, Riess H. Adjuvant chemotherapy with gemcitabine and long-term outcomes among patients with resected pancreatic cancer: the CONKO-001 randomized trial. JAMA. 2013 Oct 9;310(14):1473-81

Randomized trial to evaluate the efficacy and toxicity of gemcitabine in patients with pancreatic cancer after complete tumour resection. Patients were randomly assigned to either adjuvant gemcitabine treatment for 6 months or to observation alone.

354 patients were eligible for intention-to-treat-analysis. The median follow-up time was 136 months. The median disease-free survival was 13.4 months in the treatment group compared with 6.7 months in the observation group. Patients randomized to adjuvant gemcitabine treatment had prolonged overall survival compared with those randomized to observation alone, with 5 year overall survival of 20.7% versus 10.4% respectively, and 10 year overall survival of 12.2% versus 7.7%.

Nordlinger B, Sorbye H, Glimelius B, Poston GJ, Schlag PM, Rougier P, Bechstein WO, Primrose JN, Walpole ET, Finch-Jones M, et al. Perioperative chemotherapy with FOLFOX4 and surgery versus surgery alone for resectable liver metastases from colorectal cancer (EORTC Intergroup trial 40983): a randomised controlled trial.Lancet. 2008;371:1007–1016

Randomised control trial comparing perioperative chemotherapy and surgery versus surgery alone for patients with initially resectable colorectal liver metastases. 364 patients with histologically proven colorectal cancer and up to four liver metastases were randomly assigned to either six cycles of FOLFOX4 before and six cycles after surgery or to surgery alone (182 in perioperative chemotherapy group versus 182 in surgery group).

In the perioperative chemotherapy group, 151 (83%) patients were resected after a median of six (range 1-6) preoperative cycles and 115 (63%) patients received a median six (1-8) postoperative cycles. 152 (84%) patients were resected in the surgery group. The absolute increase in rate of progression-free survival at 3 years was 7.3% (from 28.1% to 35.4% p=0.058) in randomised patients; 8.1% (from 28.1% to 36.2% p=0.041) in eligible patients; and 9.2% (from 33.2% to 42.4% p=0.025) in patients undergoing resection. 139 patients died (64 in perioperative chemotherapy group versus 75 in surgery group). Reversible postoperative complications occurred more often after chemotherapy than after surgery (40/159 [25%] vs 27/170 [16%]; p=0.04). FOLFOX4 perioperatively increases progression free survival in eligible and resected patients.

Pending:

ESPAC4

Oesophagogastric Surgery:

Cunningham D, Allum WH, Stenning SP, Thompson JN, Van de Velde CJ, Nicolson M, Scarffe JH, Lofts FJ, Falk SJ, Iveson TJ, Smith DB, Langley RE, Verma M, Weeden S, Chua YJ, MAGIC Trial Participants Perioperative chemotherapy versus surgery alone for resectable gastroesophageal cancer. N Engl J Med. 2006 Jul 6;355(1):11-20.

MAGIC Trial: 503 patients with adenocarcinoma of stomach, OGJ or lower oesophagus randomised to perioperative chemotherapy with ECF or surgery alone. Five year survival was 36% versus 23% in surgery alone group.

Medical Research Council Oesophageal Cancer Working Group. Surgical resection with or without preoperative chemotherapy in oesophageal cancer: a randomised controlled trial. Lancet. 2002 May 18;359(9319):1727-33.

OEO2 trial: 802 patients randomised to neoadjuvant CF or surgery alone. Two year survival was 43% versus 34% for surgery alone.

van Hagen P et al (CROSS Group) Preoperative chemoradiotherapy for oesophageal or junctional cancer. N Engl J Med. 2012 May 31;366(22):2074-84.

Cross trial looking at the use of chemoradiotherapy in oesophageal and OGJ cancer. Surgery alone versus carboplatin and paclitaxel with radiotherapy for 5 weeks, then surgery. 366 patients randomised equally between groups. Median survival was 49.4 months in chemoradiotherapy and surgery group versus 24 months in surgery alone. Post operative complications were similar between groups.

Boeckxstaens GE, Annese V, des Varannes SB, Chaussade S, Costantini M, Cuttitta A, Elizalde JI, Fumagalli U, Gaudric M, Rohof WO, Smout AJ, Tack J, Zwinderman AH, Zaninotto G, Busch OR; European Achalasia Trial Investigators. Pneumatic dilation versus laparoscopic Heller's myotomy for idiopathic achalasia. N Engl J Med. 2011 May 12;364(19):1807-16..

Pneumatic dilatation versus laparoscopic Heller's cardiomyotomy for achalasia: 201 patients randomised between groups. This trial suggested comparable results. One year and two year success with dilatation was 90% and 86% with dilatation, compared with 93% and 90% with LHM. There was no difference in LOS pressure between groups. 4% of patients perforated at dilatation compared to 12% of mucosal tears with LHM.

Sjöström L, Narbro K, Sjöström CD, Karason K, Larsson B, Wedel H, Lystig T, Sullivan M, Bouchard C, Carlsson B, Bengtsson C, Dahlgren S, Gummesson A, Jacobson P, Karlsson J, Lindroos AK, Lönroth H, Näslund I, Olbers T, Stenlöf K, Torgerson J, Agren G, Carlsson LM; Swedish Obese Subjects Study. Effects of bariatric surgery on mortality in Swedish obese subjects. N Engl J Med. 2007 Aug 23;357(8):741-52.

Prospective controlled trial comparing bariatric surgery (2,010 patients) with the other conventional treatment (2,037). Average weight change in the control group was +/- 2% over the 15 year period of monitoring. Maximum weight loss in the surgical groups was at 1-2 years (32% with bypass, 25% with VBG, and 20% with bands which were stable at 10 years at 25%, 20% and 20%). 129 deaths in control group versus 101 in the surgery group over the 15 years.

Vascular Surgery:

EVAR trial participants. Endovascular aneurysm repair versus open repair in patients with abdominal aortic aneurysm (EVAR trial 1): randomised controlled trial Lancet 2005 Vol. 365, Issue 9478, Pages 2179-2186.

EVAR 1: Comparison of EVAR versus open surgery in patients fit for surgery with aneurysms of at least 5.5cm. 1,082 patients randomised between groups. All cause mortality was similar at 4 years, although there was reduction in aneurysm related deaths in the EVAR group (4% versus 7%). Postoperative complications within 4 years was 41% (EVAR) versus 9% (Open). At 12 months negligible difference in HRQL. Open surgery was £3,311 cheaper at 4 years.

EVAR trial participants. Endovascular aneurysm repair and outcome in patients unfit for open repair of abdominal aortic aneurysm (EVAR trial 2): randomised controlled trial. Lancet 2005 365, 9478, Pages 2187-2192 .

EVAR 2: Evaluation of EVAR versus no intervention in those unfit for open surgery with aneurysms of at least 5.5cm in patients over 60. 338 patients randomised. 30 day mortality in EVAR group was 9%, whereas no intervention group had a rupture rate of 9 per 100 person years. There was no significant difference for all-cause mortality between groups and aneurysm-related mortality. Mean hospital costs over 4 years were £13,632 (EVAR) and £4,983 (no intervention).

The Multicentre Aneurysm Screening Study Group. The Multicentre Aneurysm Screening Study (MASS) into the effect of abdominal aortic aneurysm screening on mortality in men: a randomised controlled trial. Lancet 2002 360, 9345, 1531-1539

MASS study: Evaluating ultrasound screening for AAA in males 65-74 years. Population of 67,800 allocated between invitation for screening or no invitations. 80% of invited participants took part. There were 65 aneurysm deaths in the invited group and 113 in the control group (overall risk reduction 42% rising to 53% in those who attended screening.) 30 day mortality was 6% for those who attended screening and had elective surgery, and 37% for emergency procedures.

Prinssen M, Verhoeven EL, Buth J, Cuypers PW, van Sambeek MR, Balm R, Buskens E, Grobbee DE, Blankensteijn JD; Dutch Randomized Endovascular Aneurysm Management (DREAM)Trial Group. A randomized trial comparing conventional and endovascular repair of abdominal aortic aneurysms. N Engl J Med. 2004 Oct 14;351(16):1607-18

DREAM trial: Comparison of endovascular AAA repair with open repair in 345 patients with AAA of at least 5cm and were eligible for both techniques. Mortality was 4.6% (open) and 1.2% (EVAR). Mortality plus severe morbidity was 9.8% (open) versus 4.7% (EVAR).

Halliday A, Mansfield A, Marro J, Peto C, Peto R, Potter J, Thomas D; MRC Asymptomatic Carotid Surgery Trial (ACST) Collaborative Group. Prevention of disabling and fatal strokes by successful carotid endarterectomy in patients without recent neurological symptoms: randomised controlled trial. Lancet. 2004 May 8;363(9420):1491-502.

ACST 1 trial: RCT comparing carotid endarterectomy (CEA) and indefinite deferral of CEA in patients with substantial carotid narrowing but no neurological symptoms. Risk of CVA or death within 30 days of CEA was 3.1%. Excluding perioperative CVA risk of stroke was 3.8% (CEA) versus 11% (deferral). Including perioperative events net 5 year risk of CVA was 6.4% (CEA) versus 11.8% (deferral). Conclusion that in asymptomatic patients less than 75 years old with a carotid diameter reduction of >70% on ultrasound, immediate CEA halved 5 year stroke risk from approximately 12% to 6%.

ACST-2 Collaborative Group, Halliday A, Bulbulia R, Gray W, Naughten A, den Hartog A, Delmestri A, Wallis C, le Conte S, Macdonald S. Status update and interim results from the asymptomatic carotid surgery trial-2 (ACST-2). Eur J Vasc Endovasc Surg. 2013 Nov;46(5):510-8. doi: 10.1016/j.ejvs.2013.07.020. Epub 2013 Sep 17.

ACST -2 compares carotid artery stenting with CEA in asymptomatic carotid artery stenosis.

Early results from initial 986 patients randomised equally between groups indicate a low risk of morbidity and mortality (1%). This trial continues to recruit.

Bibliography

Landmark Papers in General Surgery. Edited by Graham MacKay, Richard Molloy, and Patrick O'Dwyer. Oxford University Press. 2013

The Clinical Anaesthesia Viva Book. Edited by Barker, Maguire & Mills.

Care of the Critically Ill Surgical Patient. Third Edition. 2010. Edited by Iain D.Anderson. Hodder Arnold.

Kanani, Mazyar. Surgical Critical Care Vivas. Cambridge University Press.

American College of Surgeons. 2008 ATLS student course manual. 8th ed.

Core Topics in General & Emergency Surgery: A Companion to Specialist Surgical Practice. Edited by Simon Patterson Brown. 5th Edition. Elsevier.

Sabiston Textbook of Surgery: The Biological Basis of Modern Surgical Practice. 19th Edition. Courtney Townsend & R. Daniel Beauchamp & B. Mark Evers & Kenneth Mattox. Elsevier.

Oesophagogastric Surgery: Companion to Specialist Surgical Practice. S. Michael Griffin, Simon A. Raimes, Jonathan Shenfine. 5th Edition. Elsevier.

Hepatobiliary Surgery: Companion to Specialist Surgical Practice. O. James Garden, Rowan W Parks. 5th Edition. Elsevier.

Index

Locators in **bold** refer to figures and tables